THE COUNSELING PROCESS

A Multitheoretical Integrative Approach

Sixth Edition

Elizabeth Reynolds Welfel
Lewis E. Patterson
Cleveland State University

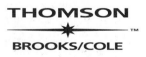

THOMSON

™

BROOKS/COLE

Australia • Canada • Mexico • Singapore • Spain
United Kingdom • United States

TO

Brandon and Fred, who bring me joy
E. R. W.

Janice, my companion in all things
L. E. P.

THOMSON

™

BROOKS/COLE

Executive Editor: *Lisa Gebo*
Assistant Editor: *Alma Dea Michelena*
Editorial Assistant: *Sheila Walsh*
Marketing Manager: *Caroline Concilla*
Marketing Assistant: *Mary Ho*
Advertising Project Manager: *Tami Strang*
Project Manager, Editorial Production:
  Candace Chen
Art Director: *Vernon Boes*

Print Buyer: *Emma Claydon*
Permissions Editor: *Stephanie Lee*
Production Service: *Shepherd, Inc.*
Copy Editor: *Karen Carriere*
Cover Designer: *Bill Stanton*
Cover Image: *Chumash Basket Tray, 1830/*
  © Planet Art
Compositor: *Shepherd, Inc.*
Text/Cover Printer: *Courier Corporation/Stoughton*

For more information about our products,
contact us at:
Thomson Learning Academic Resource Center
1-800-423-0563
For permission to use material from this text or
product, submit a request online at
http://www.thomsonrights.com.
Any additional questions about permissions can
be submitted by email to
thomsonrights@thomson.com.

Library of Congress Control Number: 2004100214
ISBN: 0-534-64032-X

Thomson Brooks/Cole
10 Davis Drive
Belmont, CA 94002
USA

Asia
Thomson Learning
5 Shenton Way #01-01
UIC Building
Singapore 068808

Australia/New Zealand
Thomson Learning
102 Dodds Street
Southbank, Victoria 3006
Australia

Canada
Nelson
1120 Birchmount Road
Toronto, Ontario M1K 5G4
Canada

Europe/Middle East/Africa
Thomson Learning
High Holborn House
50/51 Bedford Row
London WC1R 4LR
United Kingdom

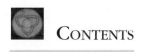

CONTENTS

Preface   vii

PART ONE: FUNDAMENTALS OF THE COUNSELING PROCESS   1

Chapter 1   *Perspectives on Effective Counseling   1*
Theoretical Foundations of This Book   2
Fundamental Precepts of Effective Counseling   4
Characteristics of Effective Counselors   12
The Joy of Helping   19
Summary   20
Discussion Questions   20
References   20

Chapter 2   *Understanding Counseling as a Process   23*
Definition of Counseling   24
Outcome Goals of Counseling   25
Process Goals in Counseling   31
Stages of the Counseling Process   32
The Three Stages of Counseling in Perspective   40
Summary   42
Discussion Questions   43
References   43

Chapter 3   *Building the Counseling Relationship and Facilitating
Initial Disclosure   45*
What Clients Bring to the Counseling Experience   46
Inviting Communication and Building the Counseling
   Relationship   47
The Core Conditions of Counseling   51
Counselor Actions That Impede Communication   65
Summary   68
Discussion Questions   69
References   70

Chapter 4   *In-Depth Exploration   71*
Goals and Methods of In-Depth Exploration   72
Advanced Empathy   77

iii

Immediacy 80
Confrontation 83
Interpretation 90
Role-Playing 94
Summary 96
Discussion Questions 97
References 97

Chapter 5   *Commitment to Action and Termination*   *99*
The Process of Goal Setting 99
Design and Implementation of Action Plans 109
Termination 119
Summary 125
Discussion Questions 126
References 127

Chapter 6   *Ethics in Counseling*   *129*
Codes of Professional Ethics 130
Ethical Principles 135
Ethical Theory 140
The Relationship Between Ethics and the Law 141
Common Ethical Violations by Mental Health
     Professionals 142
Summary 145
Discussion Questions 145
References 146

PART TWO: *COUNSELING STRATEGIES AND TECHNIQUES*   *149*

Chapter 7   *Assessment and Diagnosis in Counseling*   *149*
A Frame of Reference for Understanding
     Assessment and Diagnosis 150
Components of Effective Assessment 153
Tools for Effective Diagnosis 156
Placement of Assessment in the Counseling Process:
     Risks and Opportunities 160
Intake Interviews 161
Mistakes Counselors Make in the Assessment Process 162
Summary 164
Discussion Questions 165
References 165

Chapter 8   *Structuring, Leading, and Questioning Techniques*   *168*
Structuring 169
Leading 172
The Use of Questions in Counseling 180

Summary   182
Discussion Questions   183
References   183

Chapter 9   *Working with Ambivalent, Indifferent,*
                 and Oppositional Clients   185
                 Who Are These Hesitant Clients?   185
                 Understanding Client Reluctance and Resistance   187
                 The Counselor's Emotions Toward the Ambivalent,
                     Indifferent, or Oppositional Client   191
                 Why Work with Unmotivated and Oppositional Clients?   193
                 Working with the Client's Reluctance   195
                 Working with the Person Making the Referral   198
                 Summary   203
                 Discussion Questions   204
                 References   205

Chapter 10   *Major Theories of Counseling   206*
                 Structure for Relating Counseling Theories   207
                 Person-Centered Counseling   209
                 Gestalt Counseling   212
                 Psychoanalytic Counseling   215
                 Cognitive Counseling   221
                 Trait-Factor Counseling   225
                 Behavioral Counseling   228
                 Brief Therapy   232
                 Summary   233
                 Discussion Questions   234
                 References   235

PART THREE: *ADAPTING THE COUNSELING PROCESS TO SPECIFIC*
                 POPULATIONS   237

Chapter 11   *Working with Clients in Crisis   237*
                 Definition of Crisis   238
                 The Purpose of Crisis Intervention   240
                 Stressful Events That May Precipitate Crises   240
                 Steps in Crisis Intervention   242
                 Summary   252
                 Discussion Questions   252
                 References   253

Chapter 12   *Issues of Human Diversity in Counseling   255*
                 The Multicultural Face of America   256
                 Considerations in Counseling Culturally Diverse Clients   258
                 Counseling Women and Girls   271

Counseling Men and Boys   280
Counseling Gay, Lesbian, and Bisexual Clients   287
Summary   290
Discussion Questions   291
References   292

Chapter 13   *Working with Children and Their Parents   296*
How Children Differ from Adults   296
Communicating   299
Assessment   305
Augmenting the Socialization Process   311
Working with Parents   314
Summary   317
Discussion Questions   318
References   319

Chapter 14   *Working with Older Adults   321*
Characteristics of Older Adults as Clients   322
Experiences and Counseling Agendas of Older Adults   325
Counseling Procedures with Older Adults   330
Working with Families of Older Clients   337
Summary   340
Discussion Questions   341
References   341

APPENDICES

Appendix A   *American Counseling Association Code of Ethics
and Standards of Practice (1995)   344*

Appendix B   *American Psychological Association, Ethical Principles
and Code of Conduct of Psychologists (2002)   369*

Appendix C   *Listing of Related Codes of Ethics   392*

Appendix D   *Outline for Writing a Counseling Session Critique   395*

AUTHOR INDEX   402

SUBJECT INDEX   405

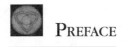 # PREFACE

The sixth edition of *The Counseling Process: A Multitheoretical Integrative Approach* is intended for use in introductory courses in professional counseling at the graduate or advanced undergraduate level. We expect that the sixth edition of the book will be used as the earlier editions have been—as a single text in a counseling methods course, along with a counseling theories text in a counseling theory and process course, or in counseling pre-practicum, practicum, or internship experiences. The text is also suitable for use in training human services workers who need basic counseling and communication skills in their work (substance abuse counselors, mental health assistants, case managers, volunteers who staff hot-lines, etc.). The previous edition was used as well in schools of theology as a guide to pastoral relationship-building and counseling.

As with previous editions of *The Counseling Process,* our purpose is to help readers develop an understanding of the universal principles of effective helping regardless of the theoretical orientation of the counselor. We emphasize counseling as a process with three major stages and delineate the knowledge, attitudes, and skills we see as essential for effective helping at each stage. Our view is that counselors and clients work together as partners to understand the issues the client faces, illuminate their causes, and then establish effective action plans to alter emotions, thoughts, and/or behaviors. For this new edition, we have labeled our approach as multitheoretical and integrative, and we have added a graphic that identifies the work of the client and of the counselor, as well as the progress that may be anticipated at each stage of the counseling process.

The broad outline of the counseling process described in the fourth and fifth edition has been retained, but the material has been reorganized and expanded. The book is now organized into three major sections: fundamentals of the counseling process, counseling strategies and techniques, and adapting the counseling process to the special populations. In this new organization, our model of the counseling process is presented in the first six chapters. The major changes in this section include a stronger emphasis on the therapeutic alliance, the graphic presentation of our model, and the inclusion of ethics as fundamental knowledge. Discussion of specific techniques and strategies is reserved for the second section, which begins with diagnosis and counseling skills that are needed in all counseling sessions and then discusses special methods for harder-to-help clients. The presentation on techniques and strategies ends with a synopsis of the variations in counseling approach espoused by the major theoretical schools of contemporary counseling. The last component of the book on adapting the counseling model to different populations now addresses clients in crisis, issues of human diversity, working with children, and working with older adults. An expanded discussion of human diversity presents perspectives on racial and ethnic minority status and gay and lesbian experience, as well as a major new component on men's issues and updated material on the status of women. The chapter on working with older adults reflects the new importance that is attached to working with elders as our population ages, and the chapter on children introduces some of the special techniques required to adapt the multitheoretical integrative model to persons with immature cognitive skills.

The book employs four learning aids to facilitate students' understanding of the material. First, case studies accompany most chapters. These cases include questions that encourage readers to place themselves in the role of helper and to consider client material as though they were the counselor. The cases are written to reflect the cultural diversity in our society. Second, the book includes several learning exercises that may be completed individually or with partners to assist in the internalization of learning and in practicing specific skills for effective counseling. Each chapter now includes discussion questions intended to stimulate student thinking about complicated or controversial issues contained in the chapter. Finally, Appendix D provides a format for counselors to use in writing critiques of their counseling sessions, along with a sample critique and supervisor feedback. We have found this format to be particularly useful in practicum and internship supervision. New for the sixth edition is a separate *Instructors' Guide* that includes essay, multiple choice, as well as true/false questions for each chapter, as well as additional case studies.

We have written the book in a personal style geared to the student interested in becoming an effective helper. After using the text in an introductory course, the reader, under careful supervision, should have sufficient knowledge to begin contact with clients. The text is also a valuable resource for internship students wishing to review principles of effective counseling as they embark on that stage of their training. The personal style also renders the book helpful for the general public interested in understanding what professional counseling is all about.

We wish to acknowledge the contributions of our reviewers, whose careful reading of the manuscript has helped us to refine our thinking and writing. They are Carolyn Dillon, Boston University; James R. Mahalik, Boston College; Paula Danzinger, William Paterson University; Pamela M. Kiser, Elon University; Leslie Brody, Boston University; Paula Helen Stanley, Radford University; Carole Campbell, CSU-Long Beach; and Tommie Miller, Pima Community College. The support and encouragement of Lisa Gebo from Brooks/Cole has been especially valuable.

We also wish to acknowledge the help of Elizabeth Patterson Supinski for creating the graphic design for our model and the help of our graduate assistants Carla Gilenko and Lalitha Prakash with research and indexing. Finally, we wish to thank our families for their support and patience during the long months we spent at the computer writing and rewriting this book.

Elizabeth Reynolds Welfel
Lewis E. Patterson

PART ONE

FUNDAMENTALS OF THE COUNSELING PROCESS

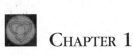 CHAPTER 1

PERSPECTIVES ON EFFECTIVE COUNSELING

People seek the services of professional counselors, social workers, psychologists, and psychiatrists when their capacities for responding to the demands of life are strained, when desired growth seems unattainable, when important decisions elude resolution, and when natural support systems are unavailable or insufficient. Sometimes the person in need of help is urged or required to seek counseling by a third party—spouse, parent, employer, teacher, or judge—who believes the individual is failing to manage some important aspect of life effectively. At other times an overwhelming trauma, a biologically based mental illness, or an unrewarding or conflict-ridden relationship motivates people to seek help.

The purpose of counseling, broadly conceived, is to empower the client to cope with life situations, to reduce emotional stress, to engage in growth-producing activity, to have meaningful interpersonal relationships, and to make effective decisions. Counseling, as we conceptualize it, is not limited to those with psychiatric diagnoses or to individuals experiencing thoughts, feelings, or behaviors that are dysfunctional, but it is also fully appropriate for those who are "symptom free" and are seeking fuller and more rewarding ways of living their lives. As a result of counseling, counselees increase their control over present circumstances and enhance present and future opportunities. Research clearly demonstrates that people who complete counseling and psychotherapy for their problems are better off than those who do not seek professional help at least 80% of the time (Lambert & Barley, 2002; Wampold, 2001).

THEORETICAL FOUNDATIONS OF THIS BOOK

People of any age, in any walk of life, and with almost any kind of problem can learn to gain power over the adversities and opportunities of their lives. Counseling to achieve client empowerment is viewed in this text as a generic process that includes essentially the same elements whether performed in a community counseling clinic, a rehabilitation center, a school, a hospital, or any other facility. Empowerment does not imply eradication of all psychological and interpersonal problems—rather it means that clients have developed the internal, interpersonal, and social resources to cope more effectively with the circumstances of their lives. Ideally, counseling provides people with tools and experiences that help them improve specific aspects of their lives, and it offers them a more positive perspective on their own self-worth and a deeper belief in their own capacity to live meaningful and productive lives. Certain methods may result in more effective work with certain clients, but the *basic* structure of the therapeutic process is the same. (See Chapter 9 for discussion of counseling reluctant clients and Chapters 11–14 for discussion of counseling clients in crisis and counseling adapted for age and cultural differences.)

The power to live effectively is enhanced by knowledge of two kinds: understandings about self and understandings about conditions of the environment. Awareness about self includes appreciation of one's own capacities, knowledge, emotions, values, needs, interests, and ways of construing self and others. Conditions of the environment include, among other factors, interpersonal contacts with family, friends, and work or school associates, social and economic factors associated with where one lives and how one earns a living, and cultural heritage. Because we believe that clients' control over their destiny is enhanced by an increased understanding of self in the environment, the generic model of counseling we present in this book must be regarded as an insight approach to counseling. We believe that clients who develop improved insights about their own needs, desires, and capacities in relation to the opportunities afforded by their own particular environment will be empowered to live more effectively. We also believe that the most effective vehicle for empowerment is the quality of the relationship that develops between the counselor and the client and the ability of the two people to work collaboratively to reach the client's goals. The context of a positive therapeutic relationship offers clients the support and structure they need to take the risks essential for insight and behavior change.

A Multitheoretical Integrative Model for Counseling

The model of counseling presented here focuses on cognitive, affective, and behavioral issues and the interaction among these three domains. We recognize that the ability to solve cognitive problems is enhanced by a positive affective state and that progress in solving cognitive problems will likely make the client feel better about himself or herself. Improvement in either the cognitive or the affective domain enhances the ability to behave more effectively. Conversely, changes in behavior frequently enhance positive thoughts and feelings. In our view, no one personality or learning theory accounts for all of human experience, and no one counseling approach embodies the "whole truth" about the helping process. Our multitheoretical model for counseling integrates ideas from most empirically supported contemporary approaches to counseling, and subsequent chapters of the text acknowledge the special contributions of the creators of those approaches. The model also relies on insights from the positive psychology movement, which proposes that attending to clients' strengths and helping them become more optimistic about the future is a path to fundamental and long-lasting change in dysfunctional patterns (Seligman & Csikszentmihalyi, 2000; Synder & Lopez, 2002).

Counseling as a Three-Stage Process

The three-stage model of helping is introduced in Chapter 2 and elaborated upon in subsequent chapters. The first stage emphasizes the quality of the counseling relationship and is rooted in the work of Carl Rogers (1942, 1951, 1961, 1980, 1986) and other authors who subsequently devised methods of teaching and evaluating relationship skills (Carkhuff, 1969a, 1969b; Egan, 2002). Recent research findings underscore the importance of that relationship, showing that the presence of an open, trusting, and empathic counselor–client relationship, along with mutually agreed-upon goals, is the *single most important factor in a successful counseling outcome,* more important than the specific counseling techniques employed (Lambert & Barley, 2002; Wampold, 2001). According to these researchers, such a relationship (also termed a *therapeutic alliance*) can be curative in itself, though it is not always sufficient for client change. Moreover, if counseling is to be successful, a strong counseling relationship must be formed early in counseling, preferably in the first few sessions (Bachelor & Horvath, 1999). Only when clients experience a sense of hope for change and a belief that the counselor really understands and supports them are they ready to engage in the difficult tasks of self-exploration and behavioral change in the next two stages of counseling (Horvath & Bedi, 2002). The second stage of counseling focuses on helping clients gain deeper understandings of self. Here we rely on psychoanalytic concepts about ego function and the defense of the ego, as well as unconscious motivation, to provide a basis for a counselor's understanding of a client's motivation. The counseling techniques suggested for promoting in-depth understanding of the self emerge from a broad literature on counseling but have special relevance to Freudian procedures (Alexander, 1963; Freud, 1923/1964) and Gestalt procedures (Perls, 1969; Polster & Polster, 1973). In this stage, the trusting therapeutic relationship becomes the foundation that allows the client to probe often painful aspects of the self. The third stage of counseling involves goal setting, action planning, and implementation of planned interventions. We have relied on the work of trait-factor counselors (Williamson, 1939, 1950, 1965), behavioral, and cognitive-behavioral counselors (Beck, 1972, 1976; Cormier & Nurious, 2002; Ellis, 2000; Ellis & Bernard, 1986; Hackney & Cormier, 2001; Meichenbaum, 1977) for some of their ideas about decision making, reinforcement of positive action, development of new skills, and evaluation of counseling progress. At this stage, the counseling relationship is a source of strength to implement the changes discussed in the safety of the therapeutic setting.

Almost every major counseling theory seems to have merit in describing some aspect of the counseling process. Although the proponents of each system tend to believe that their particular theory includes virtually all the most important elements of counseling, we believe an aggregate of the several systems to be more complete than any one alone. Of course, we do not suggest that a counselor randomly select techniques or strategies. Therefore, the title of the sixth edition has been modified to identify our approach as both multitheoretical and integrative. We have provided a rationale for selecting particular techniques according to the stage of counseling and the nature of the client's concerns so that the counselor can plan a consistent progression through the counseling process. Again we emphasize that the differences in effectiveness for one technique versus another are small, and no technique or model has a reasonable chance of success without the presence of a strong counseling relationship. A counselor always offers techniques, and those techniques cannot be separated from the personhood of the client and counselor and the quality of the relationship between them. Chapter 10 provides synopses of selected theories and identifies how each theory contributed to our multitheoretical integrative model.

FUNDAMENTAL PRECEPTS OF EFFECTIVE COUNSELING

The task of identifying the common elements that result in good outcomes for clients will never be fully accomplished, but the past 50 years of research and theory has provided a credible outline of essentials for effective counseling. This section presents a set of fundamental precepts that form the basis for our understanding of the helping process. These precepts have emerged from four sources: our study of the range of counseling theories, the research on counseling process and outcome, our experiences as helpers and counselor educators, and our collaboration as authors interested in describing the counseling process to others. The precepts (Eisenberg & Patterson, 1979/1990) are intended to orient you to some of the principles we believe to be most important in understanding the counseling process. These principles will take on deeper meaning as you assimilate subsequent chapters and should be studied again when you have finished reading the text.

Precept 1: Understanding Human Behavior in Social and Cultural Context

To be effective, the counselor must have a thorough understanding of human behavior in its social and cultural context and be able to apply that understanding to the particular problems and circumstances of each client.

Counseling is unlikely to be helpful without a clear understanding of the roots of the problems clients bring to counseling and the individual, interpersonal, and social forces that serve to maintain the problems clients want to resolve. Therefore, diagnosis and hypothesis generating are critical and inevitable parts of the counselor's work. The process of diagnosis has two interrelated functions: first, to describe significant patterns of cognition, behavior, or affective experience, and second, to provide causal explanations for these significant patterns. The process involves developing tentative hypotheses, confirming their validity, and using them as the basis for making critical decisions concerning the focus, process, and direction of the counseling experience. The process of arriving at a diagnosis is a mutual one in which the client and counselor work together to identify these patterns and their roots in the client's experience.

Understanding human behavior requires the counselor to have a set of concepts and theories that help to account for and explain significant human reactions and relate them to experiences. These concepts and principles provide the core for the counselor's diagnostic and hypothesis-generating work. Counselors use theories and concepts about human behavior to understand their own behavior as well as the concerns, actions, perceptions, emotions, and motivations of their clients.

There are four dangers in the diagnostic and hypothesis-generating process. One is that the process often becomes a game that applies labels to clients, thus putting them into categories. Once categorized, the client is stereotyped; all the general characteristics of those in that category are also attributed to the client and the uniqueness of the client as an individual may be lost. Worse, the client's other important attributes are overlooked because categorizing creates perceptual blinders for the counselor. A second danger is that counselors often make mistakes in their diagnoses, and these mistakes often result in ineffective and sometimes counterproductive counseling strategies. Third, not all counselors use the same diagnostic terms for the same client experiences. One may identify a set of problems as depression, another as a manifestation of a dysfunctional family system. Fourth, as is true of many aspects of counseling, the diagnostic and hypothesis-generating process is not free from bias based on culture or ethnicity (Sinacore-Guinn, 1995). Negative societal attitudes toward oppressed or culturally diverse groups have been shown to reduce the objectivity and fairness of the diagnosis given to clients and thereby interfere with helping the client improve.

Although these dangers are real, we firmly believe they are not inherent in the diagnostic process itself; rather they are dangers of the misuse of the process. Counselors who comprehend the role that an understanding of human behavior and its social and cultural context plays in their work and who recognize the proper function of diagnosis will work hard to avoid these dangers. It is part of their ethical responsibility.

Precept 2: Client-Defined Growth as the Definition of Successful Counseling

The ultimate purpose of the counseling experience is to help the client achieve some kind of change that he or she will regard as satisfying.

Every significant theory of counseling states that creating growth-oriented change in the client is the ultimate intended outcome of the counseling experience. Some say overt behavior change is the *sine qua non* of the experience. Others say that behavior change is just symptom change; real and lasting change comes when the client develops new perceptions on self, significant others, and life. Furthermore, some counselors take a remedial approach, with all their attention focused on alleviating presenting symptoms. Their only goal is to help the client change dysfunctional behavior to more functional patterns, such as overcoming shyness, reducing debilitating anxiety, controlling counterproductive anger, or reducing interpersonal conflicts. Others believe that the goal of counseling is to help people make important life decisions. In this case, the counselor's role is to help the client use a rational thinking process to resolve confusion and conflict. Still other counselors view their work as stimulating favorable personal and interpersonal growth. As they see it, remediating dysfunction and assisting in decision making may become important contributions to the client's overall growth experience. For these counselors, helping people to become more complete or fully functioning are the crucial outcomes of the counseling process.

Unfortunately, documenting client change is often difficult. Behavior change, if it occurs, is probably the easiest to observe because it is the most tangible. However, clients may also change their views about certain behaviors that they previously regarded as undesirable, they may change in the extent to which they experience stress related to an unwanted situation, or they may reduce their general level of emotional distress. Clients may also change their values as they progress through counseling. For example, a person may come to value family relationships more and work achievement less, or the person may become more tolerant of people with different political, religious, or social philosophies. In spite of the difficulties of assessing some kinds of change, a counselor who cannot describe the changes that the client has undergone has no basis for knowing when counseling has reached an effective conclusion.

Precept 3: Positive Relationship between Counselor and Client as Fundamental to Client Change

The quality of the helping relationship is the single most significant factor in providing a climate for growth.

When we meet new people, we decide how much of ourselves to share with them. Before sharing deeply, we assess the risk in terms of how we think the listener will react to our personal thoughts and feelings. If we do not experience trust, we remain closed and go away from the experience without benefit.

The literature in the field often describes the critical elements of the counseling relationship that promote openness: respect (rather than rejection), empathy (rather than shallow listening and advice giving), congruence or genuineness (rather than inconsistency), facilitative self-disclosure (rather than being closed), immediacy (rather than escapism to the past or future), and concreteness (rather than abstract intellectualizing) (Carkhuff, 1969a, 1969b; Egan, 2002, Rogers, 1942, 1951). Counselors must communicate respect for clients as people with rights who are trying to live the best lives they can. Genuine caring is communicated when counselors try to understand the client's world as if it were their own and give the client verbal cues about that understanding. Effective counselors share their reactions to the client with the client, using this feedback as a way of helping the client toward deeper levels of self-understanding. The goal is to develop a collaborative partnership in which the active participation of each participant is crucial to counseling success.

The quality of the relationship not only provides a safe and comforting context from which interventions that may help the client are introduced, it is often therapeutic in itself. The experience of a respectful, caring, empathic, genuine, and immediate relationship can be transforming, even if no other counseling intervention is initiated. In fact, if such a relationship is absent, clients usually drop out of counseling. If they stay, even the most brilliant counseling intervention is unlikely to succeed. Interestingly, the client's perception of the quality of the relationship is the most important predictor of the likelihood he or she will drop out of counseling—counselors' perceptions of clients' responses to the early stages of counseling are often erroneous. Therefore, counselors must be prepared to seek out clients' reactions early in the counseling process instead of relying on their own judgments and to adapt their style in ways the client views as helpful to the therapeutic alliance (Horvath & Bedi, 2002).

Precept 4: Counseling as an Intense Working Experience

The counseling experience is emotionally powerful for both client and counselor.

For the counselor, the activities of attentive listening, information absorption, message clarification, hypothesis generation, and treatment planning require sustained energy. Beyond these largely intellectual activities is the emotional experience of caring enough about another person's suffering to be affected by that person's emotions without becoming lost in those emotions. The counselor who cannot manage these emotions has diminished effectiveness as a facilitator.

For the client, the hard work comes in the effort to understand what is difficult to understand; in the endurance of confusion, conflict, and uncertainty; and in the commitment to disclose to one's self that which is painful to think about. This effort, endurance, and commitment require a level of concentration that the client may never have experienced. All clients undergo the added stresses of revealing personally felt inadequacies to another. Clients worry that their counselors will fail to understand the uniqueness of their experiences or may judge them negatively for their problems. The work of producing growth through counseling is always demanding on the client and is often painful, though at the same time fulfilling and rewarding.

Counseling is not the same thing as conversation. In conversation, two or more people exchange information and ideas in a casual and relaxed way. People leave a conversation and move easily to other things. Counseling, on the other hand, is characterized by a much higher level of intensity. Ideas are developed more slowly, encountered at a deeper personal level, and considered more carefully than occurs in casual conversation. Sometimes people leave a counseling experience mentally and emotionally depleted yet still thinking about what they discussed. At other times people are energized by the new insights they have gained in spite of the painful aspects of the new awareness.

Precept 5: Clients as Active Partners in the Counseling Process

Effective counseling is grounded in the client's commitment to be actively involved through self-disclosure, self-confrontation, and risk taking as facilitated by interaction with the counselor.

For counseling to take place, the client must disclose personal information to the counselor, who in turn tries to understand the client's world within the context of what the counselor knows about human behavior. Although clients may reveal significant personal information in their nonverbal behavior, communication in counseling is primarily verbal. Clients reveal their thoughts and feelings to a perceptive counselor by what they say, the affect with which they say it, and what they choose to obscure in their verbalizations. The more fully self-disclosure takes place, the more effectively the counselor can help the client discover new ways of coping and the more the client will understand self. The question Frank and Frank (1991) pose captures the essence of the role of self-disclosure: "How do I know what I think until I have heard what I have to say?" (p. 200).

Clients' comfort with self-disclosure varies greatly. Sometimes a client's difficulty with self-disclosure is based on cultural or family norms that dissuade discussing personal issues with strangers or with individuals from different backgrounds. In such circumstances, counselors must be particularly attentive to the establishing trust and must have a flexible repertoire of skills for facilitating client self-disclosure. At other times, difficulty with self-disclosure stems from a low level of readiness for change, a particularly common occurrence when third parties coax people into counseling or when the costs inherent in the problem behaviors are not as apparent to the client as they are to other people (Prochaska, Norcross, & DiClemente, 1994). Put another way, the client's willingness to disclose personal information acts as a gauge for both the client's commitment to be active in the process of change and for the strength of the trust in the competence and caring of the counselor. Recent research indicates that counselors who effectively facilitate client self-disclosure in the first three sessions are significantly more likely to help clients stay in counseling and achieve their goals (Lambert & Barley, 2002; Lambert et al., 2001).

Self-confrontation occurs when the client looks at self with an expanded perspective that allows him or her to develop new perceptions about self. The counselor helps clients to broaden their perspectives on self by providing honest feedback. At the simplest level, that feedback may merely be restatements of the client's own words that cause the client to reconsider a thought just expressed. Consider the following exchange between a client who sought counseling because of roommate problems:

> CLIENT: I can't believe my roommate forgot to write down my phone
> message. It was important to me. She seemed to be so absorbed
> in her own problems that she paid no attention to my needs.
> Her insensitivity really made me feel depressed this weekend,
> so depressed that I couldn't find the energy to do the laundry
> or cook dinner as I had agreed to do. I just stayed in bed
> all weekend.
> COUNSELOR: When your roommate acted in ways you found
> inconsiderate, you were unable to follow through on your
> commitments to your chores. When you look back on the
> weekend, you attribute your response to feelings of depression.
> I wonder whether other feelings were involved too.

As the counselor becomes more confident of his or her understanding of the client, he or she may choose to move to a more comprehensive form of feedback that helps the client see himself or herself from an alternative viewpoint. Because such feedback comes from the counselor's frame of reference, it frequently will be a view that the client has not previously considered. The counselor needs to be as free of vested interest as possible in using confrontative feedback as a counseling tool. If the counselor in the previous example knew the client well and had established a strong trusting relationship with her, he might have responded as follows:

> COUNSELOR: I wonder if your retreat to your bed and not doing the chores not only came from your depressed mood but also from anger at your roommate or from a desire to show her indirectly how upset you were by her forgetfulness.

Whether the counselor's feedback is at the low-risk restatement level or the higher-risk confrontation level, the client must confront self with new ways of seeing and understanding self in life situations. Through this process, a new understanding of personal needs, desires, perceptions, assumptions, and cognition emerges, and new coping skills are discovered and refined.

Precept 6: Ethical Conduct as Fundamental Professional Responsibility

Professional ethics requires counselors to place the best interests of the client as their highest priority and to follow all other provisions of the codes of conduct for their profession.

Ethical practice may be defined as providing, with care and conscientious effort, a therapeutic service for which one has been appropriately trained. Unethical practice occurs when counselors practice outside the limits of their competence, fail to place clients' interests ahead of their own needs, or fail to respond sensitively to their clients' life experiences and rights (Welfel, 2002). Because counselors present themselves to the public as persons with special skills to help people in need, they have greater burden not to do harm than other citizens who do not purport to be expert helpers. Counselors need to be aware of the great responsibility they take on when they provide services to clients. Counseling that is incompetent or insensitive or that serves the interests of the counselor not only causes harm to the clients who receive it but also damages the reputation of the counselor's employer and the profession as a whole. At its core, ethical practice means valuing each client as a person with rights to fair, dignified, and compassionate service.

Codes of ethics (see Appendixes A and B) serve to answer many questions about ethical dilemmas that present themselves in counseling practice. Understanding the ethical principles underlying the codes and broader ethical theories are necessary for resolving some complicated ethical dilemmas. In the long run, the responsibility for ethical action always rests with the judgment of the individual practitioner.

━━ *Application of the Precepts: The Case of Martina* ━━

As you read the following information, imagine that you are the counselor assigned to meet with Martina, then respond to each of the questions that follow.

Martina is a 31-year-old bookkeeper and mother of two children who enters counseling at the advice of the court. She was born in Russia but immigrated to the United States with her family when she was a teenager and now is a naturalized U.S. citizen. Her husband died of a brain aneurysm two years ago. Six weeks ago she was arrested for driving while intoxicated. In the years since her husband's death, Martina had become addicted to the prescription medications her physician gave her to help her cope with the loss. Because Martina had also left her children (ages 8 and 5) home alone while she shopped for groceries that evening, the department of children's services also became involved, and criminal charges of child neglect were filed against Martina. Because Martina had no local relatives, that agency took emergency custody of the children. She soon lost her job as a result of her arrest. Martina entered counseling feeling depressed, hopeless, wrongly treated by the child welfare system, terrified that she will become homeless without a job, and generally betrayed by life. Until her husband's death, she experienced no mental health or substance abuse problems in spite of alcoholic parents and a hard life prior to marriage. She entered counseling with an ambivalent attitude. On one hand, she wanted someone to talk to about her desperate situation and hoped to please the court by attending sessions; on the other hand, she was skeptical that a counselor could be of any real help in dealing with her practical problems. No counselor could bring her husband back, offer her a job, mandate that she get her children back, or pay her bills.

Questions for Further Thought

1. What does a contextual perspective on counseling mean to you in this case?
2. How would you define client growth in this case?
3. What do you need to do to establish a positive relationship with Martina?
4. What do you feel about Martina? How intense are these emotions and how do you think they may affect you in the counseling relationship?

5. How do you think you could help Martina become an active partner in counseling?
6. What ethical challenges do you think you would face in this case?

After you have responded to each question, we recommend that you find a partner and compare your responses.

CHARACTERISTICS OF EFFECTIVE COUNSELORS

The following exercise will help you identify the important qualities and characteristics of effective helpers. Although you can complete this exercise in private, it may have more meaning if shared with others participating in the same learning experience.

Exercise

Step 1. During your life, you have had experiences in which you were the recipient of help; you have also had experiences in which you were the provider of help. Whether or not these experiences were labeled as counseling, at important points in your life you have both given and received help. For this exercise, recall two occasions (involving different people) when you sought help from another. In either instance, the helper might be a friend, spouse, supervisor, parent, teacher, or counselor. The first occasion should be one in which the help you received was valuable to you—that is, the helper was effective in offering help to you. The second occasion should be one that did not result in success—you did not receive the help you needed.

Step 2. Think of the first experience and write down your responses to the following questions:

- What kind of help were you seeking?
- What were you concerned about?
- What did you hope to accomplish as a result of your discussion?
- How did the helping person treat you? What were his or her basic attitudes toward you and your concerns?
- What response patterns did you notice about the person who offered to help you?

- What were the most memorable characteristics of the person who offered to help you?

Step 3. Respond to the previous questions again with the second (less successful) helping experience in mind. Do not proceed until you have completed this step.

Step 4. Now, compare and contrast the two helping experiences and the helpers who were involved. What factors were present during the first helping experience that were missing during the second? How did the helpers differ from each other? Write down these comparisons. Again, please do not proceed until you have completed this step.

Step 5. Once you have completed your comparisons, share your findings with other students. Then see if you can verify from your experiences the observations that follow.

Through the years, a substantial body of research on the characteristics of effective counselors and therapists has developed (see Sexton, Whiston, Bleuer, & Walz, 1997, for a summary of this research). Most studies attempt to relate particular characteristics, such as dogmatism or experience in the profession, to counselor effectiveness. Because counseling is so complex, each study contributes but a small part of the total picture of what makes an effective counselor. Counseling theorists and practitioners have also added their clinical observations about the characteristics of effective helpers. This section summarizes several of the most important qualities possessed by effective helpers.

Effective counselors are skillful at reaching out. Through their demeanor and underlying views about others, effective counselors are able to encourage others to communicate openly and honestly with them. By actively listening for the client's feelings, beliefs, assumptions about self, significant others, and life circumstances, effective counselors avoid responding in ways that create defensiveness and block communication. They are able to concentrate fully on what a client is communicating to them, not only to understand the content of what the client is saying but also to appreciate the significance of that verbalization to the client's present and future well-being. They are able to control their own feelings of anxiety while hearing of another person's concerns and anxieties. They are also able to vary their communication patterns based on the client's personality, interpersonal style, and sociocultural background.

Effective counselors inspire feelings of trust, credibility, and confidence from people they help. In the presence of effective helpers, clients quickly sense that it is safe to risk sharing their concerns and feelings openly and that they will not be ridiculed, embarrassed, or criticized for their disclosures. Nothing bad will happen as a consequence of sharing, and there is a real chance that something productive will come of it. Effective counselors are also credible. What they say is perceived as believable and honest, free of hidden agendas or ulterior motives. They are viewed as honest, straightforward, and nonmanipulative, again supporting the general belief that they can be trusted. Finally, they ought to be attractive to clients, not because of their personal beauty, but because of their likability and friendliness. Clients who see their counselors as expert, attractive, and trustworthy are more likely to gain from counseling than those who fail to see these qualities in their counselors (Cormier & Nurious, 2002). Conversely, clients who experience their counselors' behavior as blaming, rejecting, or ignoring them are less likely to reach their goals for change (Najavits & Strupp, 1994).

Effective counselors communicate caring and respect for the persons they are trying to help. By their demeanor, effective counselors communicate to their clients the following unspoken statement: "It matters to me that you will be able to work out the concerns and problems you are facing. What happens to you in the future also matters to me. If things work out well for you and you achieve success, I shall be happy about it. If you encounter frustration and failure, I shall be saddened." The opposite of caring is not anger, but indifference. Effective helpers are not indifferent to the present and future of the people they try to help. On the contrary, effective helpers agree to offer time and energy to others because the future well-being of the people to whom they are reaching out matters to them.

To respect another person means to hold that person in regard and esteem. It means to have a favorable view of that person—to acknowledge his or her talents and not think less of that person because of human limitations. Applied to effective helping, respect means believing that the client is capable of learning, of overcoming obstacles to growth, and of maturing into a more responsible, self-reliant individual. With this perspective, effective helpers communicate regard for others by offering their time and energy and by active, attentive listening that shows involvement. They also show respect by not treating the individual as if he or she were stupid or ridiculous, incapable of sensible thinking and reasoning. They respect the role of social factors and cultural heritage in the client's experience and actively work to express their caring and respect in ways that are consistent with the client's cultural and social background. Effective helpers are neither arrogant nor conceited and thus do not act in a condescending way toward the people they are helping.

Effective counselors are able to reach in as well as to reach out. Effective helpers do a lot of thinking about their actions, feelings, value commitments, and motivations. They show a commitment to nondefensive, continuous self-understanding and self-examination. They are aware of the feelings they experience and the sources of those feelings. They are able to manage anxiety by being aware of it and its sources rather than blotting it from awareness. They are able to respond with depth to the question, "Who am I?" They can help others think openly and nondefensively about themselves and their own concerns because they are not afraid to participate in these experiences themselves.

Effective helpers also like and respect themselves and do not use the people they are trying to help to satisfy their own needs. All human beings want to be accepted, respected, and recognized by significant others and to be acknowledged for their special talents and achievements. However, some people are especially dependent on others for recognition and acknowledgment. They purposely respond to "you're okay and likable" feedback from others. They are responding in these situations to satisfy their own needs. People who do this excessively eventually alienate others and make them afraid. This interpersonal pattern blocks honest communication and instead leads to game playing. Truly effective helpers feel secure about themselves and like themselves and thus are not dependent on the people they are trying to help for respect, recognition, and acknowledgment.

Counselors who are under great stress in their personal lives are at risk of focusing on their own needs rather than the client's needs during counseling sessions. Thus, they ought to monitor carefully their effectiveness with clients. If personal stress is compromising one's effectiveness as a counselor, then the counselor needs to seek help and arrange for alternative care for his or her clients until the stress is reduced. A counselor who is needy and unable to focus on the client's best interests is commonly referred to as an "impaired" counselor or a "wounded healer" (Stadler, 2001). Under such circumstances counselors can do more harm than good. These helpers have either temporarily succumbed to overwhelming stress or have long-standing emotional difficulties that prevent them from relating positively to others. The most common reasons for professional impairment are relationship problems and alcohol abuse (Deutsch, 1985; Thoreson, Miller, & Krauskopf, 1989).

Even counselors who have worked through their own emotional difficulties or who are not overwhelmed by stress in their personal lives are at some risk for impairment. They can develop burnout, an experience of emotional depletion, alienation from clients, and a sense of futility in their work (Maslach, Jackson, & Leiter, 1996). Burnout happens when counselors let their work become the only focus in their lives and when they work under conditions that make the job itself more stressful. This combination of circumstances puts counselors at risk for losing perspective on their effectiveness and their clients. To avoid burnout, counselors must take time away from work to care for themselves, nourish their own personal support system, and get a clearer perspective on their accomplishments as professionals. Attending to the day-to-day working conditions and acting to make them as stress free as possible also reduces the risks of burnout. See Skovolt (2001) for a detailed description of strategies for good self-care to avoid burnout.

Effective counselors manage conflict between client and counselor effectively. Because counselors must often encourage clients to face painful emotions, irrational thoughts, and counterproductive behaviors, conflict or strain in the relationship may arise in the course of the process. Clients sometimes feel angry at their counselors for this focus or because the counselors are safer targets for their anger than other people in the clients' lives. The ways in which counselors navigate this conflict are important for achieving a positive result from counseling. Theorists refer to these conflicts as "therapeutic ruptures" and suggest that counselors skilled in dealing with these conflicts directly, but sensitively, are the most likely to resolve them and continue making progress on the client's therapeutic goals (Safran, Muran, Samstag & Stevens, 2002). If these ruptures are avoided or mishandled, the risk that a client will drop out of therapy increases greatly. The keys to effectively managing such conflicts are (1) the counselor's awareness that clients who develop negative feelings are likely to have difficulty expressing them directly, (2) the counselor's skill in initiating discussion about such feelings with clients, and (3) the counselor's openness and nondefensiveness in response to such client disclosures.

Effective counselors attempt to understand the behavior of the people they try to help without imposing value judgments. People have a tendency to make value judgments about the behavior of others—to judge the behavior of others by one's own standards. Though appropriate when casting a vote, this value-judging tendency seriously interferes with the process of effective helping. Effective helpers work hard to control the tendency to judge the values of their clients. Instead, they accept a given behavior pattern as the client's way of coping with some life situation, and they try to understand how the pattern developed. The helper will develop opinions about whether the behavior pattern is effective or ineffective in serving the client's goals but will refrain from classifying the client's values as good or bad. When counselors appreciate that behavior does not simply occur randomly, but that all behavior is purposeful and goal directed, they are less vulnerable to such value judgments about the actions of their clients.

Effective counselors recognize clients' self-defeating behaviors and help them develop more personally rewarding behavior patterns. People frequently do things that are counterproductive and goal disruptive rather than goal enhancing. Some communicate ridicule and hostility when they want respect and friendship. Others run away from frightening situations rather than confront the aspects of a situation that cause anxiety. Still others do things to betray trust and cannot understand why others do not trust them. There are others who are afraid to respond assertively when people make unreasonable demands on them. Effective counselors are capable of seeing such patterns and of assisting clients in developing alternative patterns.

Effective helpers have a model or image of the qualities and behavior patterns of a healthy and effective, or fully functioning, individual. Included in this model is an elaborate image of effective and ineffective ways of coping with the stressful situations of life. Effective helpers are skillful at helping others look at themselves and respond nondefensively to the question, "Who am I?" It is easy to describe aspects of self that are likable and admirable. It is difficult and painful to look at aspects of self that are not admirable. Yet self-improvement and growth require an honest, open awareness of those aspects of oneself that a person would like to change. Effective counselors are also able to help others to look at themselves, at both their likable and less admirable aspects, without debilitating fear, to identify personal changes that would promote growth and improvement, and to develop approaches to bring about those improvements.

Effective counselors have expertise in some area that will be of special value to the client. If counselors do not have some special competence, they have no business offering their services to clients. When people need help, they turn to people whom they believe have knowledge about and expertise in the problem of concern. When faced with a personal problem, people who need help turn to whomever they can identify as having an especially strong knowledge of human behavior. Counselors have a responsibility to develop expertise in areas where their clients need help and to update their knowledge through continuing education and consultation with other professionals. They also have a responsibility to practice within the boundaries of their competence and to avoid trying to deal with client concerns for which they have no training or experience. For example, only those with a background in career counseling should try to help clients with career problems, and only those with training in counseling young children should offer their services to this population.

Effective counselors are able to reason systematically and to think in terms of systems. A system is an organized entity in which each component relates to the others and to the system as a whole. Examples of systems include the human body, the organizational setting in which a person works, and the family unit. In high-entropy systems, components work cooperatively with each other and contribute favorably to the goals of the total system. In low-entropy systems, components do not work cooperatively and sometimes work against each other. Effective counselors are aware of the different social systems of which clients are a part, how clients are affected by those systems, and how they, in turn, influence those systems. In other words, effective helpers are aware of the forces and factors in a client's life space and the mutual interaction between the client's behavior and these environmental factors. Effective helpers realize that a client's concerns and problems are influenced by many complex factors that must be identified and understood as an inherent part of the helping effort.

Effective counselors are culturally competent; they are able to understand the social, cultural, and political context in which they and all other people operate. Counselors are aware of important present-day events in all the systems affecting their lives and the lives of their clientele. They are aware of the significance and possible future implications of these events. The counselor has a thorough understanding of current social concerns and an awareness of how these events affect the views of clients—especially their views about the future. The converse of being contemporary is to be encapsulated—to be unaware of what is happening in the systems and environments that make up one's life space (Wrenn, 1973, 1985). Among the important contemporary issues to which a counselor must attend is how bias and discrimination against some groups in society affect their personal well-being and progress toward self-actualization.

━━━━━━━━━━━━━━ *Exercise Continued* ━━━━━━━━━━━━━━

The previous section presented nine characteristics of effective helpers. How did they compare to the characteristics you identified in the personal learning activity? Did you identify some characteristics that were not discussed in the section you just read? The observations you made through this experience will contribute to your personal image of effective helping. Were there characteristics discussed in the previous section that you did not identify? Reading about the ones you did not see should cause you to think about how those qualities might have fit your personal helping situation.

Although some of the characteristics discussed may have seemed obvious to you, others may have seemed controversial. You probably observed, for example, that terms such as *empathy, genuineness, positive regard, self-disclosure,* and *concreteness* were not used. However, if you observe closely you will find these concepts presented in other words, such as *reaching out, credible, reaching inside of self,* and *reasoning systematically.* As you consider the characteristics of effective helpers you (and possibly those in your group) have known, you will find that everyday language may be used to describe the effective helper.

As a final step in the personal learning experience, reflect on your own personal qualities as they relate to being an effective helper. Do your qualities resemble those of effective helpers you have known and those described in the previous section? Do you see special strengths? Do you see limitations that may be remedied through study and practice? Do you see limitations that might cause you to question your choice about becoming a professional helper? If you experience confusion or stress about your own potential to be a helper, discuss your concern with your professor or a qualified professional helper.

THE JOY OF HELPING

Throughout this volume we repeat over and over that counseling must always serve the purposes of the client, that the focus of the talk must be on the client's issues, and that the counselor should make every effort to be intellectually and affectively available to the client throughout the process. We would be remiss if we did not also address the great satisfaction that comes from helping others change their lives and their attitudes toward life. Fifty years of research has amply demonstrated that counselors' optimism about the value of their work is justified; counseling really helps people alleviate their problems and approach life with greater satisfaction (Lambert & Barley, 2002; Wampold, 2001).

There is also the fascination of learning firsthand how others experience the world, indeed, how two people can participate in the same event and experience it differently. There is the wonder of seeing the human spirit in action as clients overcome adversity and grow toward new meanings in their lives. There is the great joy that comes from being the catalyst who helps clients escape from the miseries of emotional constriction and distress, indecision, and hopelessness. It is a privilege to be allowed to share the private worlds of others not only because it is essential to the helping process but because it also enriches our lives as counselors. We encourage you to reflect on the rewards that come to the professional in the counseling process and to find a personal sense of worth in the work that is accomplished. Although counseling is for the client, the counselor gains too.

OVERVIEW OF THE BOOK

In Chapters 2 through 6, we present a detailed description of our three-stage generic model of counseling and the ethical responsibilities related to counseling Technical terminology is introduced so that you can relate this work to the broader literature in the field. We describe counseling skills involved in building trust, structuring and leading client self-exploration, diagnosing problems, goal setting, action planning, and termination. Chapters 7 to 10 explore the theories, strategies, and techniques associated with the three-stage process and discuss the ways in which those techniques need to be modified for reluctant clients. Chapters 11–14 describe adaptations of the counseling process for specific populations: those in crisis and those who are diverse in culture, ethnicity, or life stage.

We describe the ways in which the counseling process should be adapted when working with children and with older adults.

SUMMARY

This chapter presented the theoretical background of our thoughts about effective counseling, some fundamental precepts that describe the essential elements of the counseling process, and a description of the qualities of the effective counselor. Inevitably, the qualities of the effective helper derive from and feed into the fundamental precepts of effective helping, because the counseling process cannot be understood apart from the person of the counselor. Finally, those who are thinking of becoming professional counselors are encouraged to take an introspective look at themselves to identify the presence or absence of qualities that have been associated with effective helping. It has been our experience that people who want to tell others how to live effectively are rarely good counselors; people who want to help others gain control over their own lives usually do well as counselors and experience personal satisfaction in their work.

≈≈≈ DISCUSSION QUESTIONS ≈≈≈

1. What strategies can counselors use to be empathic, caring, and committed to client welfare without becoming overinvolved in client problems?
2. Because the person of the counselor and the quality of the counseling relationship are so important to effective counseling, do you think that all counselors should be required to undergo counseling themselves before entering the profession?
3. The research on the importance of the therapeutic relationship seems to be in direct conflict with the emphasis in managed care on quick intervention and short-term counseling. Why do you think this discrepancy exists, and what steps can the profession take to deal with this problem?
4. Do you agree with the authors' perspective on the role of diagnosis in understanding human problems? If not, what would you change?
5. In light of the precepts and characteristics of effective counselors identified in this chapter, what procedures would you use if you were responsible for screening applicants for a training program in counseling?

REFERENCES

Alexander, F. M. (1963). *Fundamentals of psychoanalysis*. New York: Norton.
Bachelor, A., & Horvath, A. (1999). The therapeutic relationship. In M. A. Hubble, B. L. Duncan, & S. D. Miller (Eds.). *The heart and soul of change: What works in therapy* (pp. 133–178). Washington, DC: American Psychological Association.

Beck, A. (1972). *Depression: Causes and treatment.* Philadelphia: University of Pennsylvania Press.

Beck, A. (1976). *Cognitive therapy and emotional disorders.* New York: International Universities Press.

Carkhuff, R. R. (1969a). *Helping and human relations* (Vol. 1). New York: Holt, Rinehart and Winston.

Carkhuff, R. R. (1969b). *Helping and human relations* (Vol. 2). New York: Holt, Rinehart and Winston.

Cormier, S., & Nurius, P. S. (2002). *Interviewing strategies for helpers* (4th ed.). Pacific Grove, CA: Brooks/Cole.

Deutsch, C. J. (1985). A survey of therapists' personal problems and treatment. *Professional Psychology: Research and Practice, 16,* 305–315.

Egan, G. (2002). *The skilled helper: A problem-management and opportunity development approach to helping* (7th ed.). Pacific Grove, CA: Brooks/Cole.

Eisenberg, S., & Patterson, L. E. (1979). *Helping clients with special concerns.* Boston: Houghton Mifflin. Reissued (1990). Prospect Heights, IL: Waveland Press.

Ellis, A. (2000). Rational-emotive therapy. In R. J. Corsini & D. Wedding (Eds.). *Current psychotherapies* (6th ed., pp. 168–204). Itasca, IL: Peacock.

Ellis, A., & Bernard, M. E. (1986). What is rational-emotive therapy (RET)? In A. Ellis & R. Grieger (Eds.), *Handbook of rational-emotive therapy* (Vol. 2, pp. 3–30). New York: Springer.

Frank, J. D., & Frank, J. B. (1991). *Persuasion and healing* (3rd ed.). Baltimore: Johns Hopkins University Press.

Freud, S. (1964). The ego and the id. In J. Strachey (Ed. and Trans.), *The standard edition of the complete psychological works of Sigmund Freud.* London: Hogarth Press (original work published 1923).

Hackney, H., & Cormier, L. S. (2001). *The professional counselor: A process guide to helping* (4th ed.). Boston: Allyn & Bacon.

Horvath, A. O., & Bedi, R. P. (2002). The alliance. In J. C. Norcross (Ed.), *Psychotherapy relationships that work* (pp. 37–69). New York: Oxford.

Lambert, M. J., & Barley, D. E. (2002). Research summary on the therapeutic relationship and psychotherapy outcome. In J. C. Norcross (Ed.), *Psychotherapy relationships that work* (pp. 17–32). New York: Oxford.

Lambert, M. J., Whipple, J. L., Smart, D. W., Vermeersch, D. A., Stevan, L., & Hawkins, E. J. (2001). The effects of providing therapists with feedback on patient progress during psychotherapy: Are outcomes enhanced? *Psychotherapy Research, 11,* 49–68.

Maslach, C., Jackson, S. E., & Leiter, M. P. (1996). *Maslach Burnout Inventory: Manual* (3rd ed.). Palo Alto, CA: Consulting Psychologists Press.

Meichenbaum, D. (1977). *Cognitive behavior modification: An interactive approach.* New York: Plenum.

Najavits, L. M., & Strupp, H. H. (1994). Differences in the effectiveness of psychodynamic therapists: and process and outcome study. *Psychotherapy: Theory, Research, Practice, Training, 31,* 114–123.

Perls, F. (1969). *Gestalt therapy verbatim.* Moab, UT: Real People Press.

Polster, E., & Polster, M. (1973). *Gestalt therapy integrated.* New York: Bruner/Mazel.

Prochaska, J. O., Norcross, J. C., & DiClemente, C. C. (1994). *Changing for good.* New York: Avon.

Rogers, C. R. (1942). *Counseling and psychotherapy.* Boston: Houghton Mifflin.

Rogers, C. R. (1951). *Client-centered therapy.* Boston: Houghton Mifflin.

Rogers, C. R. (1961). *On becoming a person.* Boston: Houghton Mifflin.

Rogers, C. R. (1980). *A way of being.* Boston: Houghton Mifflin.

Rogers, C. R. (1986). Carl Rogers on the development of the person-centered approach. *Person-Centered Review, 1,* 257–259.

Safran, J. D., Muran, J. C., Samstag, L. W., & Stevens, C. (2002). Repairing alliance ruptures. In J. C. Norcross (Ed.), *Psychotherapy relationships that work* (pp. 235–254). New York: Oxford.

Seligman, M. E. L., & Csikszentmihalyi, M. (2000). Positive psychology: An introduction. *American Psychologist, 55,* 5–14.

Sexton T. L., Whiston, S. C., Bleuer, J. C., & Walz, G. R. (1997). *Integrating outcome research into counseling practice and training.* Alexandria, VA: American Counseling Association.

Sinacore-Guinn, A. L. (1995). The diagnostic window: Culture and gender sensitive diagnosis and training. *Counselor Education and Supervision, 35,* 18–31.

Skovolt, T. M. (2001). *The resilient practitioner: Burnout prevention and self-care strategies for counselors, therapists, teachers, and health professionals.* Boston: Allyn & Bacon.

Snyder, C. R., & Lopez, S. J. (Eds.). (2002). *Handbook of positive psychology.* New York: Oxford.

Stadler, H. A. (2001). Impairment in the mental health professions. In E. R. Welfel & R. E. Ingersoll (Eds.). *Mental health desk reference* (pp. 413–418). New York: Wiley.

Thoreson, R. W., Miller, M., & Krauskopf, C. J. (1989). The distressed psychologist: Prevalence and treatment considerations. *Professional Psychology: Research and Practice, 20,* 153–158.

Wampold, B. E. (2001). *The great psychotherapy debate: Models, methods and findings.* Mahwah, NJ: Erlbaum.

Welfel, E. R. (2002). *Ethics in counseling and psychotherapy: Standards, research and emerging* issues (2nd ed.). Pacific Grove, CA: Brooks/Cole.

Williamson, E. G. (1939). *How to counsel students.* New York: McGraw-Hill.

Williamson, E. G. (1950). *Counseling adolescents.* New York: McGraw-Hill.

Williamson, E. G. (1965). *Vocational counseling.* New York: McGraw-Hill.

Wrenn, C. G. (1973). *World of the contemporary counselor.* Boston: Houghton Mifflin.

Wrenn, C. G. (1985). Afterword: The culturally encapsulated counselor revisited. In P. Pedersen (Ed.). *Handbook of cross-cultural counseling and therapy* (pp. 323–329). Westbrook, CT: Greenwood.

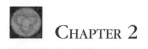

CHAPTER 2

UNDERSTANDING COUNSELING AS A PROCESS

Counseling is a term that has connoted many different activities. The word has been applied to the activities of attorneys, insurance advisors, and personal athletic trainers. Implicit in each of these is a definition of counseling as advice giving and that assumes an active, dominant expert who instructs a passive uninformed person on what he or she ought to be doing. In reality, counseling is an activity that rarely involves advice giving and demands an active collaboration between two people with equal, though different, expertise. The counselor has knowledge of human development, human behavior, and the change processes that usually help people achieve the goals they seek. The counselor is also a person who believes in the freedom and dignity of all people, who is capable of compassion for human frailties, and who has the skill to communicate that compassion and respect to the client. The client is an expert on his or her own experience, background, and personal resources for change and also knows the numerous attempts to change already used prior to entering counseling. Adopting the view first expressed by the pioneering work of Carl Rogers (1942), we also believe that the client engages in an active process of self-development during the course of counseling for which the counselor is the catalyst and facilitator. Counselors who fail to recognize clients' partnership in the process and who attempt to impose counseling goals and interventions on clients are likely to alienate the very clients they seek to help. In fact, the view that counseling is a collaboration between an active, generative client and a knowledgeable counselor whose primary role is to help client use his or her internal resources for growth has been increasingly supported by research on counseling and psychotherapy (see Bohart & Tallman, 1999, and Hubble, Duncan, & Miller, 1999, for an analysis of this research).

The term *psychotherapy* is closely related to counseling as we use the word in this book. Psychotherapy has its roots in the medical and psychological tradition that views most suffering that people bring to professional helpers as mental illness paralleling physical illnesses patients bring to physicians. In recent years, psychotherapy has come to denote a wider range of activities than just treatment for mental illness, although it retains some focus on mental illness. As described in the current literature, the outline of the process of psychotherapy closely parallels the model in this book. We have retained the word *counseling* instead of using *psychotherapy* because we believe that the former omits the connotation of a central focus on mental illness and because it more easily encompasses activities in educational as well as mental health settings.

Counseling and psychotherapy are both professions that require extensive training and experience. Currently, 48 states (along with Puerto Rico and the District of Columbia) require that individuals who represent themselves as professional counselors possess licenses to practice (Welfel, 2002). All states mandate that psychologists and school counselors be licensed or certified. The requirements for licensure or certification typically include a graduate degree in counseling or psychotherapy from an accredited university, an acceptable score on a licensing examination, and evidence of an internship or other supervised experience in the field (along with no felony convictions). The laws mandating that one have a professional credential before offering counseling services to the public underscore the high level of competence needed to succeed in helping clients and the power of the counseling process to do good or, if used incompetently, to do harm.

Because professional counseling as a helping activity is much more complex than the conventional use of the word, we need to provide a comprehensive definition of counseling. The following definition addresses both the outcome goals and the process goals of counseling. A discussion of the goals follows the definition and serves as an orientation to Chapters 3 through 5, which describe the stages of counseling in detail.

DEFINITION OF COUNSELING

Counseling is an interactive process characterized by a unique relationship between counselor and client that leads to change in the client in one or more of the following areas:

1. Behavior (overt changes in the ways clients act, their coping skills, decision making skills, and/or relationship skills)
2. Beliefs and values (ways of thinking about self, others, and the world) or emotional concerns relating to these perceptions
3. Level of emotional distress (uncomfortable feelings or reactivity to environmental stress)

The desire for change can stem from identified problems, such as loneliness, uncontrollable anxiety, or poor social skills, or from a desire for a fuller life, even in the absence of identifiable problems in functioning. In the latter case, a couple might enter counseling seeking a more intimate relationship even though their existing relationship is free of open conflict, or a worker might consult with a counselor prior to an important job change. In all cases, counseling should result in free and responsible behavior on the part of the client, accompanied by more insight into self and others and an improved ability to understand and better manage negative emotions.

OUTCOME GOALS OF COUNSELING

Change Must Occur

The first element of the above definition that alludes to goals is that counseling "leads to change in the client." This is true of individual, group, or family counseling and remains true whether the expressed intent of the counseling is developmental (oriented to personal growth) or remedial (oriented to the resolution of problems). The change that occurs may be overt and dramatic, or it may be imperceptible to anyone but the client. For instance, a person formerly incapacitated by a fear of flying may become a qualified pilot, or someone who had difficulty accepting credit for accomplishments may begin to take pride in those achievements. The awareness that counseling is supposed to lead to change diminishes the temptation to think of counseling as "just a nice conversation" and sets the tone for the hard and sometimes painful work that effective counseling requires. Successful counseling can result in gratifying, even exhilarating, changes for the client, but these positive results don't happen by magic or without real commitment by both participants. Comprehension of this fact is fundamental to change in any of the following categories.

Categories of Possible Change

Change in counseling can take several forms: overt behavior change, improvement in decision-making or coping skills, modification of beliefs or values, or reduction of the level of emotional distress. The counseling model we present in this book is labeled as multitheoretical and integrative precisely because change occurs in many domains and is derived from a variety of interventions to help achieve that change. This section examines each category of change, beginning with behavior change.

Behavior change is probably the easiest type of change to recognize because it is overt and observable. A behavior change might be the solution of a problem, as in the case of a child who learns to get what he wants from others through verbal requests and negotiation rather than through physical aggression. A behavior change might also enhance one's potential for personal growth, as in the case of a middle-aged person who returns to school or embarks on a new career. Many counselors believe that changes in thoughts and attitudes must precede changes in behavior, and they work to understand those changes. Counselors of the traditional behaviorist school maintain that a counselor can never really know a client's inner thoughts and attitudes and that only observable behavior changes indicate the success of counseling. Modern behaviorists tend to consider changes in thinking as a mediating factor in behavior change (for example, see Kazdin, 2000).

Counseling may also enhance an individual's ability to cope with life situations. Certain life events are both painful and difficult to change, but learning how to manage in the face of such adversity creates an opportunity for accomplishment and enjoyment in spite of such events. For example, some people with terminal illness refer to the period after they got sick as one of the best of their lives because of the closeness to and honesty with loved ones that their impending death has brought. Clearly, they are not glad they got sick; rather they are able to appreciate the precious gains the illness provided, in spite of its devastating consequences.

Coping ability depends on the individual's skill in identifying the questions to be resolved, the alternatives available, and the likely results of acting on each alternative. Sometimes coping means learning to live with what one cannot change. For example, a person who has suffered a permanently disabling injury in an automobile accident may use counseling to learn to adapt to his or her new situation. Learning to cope with an alcoholic parent requires that certain questions be resolved: What can I change, and what must I accept? Who can help me? Am I responsible for my parent's behavior and well-being? What do I want to do? What are the likely results of available actions? A counselor can help by encouraging the client to define dimensions of the family system as a basis for predicting what may work and what risks are worth taking. Depending on the analysis, the conclusion might range from staying away from the parent when he or she is drunk to arranging for the parent to seek treatment for his or her problem. Changes in ability to cope usually include both behavior change and change in beliefs and attitudes.

Counseling may also contribute to a client's ability to make important life decisions. The counselor typically teaches the client self-assessment procedures and coaches the client on how to use information to arrive at personally satisfying answers. Career counselors frequently engage in this work, and assisting students with career decision making is still a major focus of school and college counselors. Counselors prepared in contemporary career development methods focus heavily on helping clients identify relevant sources of information. They generally refrain from giving advice and see career decision making as a lifelong process rather than a single decision made during young adulthood.

Though not directly observable, a change in beliefs (also called personal constructs) may occur in counseling and can be assessed from the words of the client. A common goal of counseling is that the client will improve his or her self-concept and come to think of himself or herself as a more competent, lovable, or worthy person. Kelley (1955) describes personal constructs as an individual's particular view of reality and states that people's behaviors are based on what they believe to be true. Therefore, people who think they are incapable and feel embarrassed about performing in front of others will act on those personal constructs by avoiding anything challenging. Changes in beliefs often lead to behavior change, but they can also make present behavior more satisfying. For example, a parent who changes his viewpoint about his adolescent daughter's behavior, coming to see her mildly rebellious behavior as normal rather than pathological, may be less upset by it and more likely to react in ways that facilitate the teen's healthy development. Ellis (1994, 2000) has developed a system for understanding how one's personal thoughts can lead to dissatisfaction with the state of one's life. He explains that people acquire irrational thoughts that lead to expectations that can never be fulfilled, for example, "I must be perfectly competent in all that I do, or I am not a good person." Through counseling, the client may learn to give up such thinking and instead appreciate what he or she does well while working toward competence in other areas. Beck (Beck, 1976; Beck & Emery, 1985; Beck, Rush, & Emery, 1979) presents a similar model that describes the impact of negative belief systems on feelings and behaviors. Meichenbaum (1977) refers to this process as the internal dialogue and defines one goal of counseling as modifying the content of the dysfunctional internal dialogue. Using the term *stress inoculation,* Meichenbaum (1985) also incorporates strategies for coping more successfully with stress into the cognitive therapy process. No change, whether cognitive, behavioral, or emotional, comes about as a result of things counselors impose on clients; instead, all change stems from engaging with clients in their quest to improve their lives in ways that make sense to them.

In the case study that follows, the client eventually changes both his thinking and his behavior. Observe how his changes in thinking free him to behave more effectively.

The Case of Thad

Thad, a young man of 22, sought a counselor at the university counseling service because he had trouble concentrating on his studies and felt constant tension. Two months earlier, he had moved into his own apartment, leaving his parents' home for the first time. He felt guilty about "deserting his parents when they needed him." His father had a serious degenerative health problem and required some special care, though he was not an invalid. His mother was a vigorous and healthy woman who was able and eager to help make her husband's life comfortable.

As counseling proceeded, Thad came to understand that his parents needed his affection and involvement but not his physical help and daily presence. His daily visits were actually interrupting other things they wanted to do. In other words, his belief that his parents needed him to come home each day and that if he did not come home he could not call himself a good son was amended by his realization that his physical presence was not the critical factor in their perception of him as a good son. Thad changed his personal perception of his role in the family, and his new perception allowed him to live away from home without guilt. He began to make special occasions of his visits to his family, and he and his parents began enjoying each other's company once more. Thad's feelings of tension receded and he was able to refocus on schoolwork and other elements of his personal life.

Questions for Further Thought

1. What other irrational thoughts may have led to Thad's feelings of guilt about his treatment of his parents?
2. What rational thoughts do you believe replaced them as counseling proceeded?
3. How did Thad's changed thinking affect his behavior?
4. How do you think this new perception of self and family might affect his other relationships?

An additional function of counseling is the relief of emotional distress (Brammer & McDonald, 2002). Many clients enter counseling because they feel sad, angry, or frightened and need a place where they can safely vent those feelings and feel sure that they will be accepted and understood. Their level of emotional distress may be interfering with their daily activities, and they need relief from their psychic pain. Many times, the relief of emotional distress is only one piece of the necessary change, and attention to irrational thoughts, inadequate coping skills, or dysfunctional behaviors that perpetuate the emotional distress is critical to lasting change. At other times, individuals have been overwhelmed by a loss or tragedy in their lives and benefit largely from the emotional release. A person whose house has been destroyed in a hurricane may appropriately use counseling to vent the fear experienced during the storm and the sad and angry feelings about the losses due to it. Once the trauma has been processed, preexisting coping skills may be sufficient for moving on in life.

Change that occurs in counseling can influence feelings, values, attitudes, thoughts, and actions. Among the broad variety of potential changes, some will be obvious and others subtle. Because the scope of possible change covers essentially all dimensions of human experience, it can correctly be stated that if change in at least one dimension does not occur, counseling has not succeeded. The result of counseling may be inner peace with little outward sign of change. At other times, behaviors will change markedly, and the client may then need help in understanding the reactions of others to the changed behavior.

Free and Responsible Behavior

Freedom is the power to determine one's own actions, to make one's own choices and decisions. But freedom is fragile, and some of it must be sacrificed as the price for living in any kind of social system. Freedom is limited by the responsibility to consider the freedoms of others as one determines one's actions; it is not license to do exactly as one pleases. One role of counselors is to help clients assess the true margins of their freedom by focusing clients' attention to the consequences of their actions. Clients who feel that freedom is license must be helped to see that family, friends, teachers, employers, or the society at large will exact a price for behaviors that are perceived as threatening to the client's self-interest or the interests of others. Other clients may be all too willing to give away their freedoms to others (especially parents or spouses), abdicating the right to make decisions that will have major effects on the rest of their lives for the short-term gain of pleasing others. In either case, the counselor works with the client to come to a more balanced perception of personal freedom. Free and responsible behavior leaves people in charge of their own lives but also recognizes that they are members of social and cultural groups.

Counselors raised in cultures that place strong emphasis on the rights and freedom of the individual must also understand that not all cultures emphasize individual freedom to the same degree. Hence, counselors need to respect the values of clients who place the good of the group or the family ahead of the desires of an individual. Counselors are obligated to show respect for community along with their encouragement of personal growth. For example, when clients come from cultures that have the custom of arranging marriages for their young adult children, counselors may experience that custom as "wrong" or as abnormal or pathological. They may even express this view and try to discourage clients from accepting such marriages. Those actions fail to recognize the cultural variations in individual rights and freedom. Additionally, they are not likely to be helpful to the client unless the reasons the client entered counseling were related to discomfort with that custom or problems related to it. As long as the client is not coerced into the choice and understands the consequences and implications of his or her behavior, individual freedom includes the freedom to waive the right to choose a life partner oneself as much as it means the freedom to make that choice independently.

Counselors who deal with children and adolescents face conflicting guidelines about how far they may go in supporting free choice. The issue becomes one of children's rights versus parents' rights, in a context where both children and parents are capable of making very faulty judgments. Conventional belief associates wisdom with maturity, so counselors may feel little support for respecting children's rights. The younger the child, the smaller the measure of autonomy he or she can reasonably be given. A counselor can help adolescent clients protect their freedoms by helping them consider alternatives carefully so that they can make well-examined decisions about their behaviors. Unfortunately, no absolute rule exists to help the counselor know when a minor client is sufficiently wise and mature to assume responsibility for herself or himself and careful professional judgments must be made in each case with careful consideration of the rights and responsibilities of parents. Ethics codes and scholarly writings can be invaluable (Welfel, 2002) in these circumstances.

Understanding and Managing Negative Feelings

One common misunderstanding of counseling is that it eliminates negative feelings. Beginning counselors and clients are tempted to set the eradication of anxiety, sadness, or anger as one of their missions, but counselors need only look within themselves and loved ones to realize that negative feelings are often present even in people who are leading fulfilling and productive lives. Thus, a more appropriate goal of counseling is to help people understand negative feelings and to reduce debilitating anxiety, overwhelming sadness, or extreme anger.

Moreover, clients need to recognize that negative feelings are not only unavoidable given the vicissitudes of life, but also to understand that they are healthy, much in the same way that physical pain is healthy—negative feelings alert the person to a problem or circumstance that demands the individual's attention. Consequently, a better way to define the goal of counseling is to leave clients with *situation-appropriate* levels of negative feelings. Feeling anxious about an important decision or event is normal. Indeed, clients who exhibit no fear of life-threatening events (such as cardiac bypass surgery) or no concern about events that are in reality worrisome (such as a child left unattended in a room with a space heater) are often seen as in special need of counseling. Similarly, it is normal to feel sad after a loss and angry at someone who has robbed one's home or hurt a child. What clients need is the skill to cope with such emotions, the permission to experience their pain, and the capacity to express such feelings without harming others or themselves.

Professional counseling exists to help people sort out the meaning of their lives in the face of loss and pain. Again, our approach is that counselors cannot impose their meanings or values on clients; rather, clients need to use counseling as a means of sorting out for themselves issues of meaning in spite of loss, disappointment, or fear. Existential theories of counseling focus largely on apprehending meaning and purpose in spite of pain (e.g., Yalom, 1980).

PROCESS GOALS IN COUNSELING

Our definition asserts that counseling is an interactive process characterized by a unique relationship between counselor and client. The remainder of this chapter is devoted to an overview of the counseling process
and an introduction to the nature of that special relationship. To understand
counseling as a process, one must distinguish between outcome goals and
process goals. Outcome goals (described in the previous section) are the
intended results of counseling. Generally, they are described in terms of
what the client desires to achieve as a result of his or her interactions with
the counselor. In contrast, process goals are those events within the counseling sessions that the counselor considers helpful or instrumental in bringing
about outcome goals. Outcome goals are described in terms of change in the
client that will be manifest after the counseling and outside the counselor's
office. Process goals are sometimes described in terms of the counselor's
actions and at other times in terms of effects to be experienced by the client.
For example, a counselor may think, "If I am to help this client, I must
actively listen to what he is saying and understand the significance of his
concerns for his present and future well-being. I must understand how the
attitudes he is describing influence the way he behaves toward significant
others. I must understand the surrounding circumstances (including cultural
background) that relate to his concerns, and I must understand the reinforcing events that support his behavior." All of these statements are process
goals that relate to the counselor's behavior.

When reviewing a tape recording of the first session with a client, a
counselor may think, "If I am to help this client, I believe she must feel a
greater trust for me than she now appears to be experiencing. The client
seems to be talking a good deal about issues and events that do not relate
to her primary concerns. If our sessions are to be worthwhile, I think she
must focus more intently on these concerns. If the client is afraid to think
about or talk about them, it will be important to help her gain control over
these anxieties. How can I help the client feel more trust and less anxiety?"
Experiencing trust, focusing more fully on primary concerns, and controlling
fear are all process goals described in terms of effects the client should
experience. The last sentence in the counselor's thinking raises the crucial
questions "What can I do?" and "How can I behave so as to facilitate these
important process goals?"

Another kind of process goal relates to the way the counselor can act
as a model for new ways of behaving. By modeling appropriate responses
to frustration, disappointment, or negative feelings, the counselor indirectly
teaches the client alternatives to accustomed ways of responding. For example, a counselor who deals assertively (not aggressively or sarcastically) with
a chronically late client is demonstrating to the client an alternative way to
cope with feelings of frustration and interpersonal stress. In such a situation,

the client learns that there are words that can express uncomfortable feelings without alienating the other person or breaking the relationship bond. Ideally, when counselors model good communication, clients will come to understand that dealing directly but sensitively with negative affect can actually enhance personal relationships.

Some process goals appear essential for all counseling relationships and in fact define the steps in the counseling process. Other process goals are specific to particular clients. The concern about trust described in the prior section illustrates a common process goal in all counseling, whereas the example of the client who was avoiding discussion of primary concerns is particular to her. Even though other clients may show the same tendency, such behavior is not expected in all clients. Elements of the counseling process that are common to essentially all counseling interactions are introduced in the following discussion of the stages of counseling.

STAGES OF THE COUNSELING PROCESS

The word *process* helps to communicate much about the essence of counseling. A process is an identifiable sequence of events taking place over time. Usually there is the implication of progressive stages in the process. For example, there are identifiable stages in the healing process for a serious physical injury such as a broken leg. Similarly, there are identifiable stages in the process of human development from birth to death. Although the stages in this process are common to all human beings, what happens within each of these stages is unique for each individual.

Counseling also has a predictable set of stages that occur in any complete sequence. Initially, the counselor and the client must establish contact, define together "where the client is" in his or her life, and clarify the client's current difficulties. If successful, the client commits to using counseling as a tool for personal growth. This stage is followed by conversation that leads to a deeper understanding of the client's needs and desires in the context of his or her interpersonal world and to a mutually acceptable diagnosis of the problems. Finally, the participants agree on goals for change and design and implement action plans to accomplish the identified goals. When a client comes to a counselor to discuss a concern that is fairly specific and compartmentalized (such as which of two job offers to accept), the entire sequence of stages may be accomplished in a single session. In contrast, when a client comes to a counselor with highly disruptive, distressful, or long-standing concern (such as learning how to live as a single parent or how to cope with an eating disorder), the stages may be accomplished over many sessions. Once rapport has been established and in-depth exploration has been undertaken, the participants will define each problem or issue more fully and develop goals for resolving the problems. Next, the client and counselor devise a plan of action for change that the client carries out and modifies depending on its success. If new information emerges that changes either the understanding of the problems or the goals for counseling, the process is adapted to meet these new circumstances. The figure on the inside front cover provides a thorough graphic summary of the counseling process with special attention to the work of the client and the counselor at each stage. It also illustrates the product that they mutually develop marked by the central arrows.

The First Stage: Initial Disclosure

At the beginning of counseling, the counselor and the client typically do not know one another. Perhaps the client has seen the counselor in a community education program, a presentation in a residence hall on campus, or a group guidance session at the high school, but most often in community counseling and mental health agencies, client and counselor have had no contact prior to the first counseling session. Perhaps the counselor has some basic information about the client collected from an intake form or a school record. Because neither participant can know in advance the direction their discussion will ultimately take, the client is probably anxious about disclosing concerns because he or she is not sure how the counselor will receive the disclosures. Hackney and Cormier (2001) describe two sets of feelings clients have at the beginning of counseling: "I know I need help" and "I wish I weren't here" (p. 25). Their description captures well the fundamental ambivalence clients often feel in their initial encounters with a counselor. One central task of the counselor in the first stage of counseling is to allay the client's fears and encourage self-disclosure. Without honest self-disclosure by the client, counseling is an empty enterprise.

Carkhuff (1973) and Egan (2002) both describe *attending* as an important counselor behavior at the outset of counseling. Attending is simply paying careful attention to the client's words and actions. One demonstrates attending by posture, facial expression, eye contact, and even by the placement of one's chair relative to the client. As a part of attending, counselors observe clients' behavior for indications of content and feeling that may not be included in their verbal messages. Signs might include fidgeting, tone of voice, flushing of the complexion, changes in breathing rhythms, failure to maintain eye contact, and so on. We include attending behavior as a part of the initial disclosure stage of counseling because it begins when the first contact between client and counselor occurs but it remains important throughout all stages of the counseling process.

In the initial disclosure stage of counseling, based on their expectations for counseling and their perceptions of the receptiveness of the counselor, clients decide whether to articulate their personal concerns and the context in which they have arisen so that the counselor can understand the personal meanings and significance the client attaches to them. Older counseling literature described the first stage as "definition of the problem," but such terminology fails to describe the essence of the initial disclosure process and the active decision making of the client about what to disclose. Without a trusting relationship and substantial disclosure from the client, both of which require time to obtain, counselors will simply not learn enough about the client to accurately define any problems.

To encourage client disclosure, the counselor must offer a climate that promotes trust in the client and encourages clients to put their own resources to use to address the issues they bring to counseling. Carl Rogers (1951) described these trust-promoting conditions as the characteristics of the helping relationship:

1. Empathy—understanding another's experience as if it were your own, without ever losing the "as if" quality
2. Congruence or genuineness—being as you seem to be, consistent over time, dependable in the relationship
3. Unconditional positive regard—caring for your client without setting conditions for your caring (avoiding the message that "I will care about you if you do what I want")

Only counselors who actually feel empathic, compassionate, and open to their clients will be able to show these qualities to clients. One cannot take on these qualities as a role to be acted out. To effectively *communicate* empathy, genuineness, and caring to the client, the counselor must also learn to respond in words that are meaningful to the client. In other words, both motivation to help and verbal skill are prerequisites for success. At this stage, the most frequent kind of response is referred to as *restatement, paraphrasing,* or *interchangeable responding.* The counselor keeps the focus of attention on what the client is saying and on the meaning the client attaches to events in his or her life. When a client says, "When my husband goes out at night without a word to me about his destination or schedule, I feel as though I want to scream at him," a typical counselor response might be "You are very angry about the times when your husband goes out and doesn't tell you where he's going or when he will be back." Such a statement tells the client that the content and the feeling of her statement have been heard. If expressed with appropriate tone, even straightforward restatements can communicate attention to the client and genuine caring for her difficult situation.

Egan (2002) adds another condition that has relevance throughout the counseling process:

4. Concreteness—using clear language to describe the client's life situation

It is the counselor's task to sort out ambiguous statements and help the client find descriptions that will accurately portray what is happening in his or her life. Concreteness promotes clearer insight by the client into his or her life and provides the counselor with a fuller sense of the uniqueness of the client's experience. The following example contrasts a concrete counselor response to a client statement with a vague one.

> CLIENT: I am tired of living this way, but I feel as though there is no way I can get out of caring for my aging father. It all feels pretty hopeless and like no one cares about my needs.
>
> COUNSELOR A: You sound depressed by your situation.
>
> COUNSELOR B: The responsibility of caring for your father has worn you out and left you feeling isolated, unsupported, and without alternatives.

The response of Counselor B is more concrete because it tells the client that her words were heard exactly. The response of Counselor A could have been made to any number of client statements and does not relate in any specific way to the unique concerns of this client.

If these conditions are present in the initial disclosure stage of counseling, clients will be encouraged to talk freely and to elaborate on their concerns. Essentially what counselors are doing when they communicate in these ways is giving clients permission to use their tendency to active self-improvement in this relationship. Gelso and Carter (1985) refer to this point in counseling as the establishment of a "working alliance" (p. 161). In the process, clients don't simply tell the counselor what the problem is, they begin to clarify the dimensions of life concerns, rethink their problem and its relation to other parts of their lives, and consider the potential for the counselor to help and support change. In other words, as clients work to try to communicate their ideas and feelings to another, they also reach greater personal understanding and become aware of possibilities for change in a problem that seemed insoluble prior to counseling. (Chapter 3 presents a detailed analysis of the initial disclosure stage of counseling, along with case material for illustration. Also see the inside front cover for a concise review of client and counselor work in the disclosure stage with the resulting specification of the client's concerns and the establishment of a productive working relationship.)

Research by Michael Lambert and his colleagues (2001, 2002) highlights the importance of the first stage of counseling. Their work suggests that clients decide in the first three sessions whether they believe that counseling with this particular counselor will help them reach their goals for change. They make this decision based largely on the effectiveness of the counselor in forging a therapeutic alliance, in conveying real interest in them as unique people, and in a communication style that eases the difficulty of discussing painful and sensitive issues. When clients are not positively disposed toward the counselor in the first few sessions, they are at risk for dropping out of counseling before they reach their goals. Thankfully, this research also reveals that counselors who are aware that clients are not feeling satisfied with counseling can change their behavior to retain these clients and help them experience success from counseling.

One cautionary note is required here. Though we clearly believe that counseling is a powerful intervention for change, it is not necessarily the best option for every person who schedules a counseling appointment. Education or support groups, for example, may be more therapeutic for particular client concerns. The newly widowed person may benefit more from a support group of others coping with the loss of a spouse than from individual counseling. Sometimes clients define their problems as psychological when, in fact, other factors are at the foundation. Clients may misinterpret symptoms of physiological problems as psychological. For example, aging clients who are experiencing side effects of medications prescribed for them are more likely to immediately benefit from changes in the medical care than from counseling. For clients in extreme distress or experiencing psychotic symptoms, a regimen of psychotropic medications may be needed before productive counseling can take place. The counselor may realize that counseling is inappropriate in either Stage 1 or Stage 2 of the counseling process. In confusing or complex situations, careful assessment will provide the counselor and the client with the data necessary to make a determination about whether a referral to another resource is appropriate.

Counseling is not always appropriate for other reasons. The client and the counselor may have incompatible personalities or values (Corey, Corey, & Callanan, 2002; Goldstein, 1971), the client's difficulties may be beyond the counselor's helping skills, or the client's difficulties may require special modes of intervention (e.g., in cases of incest or chemical dependency). Under such conditions, referral is also an appropriate choice for the counselor. On the part of the counselor, referral requires both an honest acknowledgment that some other person or resource in the community may be more helpful to the client and a willingness to help the client make contact with these resources. Effective referral requires that the counselor have accurate information about resources in the community, including knowledge about the scope and quality of their services. Since it can be very hard to tell one's story to a stranger whose qualifications are unknown, having personal contacts and the names of specific people in an agency can make the transition easier for the client. It is important for the counselor to recognize that not every person who enters his or her office is necessarily a good candidate for counseling services.

The Second Stage: In-Depth Exploration

In the second stage of counseling, the client should reach clearer understandings of his or her life concerns and formulate a stronger sense of hope and direction. It is a useful rubric to think of these emerging goals as the flip side of problems. That is, as problems are more fully understood, the direction in which the client wishes to move also becomes clearer. At this stage, the goals are not precisely defined and the means to reach them are still undifferentiated, but an outline of the pattern of desired change is emerging.

The process that facilitates formulation of a new sense of direction builds on the conditions of the initial disclosure stage and becomes possible only if the trust and client engagement that were built in that first stage are maintained. But the therapeutic alliance has become less tenuous and fragile than it was at the beginning, so the counselor can use a broader range of actions and comments without increasing the client's tension beyond tolerable limits. The first stage merges into the second stage as the client's readiness for deep self-exploration is perceived by the counselor and his or her active engagement in the process is more visible.

The empathic responses of the counselor now include material from prior sessions and focus more on the client's awareness of the unsatisfying nature of old ways of thinking and responding. Such advanced-level empathy statements reassure the client that the counselor has an understanding of his or her world and provide an impetus for still deeper exploration. They also deepen the client's awareness of issues previously unconscious and insight into the connection between issues previously experienced as separate or random. For example, in the case study presented earlier in this chapter, Thad, who was in conflict about his responsibilities to his parents, was helped by statements that focused on his apparently conflicting desires for independence and dependence. His problem was a special case of a classic young adult struggle, and the counselor was able to infuse the conversation with a high level of empathy because she knew how important such struggles are for many young people.

As the relationship becomes more secure, the counselor also begins to share with the client observations about incompatibilities between his or her goals and current behavior. These statements are usually termed *confrontations*. In the case of Thad, the following confrontive statement was made: "You say you yearn for independence, yet you stop at home every evening and end up staying there all evening when you really want to be with friends. Do you think you will establish the kind of independence you hope for that way?" Broadly speaking, constructive confrontation provides the client with an external view of his or her behavior, based on the counselor's observations. The client is free to accept, reject, or modify the counselor's impression. In fact, effective counselors encourage clients to actively consider and discuss the "fit" between the counselor's perception and the client's awareness. In the process of considering how to use the counselor's statement, the client arrives at newly challenged and refined views of self and the counselor clarifies further his or her impressions of the needs and goals of the client. (Other variations on the theme of constructive confrontation will be offered in Chapter 4.)

Immediacy is another quality of the counselor's behavior that becomes important in the second stage of counseling. According to Egan (2002), immediacy can be defined in three distinct ways. First, it can refer to general discussions about the progress of the counseling relationship. Questions such as "Is the counseling process progressing in a way that is satisfactory to you?" fall into this category. Second, immediacy refers to any statements in which the counselor tells the client some of his or her immediate reactions to the client's statements or asks the client to disclose current thoughts about the counselor. For instance, a counselor who says, "I am wondering about your reaction to my comment about your father; you have had difficulty establishing eye contact with me ever since" or "I get the sense that you were really touched by my concern for your wife's illness" is also using an immediacy response. The third kind of immediacy response is a self-involving statement that expresses the counselor's personal response to a client in the present. "I'm amazed by all you have accomplished in just a few counseling sessions" is an example of a self-involving response. Such a response often communicates genuineness as well as immediacy.

Immediacy responses often begin with the word *I* rather than *you* so as to identify the content with the counselor, not the client. Immediacy responses can be openly supportive or confrontive. When they are confrontive, counselors monitor the client's behavior within the counseling session in order to understand how the client characteristically deals with other people and then shares some of those observations with the client. Here is one example of such an immediacy response: "You seem to be avoiding a decision and acting helpless. When you do this, I have a tendency to want to make your decisions for you." If the client then affirms that this seems to be an accurate observation, it might be followed with a confrontive comment such as "Do you suppose this is what you do with your father, even though you say you wish he would stop trying to tell you what to do?" Immediacy responses work best when the therapeutic alliance is strong enough that the client is unlikely to interpret the statements as overly critical or unduly supportive.

Because the focus of counseling is clearly on the client by the second stage, the counselor may begin sharing bits of his or her own experience with the client without fear of appearing to oversimplify the client's problems or seeming to tell the client, "Do as I did." Incidents in the counselor's life may be shared if they have direct relevance to the client's concern. Such self-disclosure can help to establish a human connection between counselor and client and suggest to the client that he or she is not alone in facing a particular concern. Although some information about how the counselor coped with a similar situation might be relevant to the client's solution, the counselor must exercise care in looking for the differences in the client's situation and permitting the client to use the counselor's experience only if he or she sees clear application.

The second stage of counseling frequently becomes emotionally stressful, because the client must face the inadequacy of habitual behaviors and must resolve to give up the familiar for the unfamiliar in order to obtain the desired goals. This stressful task is best accomplished within a caring relationship in which it is clear that the counselor is not criticizing the client's past behavior. The thrust is toward helping clients to realize more fully what they find unsatisfying or counterproductive in their responses to present situations and to gain a sense of what kinds of responses might be more rewarding.

In the second stage, the counselor and client come to a mutually acceptable assessment and diagnosis of the problem(s). Assessment is a process of information gathering and hypothesis testing that results in a diagnosis of the problem(s) that takes into account the client's history, life circumstances, and strengths. The diagnosis is determined primarily through careful analysis of the issues presented in the counseling session itself, but it often also includes the use of behavioral observations, data from others connected to the clients, and findings from standardized tests that focus on academic, career, or personality variables. Once a diagnosis is established, the counselor and client can move on to the third stage, the identification of specific goals for change, and the selection of action plans to implement those goals. Note that in this part of the process the counselor shares impressions but does not proclaim a diagnosis arrived at independent of the client's collaboration. Duncan, Hubble, and Miller (1997) quote a client's negative reaction to pronouncements of diagnosis by mental health professionals: "My other therapists never asked me what I wanted to work on. . . . It is like they think that they are some almighty power or something. . . . It's like hang on, *I am also somebody*" (p. 28, italics in the original). (See Chapter 4 for an elaboration of the in-depth exploration stage of counseling. Also see the inside front cover for a review of client and counselor work in Stage 2 leading to a mutual assessment of the client's problems.)

The Third Stage: Commitment to Action

In the third and final stage of counseling, the client must decide how to accomplish any goals that have emerged during the previous two stages. Concerns have been defined and clarified within the context of the client's life situation. The client has considered how his or her own behavior relates to accomplishing the goals that have been identified through the counseling process. What remains is to decide what, if any, overt actions the client might take to alleviate those problems. If no action is indicated, then the third stage of counseling can focus on increasing the client's commitment to a view that he or she has done everything possible or desirable in the given situation.

Typically though, the third stage includes identifying possible alternative courses of action (or decisions) the client might choose and assessing each of these in terms of the likelihood of outcomes. Ideally, various courses of action are developed by the client with encouragement from the counselor, although it is acceptable under most circumstances for the counselor to suggest possibilities the client may have overlooked. Possible courses of action and the related outcomes are evaluated in terms of the goals the client wants to attain and the client's value system. Once an action plan is chosen, the client usually tries some new behaviors while remaining in touch with the counselor. Together, counselor and client monitor the initial steps of the change process. Often the client needs to be reinforced to behave in new ways, both because the old behaviors are habitual and because new behaviors may not bring about immediate results. Particularly when the goals involve improving interpersonal relationships, the other parties usually do not respond instantly to the client's new behavior, and this can be discouraging. If the client decides that no new action is needed, the decision may be that "I don't need to let myself get so upset by the behavior of another." In such an instance, the reinforcement process supports the client's ability to manage emotions better when "red flag" experiences occur.

To summarize, the third stage is a decision-making and action time. The client considers possible actions and then chooses some to try out. The counselor gives support for trying new behaviors and helps the client evaluate the effectiveness of new behaviors or new conceptions of reality as they may relate to the reduction of stress. When the client is satisfied that the new behaviors or the new constructs are working satisfactorily, counseling is finished. (See Chapter 5 for more detail on commitment to action, and see the inside front cover for a graphic synopsis of the work of the client and counselor in the commitment to action stage.)

THE THREE STAGES OF COUNSELING IN PERSPECTIVE

Common to all the stages is the recognition that the experience involves work for both participants. Applied to counseling, work refers to the experience of exploring with an effort toward understanding more deeply, clarifying what is vague, discovering new insights that relate to one's concerns, and developing action plans. In the initial disclosure stage, the work of the client involves taking the risk of disclosing information to a relative stranger and making a conscious commitment to actively engage in counseling. At this stage clients are trying to make contact with personal beliefs, emotions, and patterns of behavior related to their issues and concerns. For the counselor, the work of this stage involves developing trust, establishing the counseling setting as a place and time to work, attending intensely so as to understand the significant themes and issues that will need deeper exploration in the next stage, and making initial contact with themes projected in a client's communications. Usually the counselor's work also includes assessing the client's level of readiness for the second stage.

In the in-depth exploration stage, the client's work involves making deeper contact with themes and issues presented in the first stage. It includes clarifying goals for counseling outcomes and developing new discoveries and insights about the self and others that relate to these goals. For the counselor, work at this stage involves helping the client develop new understandings by using a creative combination of advanced-level empathy, immediacy, confrontation, interpretation, role playing, and other structured interventions. Together the counselor and client develop a comprehensive diagnosis of the problem(s).

The client's work in the third stage involves synthesizing new concepts learned in the second stage, developing specific outcome goals derived from the diagnosis, and formulating alternative courses of action. Specific courses of action must be reality tested, and some are acted on. Because the action generally involves doing something new, the work also involves gaining control of anxiety that relates to newness. For the counselor, the work involves helping the client synthesize information, formulate goals, and make choices without controlling or imposing himself or herself onto the client.

All of these functions will be described in depth in Chapters 3 through 5. We have emphasized that counseling is not simply talk, but work that requires intense energy from both participants. However, it is also true that counseling can be fun and exciting. Saying that counseling is work does not mean that it must be laborious.

Nonlinearity of Stages

As in all stage models, the process described in this chapter depicts each succeeding stage as dependent on the preceding one. That is, unless problems have been defined, it is not possible to establish goals, and unless one has established goals, it is not possible to effectively evaluate possible courses of action. This linear conception of stages is, nevertheless, an oversimplification, and it is important to recognize the limitations of such a stage model. The reverse arrows in the figure on the inside front cover represent the fluidity in the stages as new insights open doors for further exploration in previous stages as counseling progresses.

First, it is not necessary for a client to clarify all concerns that he or she may have before beginning to think about goals and actions with respect to a particular segment of his or her life. An unemployed head of a household will probably want to work quickly on securing a source of income. Even though ultimately this person may want to become involved in an extensive career-planning process, the first question might be "What can I do right now to meet my needs and the needs of my family?" A woman who is a victim of domestic violence may eventually want to consider how she can build a life that does not include her present mate, but first she will want strategies for preventing further violence. Furthermore, a client will typically clarify his or her thinking about some goals at the same time as other goals are in the process of formation. Actions may be taken with respect to the clarified goals, but the client must wait to take action on goals that are still unclear.

Particular actions cannot be evaluated for a goal that has not been defined, and a goal cannot be defined if a concern has not been explored and clarified. Even so, the segments of an individual's life cannot be fully separated and treated as independent problems. Eventually each sector must fit back into a whole picture of the individual's life, much as the pieces of a jigsaw puzzle fit together to produce a complete picture. The process of counseling may involve refining the edges of one piece so that it fits the picture, in which case counseling will take a relatively short time. It may involve the definition of many pieces and work being conducted simultaneously on two or more of them, in which case counseling will last longer. Some pieces may require reprocessing as others take shape. In such a complex case, the process of initial disclosure, in-depth exploration, diagnosis, and commitment to action occurs with each part of the problem. Of course, counseling never returns to the absolute beginning as new sectors of concern are identified, but totally new disclosures may require extensive exploration and clarification before action plans can be considered. In parallel fashion, the counseling techniques typically associated with each stage of counseling are not rigidly bound to those stages. A counselor's self-disclosure, for example, may sometimes be appropriate in the first stage of counseling, especially if the counselor shares a unique experience with the client. Substance abuse counselors who are in recovery frequently disclose their history of substance abuse to clients as a way of building trust. In another example, an advanced-empathy response may be used in the first stage when a client seems quick to trust and unusually capable of insight into self.

The counseling process also needs to be modified somewhat in certain situations, and these adaptations are reviewed in Chapters 11 through 14. The special needs of clients from diverse backgrounds, clients in crisis, minor clients, and those not competent to manage their own affairs require that counselors be flexible in their conceptualization of counseling and skilled in using a variety of methods to help clients. The ways in which the varying theoretical orientations to counseling affect the process and the ethical and legal duties facing counselors are described in the final two chapters of the book.

SUMMARY

This chapter began with a comprehensive definition of counseling that introduced the broad goal of change in the client, facilitated by discussion with the counselor. Building on the definition, both outcome and process goals were discussed. The client may change behavior, ways of thinking about self and others, or ways of coping with life and making decisions.

The stages of the counseling process were introduced as initial disclosure, in-depth exploration, and commitment to action. The flow moves from the initial meeting of counselor and client, to thorough exploration of client concerns, to goal setting and action planning. Counseling techniques appropriate to each of the three stages were briefly identified. This introduction provides a background for the next three chapters, which contain detailed descriptions of the stages.

≈≈≈ *DISCUSSION QUESTIONS* ≈≈≈

1. This model of counseling emphasizes the active role of the client in the process and the influence of the client's engagement on the ultimate success of counseling. This model also suggests that even clients with longstanding psychopathology must be viewed as partners in change with the counselor. What do you see as the strengths and limitations in such a model?
2. The chapter discusses four important aspects of an effective counseling climate in the first stage of counseling: empathy, genuineness, caring, and concreteness. Do you agree that these are essential? If you were to seek counseling tomorrow, how do you think you would respond to a counselor who expressed these qualities?
3. The chapter presents the case of "arranged marriages" and the freedom of the person to waive her or her right to choose a life partner? What emotions does this situation trigger in you? Do you agree with the authors' perspective on this issue?
4. Sometimes clients directly ask counselors to "tell them what to do." In that circumstance, is a counselor justified in giving advice? What do you think is the client's internal dynamic when such a question arises?

REFERENCES

Beck, A. (1976). *Cognitive therapy and emotional disorders.* New York: International Universities Press.

Beck, A. T., & Emery, G. (1985). *Anxiety disorders and phobias: A cognitive perspective.* New York: Basic Books.

Beck, A. T., Rush, A. J., & Emery, G. (1979). *Cognitive therapy of depression.* New York: Guilford.

Bohart, A. C., & Tallman, K. (1999). *How clients make therapy work.* Washington, DC: American Psychological Association.

Brammer, L. M., & McDonald, G. (2002). *The helping relationship: Process and skills* (8th ed.). Boston: Allyn & Bacon.

Carkhuff, R. R. (1973). *The art of helping.* Amherst, MA: Human Resources Development Press.

Corey, G., Corey, M., & Callanan, P. (2002). *Issues and ethics in the helping professions* (6th ed.). Pacific Grove, CA: Brooks/Cole.

Duncan, B. L., Hubble, M. A., & Miller, S. D. (1997). *Therapy with impossible cases: The efficient treatment of therapy veterans.* New York: Norton.

Egan, G. (2002). *The skilled helper* (7th ed.). Pacific Grove, CA: Brooks/Cole.

Ellis, A. (1994). *Reason and emotion in psychotherapy revisited.* New York: Carol Publishing.

Ellis, A. (2000). Rational-emotive therapy. In R. J. Corsini & D. Wedding (Eds.), *Current psychotherapies* (6th ed.). Itasca, IL: Peacock.

Gelso, C. J., & Carter, J. A. (1985). The relationship in counseling and psychotherapy: Components, consequences and theoretical antecedents. *The Counseling Psychologist, 13,* 155–243.

Goldstein, A. P. (1971). *Psychotherapeutic attraction.* New York: Pergamon.

Hackney, H., & Cormier, L. S. (2001). *The professional counselor: A process guide to helping* (4th ed.). Boston: Allyn & Bacon.

Hubble, M. A., Duncan, B. D., & Miller, S. D. (Eds.). (1999). *The heart and soul of change: What works in therapy.* Washington, DC: American Psychological Association.

Kazdin, A. E. (2000). *Behavior modification in applied settings* (6th ed.). Pacific Grove, CA: Brooks/Cole.

Kelley, G. A. (1955). *The psychology of personal constructs.* New York: Norton.

Lambert, M. J., & Barley, D. E. (2002). Research summary on the therapeutic relationship and psychotherapy outcome. In J. C. Norcross (Ed.), *Psychotherapy relationships that work* (pp. 17–32). New York: Oxford.

Lambert, M. J., Whipple, J. L., Smart, D. W., Vermeersch, D. A., Stevan, L., & Hawkins, E. J. (2001). The effects of providing therapists with feedback on patient progress during psychotherapy: Are outcomes enhanced? *Psychotherapy Research, 11,* 49–68.

Meichenbaum, D. (1977). *Cognitive behavior modification: An integrative approach.* New York: Plenum.

Meichenbaum, D. (1985). *Stress inoculation training.* Boston: Allyn & Bacon.

Rogers, C. R. (1942). *Counseling and psychotherapy.* Boston: Houghton Mifflin.

Rogers, C. R. (1951). *Client-centered therapy.* Boston: Houghton Mifflin.

Welfel, E. R. (2002). *Ethics in counseling and psychotherapy: Standards, research, and emerging issues* (2nd ed.). Pacific Grove, CA: Brooks/Cole.

Yalom, I. D. (1980). *Existential psychotherapy.* New York: Basic Books.

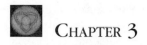 CHAPTER 3

BUILDING THE COUNSELING RELATIONSHIP
AND FACILITATING INITIAL DISCLOSURE

The previous chapter described counseling as a person-to-person interaction process to stimulate change in affect, thought, and behavior. Changes are regarded as desirable if they help the client make an important life decision, cope more effectively with developmental tasks and life stresses, achieve a sense of personal effectiveness, or learn to use freedom responsibly. Chapter 2 also described three critical interactive stages of the counseling experience: initial disclosure, in-depth exploration, and commitment to action. This chapter explains the important counselor qualities and related skills of the first stage.

In addition to encouraging the client to continue in counseling after the initial meeting, effective counseling procedures in the initial stage are aimed at facilitating and sustaining client self-disclosure. Sustained client self-disclosure is crucial for the following reasons:

- It informs the counselor about what has been occurring in the client's life and how the client thinks and feels about those events.
- It brings the client some feeling of relief through the process of talking about her or his problems.
- It encourages the client to develop a clearer definition of his or her concerns and a greater understanding about exactly what is disturbing.
- It helps the client see the connections between components of his or her situation that the client had not recognized before—that is, self-disclosure promotes client insight.

Without these data, the counselor has no information with which to try to understand the client's unique experience. Beginning counselors often overlook the importance of the other three purposes. This brief exercise illustrates the value of the other effects of self-disclosure.

━━━━━━━━━━━━━━━━━━━━━━━ *Exercise* ━━━━━━━━━━━━━━━━━━━━━━━

Reflecting on your own personal experience, try to recall a time when you talked about an important problem with someone else. Did you feel better after sharing the concern, even if no new solution was evident? This process is known as catharsis and is explained by the emotional release that comes from getting the problem out. In telling your story to someone else, did you discover that you understood more precisely what was bothering you? Finally, did you discover that by telling your story you reached new understandings of how things fit together?

Just as you became more self-aware through articulating the problem to a friend, clients frequently gain such new insights too, through the process of self-disclosure.

WHAT CLIENTS BRING TO THE COUNSELING EXPERIENCE

Counselors are wise to remember that virtually no one enters counseling at the first sign of a problem. Prior to deciding to start counseling, clients have attempted to solve their problems on their own without the level of success they hoped for. These unsuccessful attempts typically include thinking about the problem independently, reading self-help books, surfing for Web-based resources in mental health, and discussing the problem with friends and family. Even when the advice from books and Web sites or the suggestions of loved ones seem helpful, the client has probably been unable to implement these recommendations in a satisfying way. In the worst case, loved ones have minimized the client's problems or have judged the client harshly for expressing negative thoughts and feelings, leaving the client to feel more isolated and hopeless. Taken together, these experiences lead clients who have never experienced counseling before to wonder whether a stranger can do better. If the strategies offered by self-help books and Web sites (written by supposed experts) have not been helpful, the doubts clients have about counseling may increase.

Why then do they bother? Clients go forward with the appointment because they hope that the counselor will be more objective and wiser than the other people they have consulted and because they have exhausted other strategies. They are willing to risk another failure precisely because the need for change is so great. Clients ask themselves critical questions as they begin counseling, such as "What will this person do with the information I share with him or her?" "What impressions of me will the counselor develop if I honestly describe my concerns, stresses, and doubts?" "Are my concerns and feelings so unique that not even a counselor can understand me?" Some of their worry about the counseling experience stems from the unknown: "What will happen to me during this experience?" This is the context that makes the immediate communication of empathy, genuineness, and caring so important to Stage 1, even when clients volunteer to enter counseling. Even when clients are enthusiastic about the potential for counseling to help them, they may be uncertain about the ability of the particular counselor assigned to their case to assist them. Thus, virtually all clients have some degree of ambivalence at the start of the process. Some are genuinely hostile, especially if they are pushed into counseling by others or by the legal system. Examples of reluctant clients commonly include individuals who have been abusing drugs and alcohol, people whose aggressive or disruptive behavior has gotten them into trouble with others or with the law, or students who are unmotivated and unsuccessful in school. Working effectively with reluctant clients requires some special skills, which we will discuss in Chapter 9. This chapter focuses on clients who have entered counseling with some recognition that they have problems and some openness to the work needed to resolve those problems.

Hesitation to enter counseling can also result from a variety of cultural messages that suggest caution about seeking help with problems. On the one hand, there is the belief that people should be able to manage their own affairs and that seeking help is a sign of weakness. Some people may even believe that only "crazy" people need to see counselors. In addition, individuals from some ethnic groups may be reluctant to talk with a counselor outside their ethnic group, and certain cultural groups are cautious about discussing personal problems outside the family (see Chapter 12).

Regardless of the client's level of readiness for counseling, all counselors initiate disclosure with three interconnected patterns: by inviting communication, by responding to client concerns in a caring and understanding way, and by avoiding doing and saying things that block communication. Only the time devoted to initial disclosure and trust building varies, not the need for such forms of communication. The following section describes the specific skills and attitudes counselors need to demonstrate at the start of counseling.

INVITING COMMUNICATION AND BUILDING THE COUNSELING RELATIONSHIP

The Counselor's Nonverbal Messages

You can easily recall many instances when you have been with people whose body language invited communication and when you have been with others whose body language indicated disinterest and perhaps even anxiety about communicating. The active, interested listener faces and leans toward the speaker in a posture of attention and even concentration on the speaker. Active listeners focus their eyes in the general direction of the person's face.

Their arms are in an open mode in relation to the trunk, as if to say, "I am very interested in receiving, with all my sensory processes, what it is you want to say to me." The attentive listener maintains an interested facial expression and makes encouraging gestures (nods, smiles, hand gestures, etc.). The energy for offering these cues seems to come naturally and without contrived effort; an attentive posture is a bodily representation of a strongly held belief about how to receive and welcome another human being.

These skills of reception are referred to as *attending skills* and quite literally they communicate the counselor's undivided attention to the client's concerns. Egan (2002) substitutes the term "visibly tuning in." Attending requires an "intensity of presence" and acts as a nonverbal expression of empathy (p. 66). Attending behavior encourages the client to talk and therefore reduces the need for the counselor to talk (Ivey & Ivey, 2003), placing the content of the session more in the client's control.

In contrast, the listener who is disinterested and uncomfortable does not use his or her body to invite communication. Facial focus may be 45 degrees or more away from the client's face, arms folded in a self-protective position, eyes on the desktop. Body cues such as these communicate messages such as "I'm indifferent to you," "I don't care," "I don't have the energy to be available to you," or "I'm afraid to be open with you." Cues that indicate the listener is closed can be subtle, often outside the person's awareness.

Habits of attending vary somewhat from one culture to another. For example, the patterns of eye contact that have been described are typical for European Americans in a North American culture. Ivey, Ivey, and Simek-Morgan (2002) indicate that African Americans often show a pattern of greater eye contact when speaking than when listening, and that Native Americans may avoid eye contact altogether when speaking of important matters. The skilled counselor will learn to recognize and respect these cultural differences and will interpret the meaning of clients' behaviors in the context of their culture.

In addition to the nonverbal messages of body language, the counselor also communicates attending by means of voice characteristics and manner of speaking. These qualities are sometimes referred to as *paralinguistic,* because they are communicated by voice but have nothing to do with verbal content. For example, rapid speech, stumbling over words, loud tone, and tightness of voice all may signal stress. Slow, quiet, listless speech may indicate boredom or distraction. Vocal tone and emphasis can highlight certain material as important. Comfort may be communicated by a pleasant tone, purposeful but easeful pacing, and other qualities of voice.

Finally, it is important to realize that just as counselors communicate comfort and attention by their nonverbal behaviors, clients also give many clues to their emotional state and reactions to counseling by nonverbal behaviors. Brammer, Abrego, and Shostrum (1993) suggest that the counselor's nonverbal behavior should match the nonverbal behavior of the client, mirroring, for example, body posture, position, breathing, voice volume, rate of speech, and other qualities.

Though many of the attending skills seem commonsensical, unfortunately many counselors do not consistently exhibit these behaviors. Attending is compromised when counselors are distracted by other events such as worries about whether the snowstorm will cancel school for their children, are impaired by stress such as an impending divorce, or are emotionally exhausted from the demands of their work. Can you think of examples of people who were deficient in attending skills and thus made necessary communication difficult? James and Gilliland (2003) state that attending is both an attitude and a skill and that practice leads to improved performance. Not surprisingly, research by Najavits and Strupp (1994) also shows that clients who feel that their counselors are frequently ignoring them are less likely to reach their goals (or even to stay in counseling long enough to find out whether their goals are attainable).

Exercise

Form groups of three students, one who will be the client, one who will be the counselor, and one who will observe. The client should think of some issue he or she would like to discuss with the counselor. The counselor is instructed to intentionally violate the principles of good attending described previously as the client presents his or her issue. The observer notes whatever occurs. Continue this pattern for 3 minutes. Then discuss what the counselor's behavior did to the process. Did the client show any nonverbal signs of his or her reactions? This is a time when the client can share directly how it felt to be ignored while trying to talk. If this exercise is done in a classroom setting, debrief the various triads to share experience across groups.

Repeat the same process (switching roles so that each participant eventually can serve as counselor, client, and observer) for an additional 3 minutes, with the helper practicing the best attending skills possible. Discuss the contrast with the first exercise.

Finally, after switching roles again, a counselor and a client should engage in a discussion about something important to the client for a longer period—7 minutes. The counselor should maintain good attending and may offer brief verbal responses as appropriate. The observer will take written notes on the paralinguistic and attending behaviors of both the counselor and client. At the conclusion of the discussion, the observer will report

his or her findings and the triad will discuss the meanings they
attach to the behaviors that were observed. Both the counselor
and the client are encouraged to be self-disclosing about how
they felt when a particular behavior was occurring in the session.

The Counselor's Verbal Encouragement to Disclose

Encouraging communication usually begins with the counselor offering
an open invitation to communicate. A statement such as one of the following is usually sufficient: "How can I help?" What would you like to discuss
today?" "How would you like to begin?"

Most voluntary clients will respond to such invitations with the expression of a concern along with an implied need for help. Following are examples of initial client statements and of counselor responses that encourage
further clarification or development of the initial statement.

Example 1

CLIENT: My husband is an alcoholic and has been that way since before
    we were married. I can't get him to stop and I'm scared. I don't
    know what to do.
COUNSELOR: You're worried about your husband's drinking and aren't
    sure how to handle it anymore. Can you tell me more about
    specifically what has been happening that led to your decision to
    seek help now?

Example 2

CLIENT: I find that I am more sexually attracted to men than to women,
    but I really feel guilty because I know it's wrong.
COUNSELOR: It sounds as though your sexual responses aren't as you
    believe they should be, and that is troubling you. Help me
    understand more fully what has led to this concern.

Example 3

CLIENT: Tommy keeps bothering me on the playground. He pushed me
    off the jungle gym again yesterday and he punched me.
COUNSELOR: You say Tommy *keeps* bothering you during recess. It
    sounds like this has been going on for a while.

Example 4

CLIENT: It's just two weeks till graduation and I don't have any idea
    what I'm going to do next.

COUNSELOR: It sounds like you're feeling great pressure about this impending change in your life. Help me understand what you have been thinking about doing up till now.

Example 5

CLIENT: Well, my daughter really seems to be out of control. She stays out till all hours of the night and refuses to talk about what she's doing.
COUNSELOR: It sounds like you're worried about your daughter. Why don't you fill me in on exactly what has been happening.

In each example, the counselor first acknowledges the content and/or feeling in the client's statement of an initial concern. Further development and clarification are always necessary. Follow-up invitations that encourage further development take the following general form:

- "Tell me more about . . ."
- "Help me understand more fully . . ."
- "Tell me what happened when . . ."
- "Help me understand your thinking about . . ."
- "Can you talk more about how that plays itself out in your daily life?"

THE CORE CONDITIONS OF COUNSELING

In the previous section, we described some specific counselor behaviors, both nonverbal and verbal, that invite a client to begin talking about his or her concerns. Many beginning counselors are able to accomplish these first steps with ease, but then have difficulty knowing what to say when the client begins to disclose more information. It is helpful to remember that the purposes of disclosure are to help the client to articulate his or her experience, to offer a safe place for the client to release pent-up feeling in the process of telling the story, and to help to clarify the true nature of the problem or problems presented. In these ways, disclosure shows the client that counseling is a positive experience that has the potential to help solve the problems that need resolution. The counselor's goal is to come to understand the client's experience as clearly and as personally as possible, not only to lay the foundation for change but to cement the therapeutic alliance with the client. New counselors are often so predisposed to finding a solution to the problem(s) that they forget that it is ultimately the *client's* responsibility to solve the problem(s). They also are forgetting that the single most important thing that counselors offer their clients is a good relationship that energizes clients to use existing resources and assists them in developing new skills and resources to solve their problems (Bohart & Tallman, 1999). By offering premature suggestions to resolve clients' concerns prior to careful disclosure, counselors can short-circuit the counseling process, demean the client's own ability to be self-directing, and often provide solutions that don't fit the situations. Counselors must remember that the glib advice from well-intentioned people who have only half-listened to the client is one reason the client decided to come to counseling in the first place. Premature suggestions for change are the last thing they want from professional counselors.

To support clients' discussion of meaningful issues during the initial disclosure stage of counseling, the counselor maintains an attitude of receiving the client, often referred to as the core conditions of counseling. Three of these conditions—empathy, positive regard, and genuineness—were described by Carl Rogers (1957, p. 95) as "the necessary and sufficient conditions of therapeutic personality change." The fourth condition, concreteness, is the counselor's skill in focusing the client's discussion on specific events, thoughts, and feelings that matter, while discouraging intellectualized storytelling. Concreteness is a precaution against the rambling that can occur when the other three conditions are employed without sufficient attention to identifying the client's themes. Concreteness will be evident to the degree that the counselor identifies and responds to important client themes while choosing not to respond to small talk, excessive storytelling, and other client material of a social or diversionary nature.

Empathy

Rogers (1961) defined empathy as the counselor's ability "to enter the client's phenomenal world—to experience the client's world as if it were your own without ever losing the 'as if' quality" (p. 284). Bohart and Greenberg (1997) have noted a resurgent interest in empathy in psychotherapy, detailing how it is perceived in client-centered, psychoanalytic, behavioral and cognitive, postmodernist, and eclectic approaches.

They described three categories of empathy:

- Empathic rapport—"primarily kindness, global understanding, and tolerant acceptance of the client's feelings and frame of reference" (Bohart & Greenberg, 1997, p. 13).
- Experience near understanding of the client's world—"what it is like to have the problems the client has, to live in the life situation the client lives in, . . . what it is like to be him" (p. 14). This perspective includes conscious as well as some unconscious elements of the client's experience.
- Communicative attunement—"The therapist tries to put himself or herself in the client's shoes at the moment, to grasp what

they are trying to consciously communicate at the moment,
and what they are experiencing at the moment" (p. 14).

Empathy as used in this text might serve any one or all three of these
purposes at a given point in the counseling process—simple acceptance or
relationship-building, enhancement of communication, or deeper understanding of what it is like to live the client's life.

Some authors (Carkhuff, 1969; Egan, 2002; Ivey & Ivey, 2003; Patterson
& Eisenberg, 1983) have reasoned that there are different levels of empathy—
meaning that the counselor may vary in the depth of understanding of the
client's experience and may make choices about how much of that understanding is communicated in responding to the client. Sometimes the counselor will perceive attitudes and motives in the client's statements that she or
he is not yet ready to discuss directly. To stimulate client exploration, the
level of empathy communicated should match the client's level of readiness.
Primary empathy is the level that is usually facilitative in the initial disclosure
stage of counseling, and advanced level empathy is often more appropriate
for the in-depth exploration stage to be discussed in the next chapter. In this
section, we develop some overall understandings about empathy and focus
on the primary level.

Empathy involves two major skills: perceiving and communicating.
Perceiving involves an intense process of actively listening for themes,
issues, personal constructs, and emotions. *Themes* may be thought of as
recurring patterns, such as views of self, attitudes toward others, consistent
interpersonal relationship patterns, fear of failure, and search for personal
power. *Issues* are questions of conflict with which the client is struggling:
"What do I want for my future?" "How can I be sexually active and safe?"
"Why does every event in my family turn into a disaster?" "Why do I still feel
that I am fat, when I have lost a lot of weight and am, in fact, thin?" Relative
to each theme or issue, a client will have emotions of elation, joy, anger,
anxiety, sadness, confusion, and so on. Understanding the client's emotional
investments is a critical part of the perceptual element of empathy.

George Kelley (1955) described the perceptual element of empathy as
understanding the client's personal constructs. He defined *personal constructs* as the unique set of thoughts a person uses to process information,
give meaning to life events, order one's world, explain cause-and-effect
relationships, and make decisions. They include beliefs about oneself and
others, assumptions about how and why events happen in the world, and
private logic and moral premises that guide one's world. The counselor can
detect a client's personal constructs from his or her descriptions of life situations, behaviors, decisions, or even responses to tests and inventories.

Beck (1976) and Meichenbaum (1977) discuss "automatic thoughts"
and "internal dialogue," respectively, each describing how the client's cognitive structure (complex of personal constructs) predisposes him or her to

interpret events in certain ways. Emotions emanate from these interpretations. Empathy, then, includes knowing not only what events have occurred in the client's life but also how his or her cognitive structure has led to interpretation of the events and to consequent feelings.

As the client discloses information about self, some of the client's themes form quickly in the counselor's perceptual foreground while others remain in the background. Some personal constructs (for example, "The world is not a safe place," "People are phony") may emerge quickly, although others remain unavailable. Often as the counselor listens to the client's story, the counselor will see errors in the client's logic, construct different cause-and-effect relationships from the client's, and identify the basis of the client's distressed feelings. This diagnostic thinking will guide treatment planning and serve as a basis for the counselor's responses later in the counseling process.

In the *communication* component of empathy, the counselor says something that tells the client that his or her meanings and feelings have been understood. If a counselor listens carefully and understands well but says nothing, the client has no way of knowing what is in the counselor's mind. Sometimes the client may even misinterpret a counselor's lack of response as a negative judgment about what they have said. (Remember that clients may have experienced such negative judgments from the people they consulted prior to entering counseling.) It is often through hearing his or her meanings and feelings accurately repeated that the client takes another look at life events and begins to perceive them differently.

Primary empathy is most often communicated through an interchangeable verbal response (though facial expressions and other nonverbal responses can also be used). Interchangeable responses are statements that capture the essential themes in a client's statement but do not go deeper than the transparent material. A paraphrase like "You felt degraded and angry because your girlfriend criticized you in front of your friends" is a fairly typical response of this type. It captures both the feeling and the meaning of the client's previous disclosure in simple language the client can understand. Feeling understood, the client will likely trust the counselor enough to continue to elaborate on the meaning of that or related experiences. It is important to realize that statements such as "I know just how you felt" do *not* communicate empathy because they contain nothing of what the client has shared. *Advanced empathy* (discussed more fully in Chapter 4) is communicated through additive verbal responses, wherein the counselor adds perceptions that the client implied but did not state directly. The ability to hear these implied meanings grows with experience and with the quality of the counselor's diagnostic thinking.

In the first stage of counseling, primary empathy is used most because it demonstrates to the client that the counselor is listening effectively, without the threat that can occur with additive empathy statements in which the counselor seems to be seeing through client defenses too quickly. The client's sense of progress and comfort are both served at this relationship-building stage if the counselor is seen as perceptive—but not too perceptive. Practically speaking, attempts at additive empathy responses at this point in the counseling process are also likely to be inaccurate because the counselor's knowledge of the unique experience of the client is still limited.

A good example of interchangeable responding comes from a classic counselor education training film of Carl Rogers (1965) counseling Gloria, a divorced client with two young children. At one point Gloria says to Rogers, "I really don't know how my daughter (who is nine years old) will feel about me if she knows that I sleep with a man I'm not married to." Rogers restates Gloria's concern, "If your daughter knew about your actions, would she, *could she,* accept you?" Gloria affirms Rogers' understanding and goes on to describe her anxieties about being a good mother and being accepted by her daughter. Notice that Rogers identified a key theme and reflected it back to Gloria in a way that helped her look at it more deeply. He did not simply repeat the statement but focused it without adding anything to it.

Cultural sensitivity and the knowledge of cultures different from the counselor's own are important to the effective use of empathy. Okun (2002) cautions that "While there are some basic skills and strategies that cut across class, race, and culture, helpers must adapt their counseling style to achieve congruence with value systems of culturally diverse clients" (p. 10). Cultural background influences not only the personal constructs through which an individual interprets the world but also the style of expression that is experienced as empathic. For example, verbal responses that move too quickly to meanings and feelings are often considered to be rude in Asian cultures.

Effectively communicated empathy has a number of desired effects in the initial disclosure stage of counseling. First, the intellectual and emotional energy required to listen actively expresses caring and affirmation to the client. The counselor is saying, "I care enough for you that I want to work hard to understand you clearly." Second, the feedback that comes from the counselor's contact with significant themes helps the client see his or her own themes more clearly. This helps the client to understand himself or herself more deeply and to reexamine relevant perceptions, attitudes, and beliefs. Third, empathetic responses establish positive expectations about the nature of the counseling experience. Counseling is conveyed to the client as a process that involves attending to oneself—exploring, searching, and perceiving oneself more clearly. Counseling is established as an experience involving active engagement by all participants, not simply conversation. Indeed, the work of the counselor is to stimulate the client's work of self-discovery. If the counselor is careful to offer a level of empathy that is consistent with the client's level of readiness, the client will feel safe to continue the counseling experience. The client learns that nothing bad will happen as a result of communicating, and that something helpful is likely to occur.

A fourth effect is that empathy communicates to the client that the counselor has special expertise to offer. People do not routinely experience empathy in the events of daily life. A counselor who can make empathic contact establishes himself or herself as having some special skill. In turn, this helps the client experience a sense of optimism about future sessions. Bohart and Greenberg (1997) and Bachelor and Horvath (1999) report that research over the years has consistently shown correlations between therapist empathy and counseling outcomes. This evidence also supports the view that empathy is the most important of the positive counselor qualities for client success in counseling. This has proven to be true whether the empathy was rated by the clients themselves or by expert raters watching the counseling—and it has been shown to be true across a variety of clients.

Exercise

Consider carefully what it is like for the client in this example to cope with her life on a daily basis. Then consider each of the possible counselor responses, ranking them from the best to the poorest.

CLIENT: (Who is a European-American adolescent with a mixed race baby.) I got so mad at Kevin that I just jumped across the table and grabbed him by the throat. He said that Douvon (a black classmate) stole his wallet just because he is black. I hate the way kids here at this school treat black people. Sometimes I feel more like a black person myself. What right did Kevin have to make accusations? And now *I'm* the one who is suspended.

RESPONSE 1: Kevin should be more careful about what he says. I guess he was angry about losing his wallet.

RESPONSE 2: I know just how you feel. I'd be angry too.

RESPONSE 3: You don't feel that it's fair that you got suspended when it was Kevin who started all the trouble.

RESPONSE 4: You really lost control when you saw Kevin judging Douvon just because he is black. I guess that hits pretty close to home and makes you feel scared about how people will treat your baby as he grows up.

RESPONSE 5: Well, you know you can't just go attacking people when you get angry, even if they are in the wrong.

RESPONSE 6: You say you sometimes feel like a black person yourself. It seems that you are kind of confused about your identity.

Next, compare your responses with those of a classmate and discuss any differences that may have occurred. Then compare your responses to those of the authors, described next.

The authors rank the responses in the following order: 4, 3, 2, 6, 1, 5, though only Responses 4 and 3 show facilitative levels of empathy. Response 4 is best because it comes closest to stating where the client lives her everyday life, feeling sensitive about slights to black people out of concern for her son. The details of her present dilemma are secondary to acknowledging the pain and anxiety this event has caused. Response 3 picks up on the fact that the client feels that she is being treated unfairly—and it would probably sustain useful discussion because it includes elements of meaning and feeling about the incident, even though it does not get to the deeper basis for her reaction to Kevin. Response 2 reassures and placates the client but does not show empathic understanding. Response 6 picks up on part of the client's statement but shows so little understanding of the client's meaning that it would seem insensitive to the client. Response 1 takes the focus away from the client's circumstance and talks instead about Kevin, even feebly defending Kevin's accusation. Response 5 lectures the client about the inappropriateness of her behavior and would possibly end any hope the client might hold that the counselor will be helpful in resolving her problem.

Positive Regard

Positive regard is caring for your client for no other reason than the fact that she or he is human and therefore worthy of care. Positive regard is expressed by the enthusiasm one person shows for being in the presence of another and by the amount of time and energy one is willing to devote to another's well-being. The experience of being cared about by others helps develop and restore a sense of caring for oneself. It creates energy and encourages a person to respond to the demands of life. A counselor's caring can increase the client's enthusiasm for work and growth.

Rogers (1957) developed the concept that the counselor's caring for the client can be *unconditional*. Because the counselor does not have a role in the client's life outside the counseling situation, he or she can become the client's instrument for change without a lot of preconceived ideas about what behaviors the client should exhibit. The counselor's respect for the dignity and worth of the individual remains intact regardless of client behaviors. Parental love—which is probably the most important support a growing human ever experiences—is nevertheless conditional at times because parents have a vested interest in what their children do. They believe their children's behavior reflects on their effectiveness as parents and by extension on their worth as individuals. As a paid professional helper, the counselor does not have comparable ego investment in the client.

It is, of course, an ideal that the counselor can care for each client equally. All counselors, being human, meet clients who are hard to like. When this occurs, the counselor should examine and work through his or her feeling of disregard or refer the client to another counselor. If the counselor does not have a feeling of positive regard for the client, one of the necessary conditions for therapeutic change is missing.

To work through feelings of disregard for a client, the counselor must first acknowledge them and take responsibility for their existence. After recognition, the counselor's task is to identify specific characteristics of the client that she or he does not like. For many counselors, lying, defensiveness, manipulation, destructiveness to oneself and others, unwillingness to conform to reasonable social rules, and irresponsibility to others are traits that often trigger dislike. For example, some counselors may have difficulty working with a client who is known to be the perpetrator of domestic violence on a spouse. After taking whatever steps are necessary to secure the safety of the victim, the counselor's task is to become committed to helping the client get beyond a serious problem in his or her life. Though the client's behavior may be repugnant if judged through the moral imperatives by which the counselor lives her or his own life, the counselor tries to understand the meaning of the behavior in the client's life without judgment so that strategies for change can be devised.

Several parameters of human behavior may help counselors work through their own emotions. One is that the counselor may be tempted to impose *should* statements on the client. In the case of a client who is an unfaithful marriage partner, the counselor may feel that the client *should* behave more responsibly toward his or her spouse. In the case of an adolescent skipping school, many counselors may want to say the client *should* attend. But to the client, the counselor attempting to *impose* either of these *shoulds* would be perceived as uncaring. The likelihood is that the client already understands that there are negative consequences to his or her behaviors and yet has still chosen the behaviors. Rather than being rejected for those behaviors, he or she needs help in finding alternative behaviors that will have more positive consequences.

A second parameter is that anxiety often accompanies feelings of dislike for a client. This anxiety is different than the ordinary performance anxiety about doing competent work that counselors usually feel with new clients. The counselor may feel threatened by client behavior that raises concern about his or her own unresolved issues or by the fear that the client's problems are beyond his or her ability to help. Excessive resistance by the client or power struggles in the counseling sessions can also trigger counselor anxiety.

A third parameter is that some of the client's characteristics may remind the counselor of some other person for whom the counselor has feelings of anger or resentment or, on the flip side, feelings of love and attachment. In such circumstances, the counselor does not perceive the client with full accuracy but instead has some distortions in his or her image of the client. (See the discussion of this phenomenon, called countertransference, in Chapter 9.)

Keeping these parameters in mind, working through dislike for a client requires that the counselor give honest answers to the following questions:

- What characteristics of my client interfere with my ability to find him or her likable?
- What do I think my client should be doing that he or she is not?
- How are my *shoulds* affecting our relationship and my openness with the client?
- If I am imposing *shoulds,* what am I missing about my client as a result?
- Am I experiencing an anxious rather than a calm feeling with my client?
- With whom in my life might I have important unfinished business?
- Is my own unfinished business interfering with my ability to feel caring for this client?

These questions are difficult for any counselor to answer without the assistance of a professional colleague. For this reason, we strongly recommend that every counselor have his or her own resource counselor—usually either a colleague or a supervisor. Exploring feelings of disregard for a client in conjunction with another professional will help the counselor determine whether the disregard can be understood and replaced with a more helpful attitude or whether the client should be referred. The counselor may also learn that his or her own unresolved issues are intrusive in enough counseling interactions that personal therapy may be necessary.

Of course, effective counselors experience positive regard for the vast majority of their clients. Although caring is usually not expressed as directly as empathy, it will become apparent to the client through the counselor's spontaneous statements that acknowledge the validity of the client's struggle for a more satisfying life. As Ivey and Ivey (2003) state, "the counselor points out how, even in the most difficult situation, the client is doing something positive" (p. 147). Similarly, clients usually detect the absence of caring fairly quickly, so counselors are well advised to deal promptly with such feelings.

Exercise

Practice writing counselor responses that show positive regard to the following client statements. Note your emotional reaction to the client statements as you are trying to decide on what to write.

"I just can't stop myself from yelling at my grandfather. I know he's got Alzheimer's disease and doesn't know what he's doing, but I get so angry I feel like bursting if I don't express that anger. He ends up crying like a baby. It's awful."

"My life feels hopeless. No matter what I do, I can't seem to control these obsessive worries about germs and disease. My hands are red and bleeding from all the washing, and I'm embarrassed to leave the house because of them."

"All my problems stem from my husband and my boss. If they would just stop hounding me and let me do things my way I'd be a lot happier and easier to get along with."

"I know I failed organic chemistry twice and have only a 2.8 grade point average, but I'm sure I can succeed as a doctor. It's the only career I've ever wanted."

Now share your responses with a classmate and discuss what was intellectually and emotionally difficult (if anything) about expressing positive regard for each client.

Genuineness

Rogers (1942) originally defined genuineness as the characteristic of transparency, realness, honesty, or authenticity. He used the term *congruence* to suggest that a genuine counselor behaves in ways that are congruent with his or her self-concept and thus consistent across time. The counselor shares thoughts and feelings in ways that do not manipulate or control the client. Although genuineness does not give the counselor license to ventilate his or her own emotions on the client, Rogers said that a counselor who is having trouble liking a client would do well to share and try to resolve the feeling with the client rather than trying to hide it. We caution that clients with deep wounds to their self-esteem may not be able to handle such honesty from the counselor. Genuineness may have to be established through persistent congruence over a longer period of time.

Rogers believed that if the counselor behaves consistently over time, he or she eventually will be perceived as real. Having this perception of the counselor will help the client feel safer, develop a greater sense of trust, and thus be more willing to engage in the intensive exploration work of counseling. Experiencing genuineness from the counselor in a climate of safety enables the client to be more genuine and also encourages him or her to drop defenses, games, and manipulations. Transparency—that is, allowing the client to see into the counselor's thoughts and feelings—reduces the client's concern that there are hidden agendas, that the counselor is going to try to manipulate the client into behaving in certain ways.

To be fully genuine in the sense that Rogers described, counselors must know themselves well. They must have a clear picture of their personalities and how the elements of personality are expressed in significant events and relations with people. They must value themselves and be able to accept their flaws and mistakes.

The principle of genuineness dictates that the counselor should never communicate dishonestly, never present information that misleads, and never knowingly present an image of herself or himself that deceives the client. However, the principle does not require that the counselor impulsively disclose every thought, opinion, and feeling to the client. Sharing information about oneself is a decision, not an impulse, for both counselor and client. The counselor decides what and when to disclose based on perceptions of the client's need for or ability to benefit from the information. For example, describing an emotion experienced in the client's presence or an observation about what is happening right now in the relationship (such as "I feel that you are unloading on me today") is immediacy communication that the client may have trouble working with during Stage 1. In the next stage, such responding may be appropriate because the client feels safer and is more ready to work with it. Disclosing a past experience that parallels the client's experience may help to reduce distance and create a feeling of mutuality. However, going into a lot of detail about past personal experiences can quickly move into storytelling that can take the focus away from the client and block the exploration process. If the counselor chooses to disclose personal experiences she or he should disclose no more than is necessary to help the client see the parallels with his or her own experience.

How counselors respond when clients make negative disclosures about other people in their lives can influence the client's perception of the genuineness of the counseling. Clients who are experiencing interpersonal stress sometimes want confirmation that they are right and others are wrong. As a result, they may try to draw the counselor into taking a position about them or the people they are describing. For example, with couples experiencing marital disagreement, each client may seek to make the counselor an ally against the other. Because the counselor cannot know all the circumstances or motives involved, and because talking about another person's behavior is gossiping, it is wise for the counselor not to express any judgment. A counselor who makes the error of judging a third party's behavior will be seen as a counselor who will judge the client as well. It may help if the counselor explains that he or she is not in a position to judge.

━━━━━━━━━━━━━━━━━━━━━━━━━━━━ *Exercise* ━━━━━━━━━━━━━━

Think of two people in your life. Person A is an individual you perceive to be genuine. Person B is an individual you do not perceive to be genuine. Develop a clear visual image of each person. Recall one or two significant experiences you have had with each one. Now, while remembering these experiences, answer the following questions. Write down your answers or share them with another student.

1. What specific observations have I made about Person A that gives me the impression that he or she is a genuine individual?
2. What specific observations have I made about Person B that gives me the impression that he or she is not a genuine individual?
3. What differences do I note in their way of relating to me?
4. How would I describe my inner experiencing in the presence of Person A, particularly my emotions?
5. How would I describe my inner experiencing in the presence of Person B, particularly my emotions?
6. From my personal experience, what principles about genuineness seem valid for me?

━━

Concreteness

As Ivey and Ivey (2003) state, "a concrete counselor promptly seeks specifics rather than vague generalities. As interviewers, we are most often interested in specific feelings, specific thoughts, and specific examples of actions" (p. 147). Concreteness is *not* one of the Rogerian conditions of the helping relationship. In fact, the concept has emerged because it has been observed that counselors who are empathic, caring, and genuine may still encourage a client to ramble a great deal and allow the client to avoid talking about important material. If the counselor responds with equal interest to the statements "The weather has been very nice" and "The way my husband has been treating me and the kids really sucks," the client is likely to be encouraged to elaborate on either statement as though they were of equal importance.

As stated earlier in the chapter, it is the counselor's responsibility to identify which of the client's statements are central to his or her reasons for being a client, and to encourage talk about those issues. The client is still the person who determines the content of the session, but the counselor manages the process in such a way as to make it easier for the client to talk about what matters. What the counselor responds to, the client will probably follow up on; what the counselor ignores will likely be dropped. As diagnostic skills improve with experience, it will become easier for the counselor to identify important themes to be pursued, but even the beginning counselor can easily distinguish between small talk and self-disclosure. Beyond the initial social amenities that may contribute to client comfort, small talk wastes valuable counseling time.

Ivey and Ivey (2003) suggest that concreteness can be increased by asking directly for specific examples of troublesome events. For example, the frequently heard phrase "She is always picking on me" tells little, but examples of specific interactions between the client and the other person will shed much light on the relationship dynamics. "Picking on me" may actually mean that "Every time I don't have my homework done, the teacher calls attention to it in a public way and embarrasses me."

The language used by the client and by the counselor can also contribute to unfocused discussion. Vagueness, abstractness, and obscurity are the opposites of concrete communication. Therefore, the counselor should model direct communication and challenge the client to be more specific. The more fully and concretely the troublesome events in clients' lives are recreated (complete with affective tone) within the counseling session, the more likely it is that clients will come to new understandings and begin to develop more positive feelings about themselves and their lives.

Example

The following example includes three counselor responses, each of which is at least minimally responsive to the client's statement. The responses increase in their level of concreteness and thereby increase in their potential to focus the client's self-exploration.

> CLIENT: I feel so frustrated with my teenage daughter. She is completely out of control. No matter what I do she stays out till all hours and won't get up for school in the mornings. I've tried everything, but it just seems hopeless.

Response with little concreteness:

> RESPONSE 1: You seem very upset and worried.

Response with moderate concreteness:

> RESPONSE 2: You seem pretty frustrated with your daughter's behavior and are running out of ideas.

Response with a high degree of concreteness:

> RESPONSE 3: You are frightened that your daughter is harming herself and feel powerless and hopeless. At the same time you haven't given up. You are here and ready to try to work out some other way to help.

Although the first response identifies something of the client's feelings, the second includes more of the client's meaning as well. The third response includes feeling and meaning in more detail, and it begins to structure toward hope that exploration might lead to new possibilities for helping. Although any of the three responses would likely sustain the conversation, the more concrete the response, the more likely the client will focus energy productively.

Exercise

Practice writing counselor responses that show concreteness to the following client statements.

"I know I'm only 18 years old, but I'm absolutely convinced that I'm mature enough to get married in spite of what my parents think. Jonah and I love each other so much we can overcome any problem that comes our way."

"I hate my step-dad, I hate my new school, and I hate the way my mom acts now that she's married to him. Next time I go visit my dad, I'm not going to let him send me back here."

"I've lived a long life, too long at 93, and it's hard having lost so many people that I love. I know my children want me to take better care of myself, but I just don't care enough anymore to make the effort."

"I feel unloved by my husband. He never compliments me, never asks about my day at work, never even suggests that we go out to a movie. Then I'm supposed to feel romantic toward him at bedtime. It's impossible."

Now compare your responses with one other student and discuss what was difficult and what was easy about this exercise.

COUNSELOR ACTIONS THAT IMPEDE COMMUNICATION

Just as certain attitudes and behaviors can facilitate client disclosure, other predispositions and behaviors sabotage communication and build roadblocks to disclosure. Many of the ineffective responses that new counselors make are a result of carrying social behaviors and an "expert" model of helping into the counseling room. Counselor behaviors such as advice giving, lecturing, excessive questioning, and storytelling make client self-disclosure difficult.

Counselor Predispositions

People learn to avoid emotional content in social interactions with others unless the relationship is strong and the circumstances are private. For example, a couple at a party who get into a disagreement over how to manage money will be avoided by the other party guests. People learn how to give other people social distance and privacy. If a counselor employs the same approach in the counseling session, the impact is to communicate to the client that it is not safe to share emotional content. It is important to remember that the client sees the counselor as a stranger in the first session. The goal is to establish trust as quickly as possible by employing the attitudes and behaviors described in the previous sections. Another attitudinal barrier that many counselors struggle with initially is the feeling that as experts they ought to be able to solve the client's problems and relieve them of their psychological pain very quickly. This attitude will shortcut the disclosure process because the counselor adopts the client's anxiety and tries to move prematurely to solutions.

Premature Advice Giving

Even in ordinary conversation, most people are ambivalent about advice. On the one hand, people hope for good ideas, on the other hand, they want to devise their own solution in their own good time. The same ambivalence toward advice holds true in the counseling relationship, especially in the early stages when clients are still unsure that the counselor understands the uniqueness of their experience and they still feel ambivalent about the costs of change. "Why don't you . . ." or "Yeah, but . . ." (as described in transactional analysis) is a verbal game frequently played in counseling sessions when counselors are giving advice. The client enters, communicating confusion, stress, exasperation, or helplessness. Wanting to offer some relief, the counselor recommends a course of action ("Why don't you . . ."). The client responds, "Yeah, but . . . ," far from enthusiastic about the advice. Soon barriers are built in the relationship. The client begins to feel more defensive. Feelings of exasperation grow in the counselor and may cause him or her to reject the client.

In addition to impeding communication, premature advice giving has the effect of making the client feel like an inadequate, dependent child, and thus slows the development of responsible self-reliance. Indeed, clients sometimes present themselves as helpless children to entice counselors into giving advice. Giving advice under these conditions reinforces defensive manipulations and game playing. Advice also discourages the client from becoming actively involved in counseling, falsely communicating that the counselor is the active party in this action and that his or her role is as a passive recipient of information.

A counselor's thoughts about how a problem may be solved do have value, of course, but are much more appropriate later in the counseling process, after the circumstances have been thoroughly explored, a strong therapeutic alliance is in place, and the counselor *really* knows something of the client's experience. At that point, the counselor's ideas can be considered along with the client's as options that might be useful.

Lecturing

Lecturing is really a disguised form of advice giving. When lecturing, a counselor presents himself or herself as an expert, developing a few paragraphs or more of "sage wisdom." The hidden message is "You should do it my way. If you don't, you are less of a person than I thought and I will be disappointed with you." Disregard for the client is shown in several ways. In addition to conveying a message of inadequacy or immaturity, the counselor is allocating more time to his or her own ideas than to the client's. During long-winded lectures, clients frequently shut off their ears and often disregard the messenger as well as the message itself. This is especially true for clients who have been involved in power struggles with authority figures. The client should not see the counselor as just one more authority figure. *You know you are probably lecturing if you say more than three consecutive sentences to your client.*

Excessive Questioning

"How old are you?" "Where do you live?" "How many brothers and sisters did you grow up with?" "What was your family's religious preference?" "When did you reach puberty?" "Do you have satisfying interpersonal relationships?" "How do you spend your spare time?" "Why are you taking the course for which you are reading this book?" "What do you want to do with the rest of your life?"

Excessive questioning does not open communication; it conveys that the client's job is to be *passive* and *respond* to the counselor's questions. The counselor asks and the client responds. The problem is that the client has little opportunity to do any initiating. The counselor is in charge, but the client is the person who knows what the issues that need airing are. Excessive questioning results in important information being missed. (Have you ever been in a situation where you had important information to share with another, and his or her questions were focusing on something else and limiting your ability to say what you needed to say?)

"Why" questions are especially destructive because they ask the client to explain and justify his or her behavior. They put the client on the spot, raising his or her anxiety and encouraging the defenses of rationalization and intellectualization. They may also lead clients to look for the "right" answers rather than expressing their actual experience.

Sometimes counselors ask questions to stimulate interaction with a nonverbal client. Sometimes they ask questions to get information or to direct the client's attention to a specific topic, theme, or issue. All of these goals are valid, but responses in forms other than a question are usually more facilitative for accomplishing these ends in the initial disclosure stage of counseling.

To help a nonverbal client, the counselor might use alternatives such as "I can see that it is hard for you to talk comfortably with me. Please take the time to think about what you want to say if you need to. We're in no rush. Perhaps it would help to share with me what is happening in your life that creates excitement for you." Notice that this response works with, rather than against, the client's energy.

If there is information that is important to know, the counselor might try an alternative such as "I need to understand more clearly how things looked, sounded, and felt to you when your wife decided to move out. Help me understand what it was like for you then." Such responses create mutuality in the counseling experience. Before making such a request, the counselor should first establish that the information being requested is very important to his or her understanding of the client's concern.

To focus a client's attention on a specific theme, an alternative such as the following can be helpful: "You have mentioned sitting alone on a school bus a couple of times. Tell me what you think about when this happens." Again, this alternative invites exploration in a comfortable way while promoting concreteness in the content of the discussion.

Unless it probes too deeply into private space, an occasional question is unlikely to damage the client–counselor relationship. Questions are detrimental if they become the dominant mode of counselor communication or if they create a stifled rather than a spontaneous atmosphere.

Beginning counselors can control the tendency to regress into questioning by never asking two questions in a row, by following a question with a nonquestion that relates to the information received in response to the first question, and, if necessary, by using a general lead such as "Tell me more about . . ."

It also helps to distinguish between closed and open questions. *Closed questions* usually probe for specific factual information and can be answered with single or few words. *Open questions* call for ideas, beliefs, or emotions and require longer discussion for full response. "Are you living with your husband now?" is a closed question. "What do you do when your husband comes home drunk?" is an open question. Open questions provide for more client disclosure and are usually better than closed questions during the first stage of the counseling process.

Storytelling

> COUNSELOR: I remember when *I* was in the 10th grade. The kids in my
>   group were really self-centered then too. Everybody seemed
>   interested in looking out for number one. None of us knew
>   anything about being a friend. Everybody seemed to be putting a
>   lot of energy into building themselves up by putting others down.
> CLIENT: Gee, I guess life must have been pretty lonely for you at 15.
> COUNSELOR: Yea, it really was. Why I remember a time when . . .

Counselors sometimes tell stories about their own lives, ostensibly to help the client identify with them and to communicate the message "I understand what you are experiencing because I experienced it too." Though well intentioned, generally this procedure impedes rather than facilitates communication. First, it is often difficult for clients to believe that the counselor could have ever been in a situation *exactly* like theirs, and usually they are correct in their skepticism. Furthermore, an underlying presumption is that, in a similar situation, the counselor held the same beliefs and experienced the same emotions. By moving the focus of discussion from the client, the counselor interrupts the exploration process. He or she discounts the client and risks the introduction of interfering noise into the session by projecting his or her own emotions onto the client. Storytelling is often a way for the counselor to cope with his or her personal anxiety. At worst, the counselor may be using the client as an audience to gratify a need for attention.

SUMMARY

The primary task of the initial disclosure stage is to work toward the development of a relationship characterized by trust, honesty, and open communication and to promote self-examination and clarification. As the experience evolves, clients disclose progressively more information about themselves and their personal concerns. The sharing of this information helps the client gain new insights, helps the counselor understand what is occurring in the client's life, and helps both to work toward tentative goals for counseling.

Counselors need to recognize that clients who enter counseling voluntarily have already tried to solve their problems on their own and that people approach counseling with varying levels of readiness for change, ranging from virtually no recognition of a need for change to a history of significant success in most, but not all, aspects of change. Clients who acknowledge the need for change and are willing to accept the costs involved in change move through the initial stage of counseling most quickly.

As the client discloses information, the quality of the interaction with the counselor gives the client feedback about whether it is safe to continue. This interaction also establishes counseling as a process of self-examination as opposed to mere conversation. It should extinguish any client predisposition that the process is an interview in which the counselor collects information and then provides a solution.

Effective counselor contact includes encouraging communication with verbal and nonverbal initiatives and communicating empathy appropriate to the client's level of readiness as well as genuine concern about the client's welfare. Empathy can be described as the counselor's ability to perceive and understand themes and issues projected by the client's communication. It can also be defined as perceiving and understanding the personal constructs a client uses to understand and organize his or her world. Empathic skill includes a communicating as well as a perceiving component, and the most common way of expressing empathy is through interchangeable responses. Concreteness is a quality of the counselor's technique that keeps the session focused on important themes and promotes a clear and specific description of the client's life situations.

Several communication patterns that are often thought to be helpful by new counselors and untrained persons in general are advice giving, lecturing, questioning, and storytelling. In fact, these behaviors usually impede communication in the initial stage of counseling. Limited use of questions, advice, and self-disclosure (storytelling) may be appropriate and helpful later in the counseling process but usually not at the beginning. These communication styles dissuade clients from revealing sensitive personal information, erode their confidence in the counselor's genuine interest in them, and sustain the myth that counseling is a process in which someone else is responsible for their own change process. When these problematic patterns are avoided and positive skills are substituted, the development of an effective working relationship during the initial disclosure stage establishes the foundation for the next stage: in-depth exploration.

≈≈≈ *DISCUSSION QUESTIONS* ≈≈≈

1. What is the difference between the kind of caring discussed as an important counselor attribute and the kind of caring we feel toward our families and life partners?
2. Attending is a prerequisite for listening but is not all there is to listening. Based on what you have read here and what you know from your own experience, what does listening involve beyond attending?

3. Comments that invite clients to elaborate on their experiences without asking questions are important to client engagement and to client self-disclosure. What other counselor responses do you think would invite communication besides those offered by the authors?

4. The authors emphasize that the core conditions cannot be "faked" or taken on the way an actor takes on a role, but they also argue that skills related to these conditions can be learned. Are these positions inconsistent? If not, how do you reconcile them?

REFERENCES

Bachelor, A., & Horvath, A. (1999). The therapeutic relationship. In M. A. Hubble, B. L. Duncan, & S. D. Miller (Eds.), *The heart and soul of change: What works in therapy* (pp. 133–178). Washington, DC: American Psychological Association.

Beck, A. T. (1976). *Cognitive therapy and the emotional disorders.* New York: International Universities Press.

Bohart, A. C., & Greenberg, L. S. (1997). *Empathy reconsidered: New directions in psychotherapy.* Washington, DC: American Psychological Association.

Bohart, A. C., & Tallman, K. (1999). *How clients make therapy work.* Washington, DC: American Psychological Association.

Brammer, L. M., Abrego, P. J., & Shostrum, E. L. (1993). *Therapeutic counseling and psychotherapy* (6th ed.). Englewood Cliffs, NJ: Prentice Hall.

Carkhuff, R. R. (1969). *Helping and human relations* (Vols. 1 & 2). New York: Holt, Rinehart & Winston.

Egan, G. (2002). *The skilled helper: A problem management approach to helping* (7th ed.). Pacific Grove, CA: Brooks/Cole.

Ivey, A. E., & Ivey, M. B. (2003). *Intentional interviewing and counseling* (5th ed.). Pacific Grove, CA: Brooks/Cole.

Ivey, A. E., Ivey, M. B., & Simek-Morgan, L. (2002). *Counseling and psychotherapy: A multicultural perspective* (5th ed.). Boston: Allyn & Bacon.

James, R. K., & Gilliland, B. E. (2003). *Theories and strategies in counseling and psychotherapy* (5th ed.). Boston: Allyn & Bacon.

Kelley, G. A. (1955). *The psychology of personal constructs* (Vol. 1). New York: Norton.

Meichenbaum, D. (1977). *Cognitive behavior modification: An integrative approach.* New York: Plenum.

Najavits, L. M., & Strupp, H. H. (1994). Differences in the effectiveness of psychodynamic therapists: A process and outcome study. *Psychotherapy: Theory, Research, Practice, Training, 31,* 114–123.

Okun, B. F. (2002). *Active helping: Interviewing and counseling techniques* (6th ed.). Pacific Grove, CA: Brooks Cole.

Patterson, L. E., & Eisenberg, S. (1983). *The counseling process* (3rd ed.). Boston: Houghton Mifflin.

Rogers, C. R. (1942). *Counseling and psychotherapy.* Boston: Houghton Mifflin.

Rogers, C. R. (1957). The necessary and sufficient conditions of therapeutic personality change. *Journal of Consulting Psychology, 21,* 95–103.

Rogers, C. R. (1961). *On becoming a person.* Boston: Houghton Mifflin.

Rogers, C. R. (1965). *Client-centered therapy.* In E. Shostrom (Producer), *Three approaches to psychotherapy* [Videotape]. Orange, CA: Psychological Films.

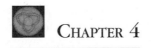 CHAPTER 4

IN-DEPTH EXPLORATION

As the counseling process continues, the client increasingly sees the counselor—at first a stranger—as a caring and genuine person who is able to understand and accept the client's problems and emotions. When the client begins to understand that the counselor will not reject him or her for what he or she says, that client begins to feel that it is safe to share more private thoughts. The counselor, having gained increasing insight into the client's personality and circumstances during Stage 1, has a base of information that provides context for understanding the client's continued disclosures. The counselor is therefore able to respond more accurately and completely to what the client says. Furthermore, as the trust level builds, the counselor can give the client feedback about his or her thoughts and actions that would have raised defenses and perhaps caused the client to terminate counseling if introduced earlier. The combination of greater client readiness and increased counselor knowledge of the client leads to the second stage of counseling—in-depth exploration—which is characterized by more emotional intensity and more complex thought processes than are present in the first stage. The client at this stage is truly engaged in the counseling process and feels more powerful to effect the desired changes, though the fear of change has not disappeared.

As the client continues to reveal his or her intimate thoughts and feelings and describes not only his or her own behaviors but also the reactions of others, both client and counselor become more aware of the following:

- Significant events that have shaped the client's present personality and circumstances
- The influence of ethnicity, culture, socioeconomic status, gender, or sexual orientation on client opportunities
- Deficiencies in the client's coping skills
- Strengths that the client has available but may not be applying to the resolution of his or her problems
- Interpersonal relationships with significant others in the client's life that affect the client's thoughts, feelings, and actions (including unfinished business from the past)
- Feelings about self and others

- Goals that have been implicit in the client's unsuccessful
  efforts to resolve his or her problem(s) and that now can be
  made explicit in preparation for action planning

These new awarenesses create insight into the client's concerns and
open up options for resolving those concerns. The counselor will frequently
develop those insights more quickly than the client because of the counselor's familiarity with personality dynamics and the patterns of behavior
that people typically employ to fulfill their needs when confronted with circumstances that block the way. These counselor insights form the basis for
assessment and diagnosis, discussed in more detail in Chapter 7.

The counselor's hypotheses about the sources of the client's problem(s)
create the basis for the additive responses of second-stage work. In additive
responses, the counselor tries to make conscious the connections between
aspects of the client's life of which the client was not fully aware before
counseling. If additive responding occurs in the context of a strong therapeutic alliance, additive responses not only assist the client in developing a
deeper self-understanding, but they also help ready the client for the implementation of actions aimed at behavior change. Counselors should continually be cognizant of the threat to the therapeutic alliance inherent in additive
responding and should regularly monitor whether additive responses are
undermining the trusting relationship so essential to any client change.

GOALS AND METHODS OF IN-DEPTH EXPLORATION

Two goals are implicit in the second (in-depth exploration) stage of
counseling for the client. The first is for both counselor and client to gain
insight into the client's strengths, deficiencies, interpersonal functioning,
"baggage" from the past, feelings, desires, and needs. The second is to use
the insights gained to begin formulating goals regarding those changes that
the client has the power to make. The belief that insight acts as the basis for
client growth and problem resolution is fundamental to this book's generic
model of counseling. When people understand what led them to their current problems, they begin to feel hope that they can change. Without
insight, problems remain overwhelming and insoluble.

With children and with adolescents and adults who are less intellectually
capable, the fostering of extensive insight may sometimes be an unachievable
goal. Looking inside is not a capacity that all clients possess in equal measure.
Even so, helping clients to develop a more internal orientation—to consider
the thinking behind their behaviors—is a worthy endeavor even when deep
insight is not possible.

Some clients may experience emotional release (catharsis) through
counseling that leads to more satisfactory feelings and behaviors *without*
ever achieving a thorough understanding of the roots of their difficulties or

the thoughts and behaviors that serve to maintain those difficulties. Other clients who achieve insight into the nature of their difficulties may never formulate goals or take any action. Such individuals are less likely to experience sustained benefit as a result of the counseling experience.

Not all clients need the same depth or breadth of insight. Some may need a clearer picture of interests and ability patterns that relate to career choice. Some may require clarification about how their behavior affects others. Confused clients may need to understand internal beliefs and perceptions that create conflict. Still others may benefit from becoming aware of their inner emotions and how these emotions are expressed, disguised, or stifled.

Insight (or interiority) is gained through the process of exploring significant themes, patterns, concerns, and issues. During the first stage, some initial nuclei of these themes are identified. In the second stage, they become the focus of attention and are explored in depth. As the client explores and the counselor provides feedback, elements of the client's thoughts that have been in the background emerge into perceptual foreground. During the process, assumptions, beliefs, emotions, motivations, and inconsistencies become clearer to the client. The experience can be enlightening and produce tension at the same time. Therefore, the counselor should continue to use the core skills of the first stage that create and maintain closeness and trust while interspersing the more challenging skills of the second stage.

As the figure on the inside cover indicated, counselor skills associated with the process of deeper exploration include advanced-level empathy, immediacy, constructive confrontation, interpretation, and role-playing. The common characteristic of each of these techniques is that they provide potentially beneficial feedback to the client about the factors that caused their problems and the factors that make those problems difficult to change independently. To understand these skills and their relationship to the counseling experience, we first need to understand the experience of receiving and giving feedback. "Feedback is concerned with providing clients with clear data on their performance and/or how others view them" (Ivey & Ivey, 2003, p. 284).

Exercise

Everyone receives feedback throughout his or her life. Some of it is encouraging and rewarding—as, for example, when a significant other makes a statement such as "I like how you look" or "I appreciated your observations at our staff meeting." Other feedback takes the form of criticism—for example, "You would have been more effective if you had listened instead of changing the topic."

List on a piece of paper three recent experiences in which you have received feedback you regarded as critical, leaving space after each entry to write the answers to these three questions:

1. What did you notice about the giver's tone of voice and attitude toward you?
2. What were you aware of inside yourself while you were receiving the feedback?
3. What, if anything, did you do as a result of the feedback?

Repeat these steps as you recall three instances of receiving positive feedback. Then before proceeding to the next section, generate three to five principles (based on your experience) that describe how you think that people respond to feedback. If possible, share your thoughts with other students in a small group discussion. Finally, identify an experience when you received feedback that was essentially negative but felt significantly less uncomfortable. For example, a teacher once identified the following negative feedback as less uncomfortable than other criticism of her teaching: "You seemed unusually impatient with your students' questions in class today." Then examine what features of that experience made it less problematic.

Principles Governing the Use of Feedback

Eight principles govern the counselor's use of feedback. First, *feedback is hard to receive.* All feedback, even when supportive, can meet with some resistance. When receiving supportive feedback, people often have mixed emotions: they appreciate the good words yet feel uncomfortable in the spotlight of attention. Critical feedback identifies behavior that an observer has found to be inappropriate, and it is even harder to accept. When others are critical, one feels that one's judgment is being questioned—and this is especially difficult if one is already feeling uncertain or guilty about some action.

Second, *feedback that does not fit a person's self-image will be harder to receive than feedback that is consistent with self-image.* Consider, for example, a client who has just finished his first semester in college with a grade point average of C and a failure in chemistry. He has also felt lonely because he has not established many new friendships and has no steady romantic relationship. When a counselor attempted to be encouraging by providing feedback that the client is bright and attractive to others based on his experiences in high school, the client simply became more insistent that he was a failure who would never reach his goal of becoming a doctor. At that moment, success was not a part of the client's self-image, and he could not accept factual feedback of a more hopeful nature regardless of its essential validity.

Third, *feedback is never fully internalized at the time it is received.* Elements that are consistent with the self-concept are quickly acknowledged, other elements are rejected or discounted, and still others are reviewed many times before they are recognized as valid and incorporated into a revised self-concept. Even when we want feedback, we resist it (Harrison, 1977).

The fourth principle emphasizes the importance of trust. *Feedback is easier to receive if it comes from a trusted source.* As discussed in the previous chapter, trust develops in the context of a genuine, caring relationship where the counselor shows respect for the client. Trust is also a function of the client's assessment of the counselor's credibility. If the client sees most of the counselor's observations, perceptions, and judgments as valid, he or she will work harder to accept new feedback that may initially seem incongruent with self.

Next, *feedback is easier to receive when the giver offers it with a calm presence.* The calm presence of the counselor helps the client feel confident about the feedback. A counselor who is anxious, angry, or embarrassed will cause the client to feel insecure and will block assimilation. Counselors may have special difficulty with giving feedback when they project themselves into the role of the client and in essence say to themselves, "I would not want to receive what I am giving." Remembering that the client's goal is change and that the client is quite distressed by his or her current situation helps counselors take the risk of offering uncomfortable feedback. It can be a short-term cost for a long-term gain.

The sixth principle is concerned with the clarity of the communication of feedback. *Feedback is more effective when it is communicated clearly and specifically.* This principle derives from the concept of concreteness discussed in Chapter 3. To offer feedback clearly, the counselor must know what information she or he wants to give and be comfortable about giving it. This requires careful thought prior to verbalizing the feedback. If the counselor knows what he or she wishes to say but feels uncomfortable about saying it, the language will often be obscured in the counselor's effort to take the edge off the message, and the client is deprived of the counselor's accurate insight. Specific feedback promotes more effective exploration than vague feedback (Ivey & Ivey, 2003). It is much more helpful to say, "You feel that your husband does not respect your career and this angers you," than it is to say, "You feel that your husband keeps putting you down." The first response encourages discussion of specific hurtful exchanges between husband and wife that can be brought into the here and now; the second response does little to focus the discussion.

Seventh, *feedback can only be absorbed in small doses.* Although most people may have many areas that would profit from change, they cannot work on all of them at one time (Ivey & Ivey, 2003). It is important not to overwhelm the client. The urge to present the client with a litany of short-comings is greatest when the counselor is feeling frustration with the progress of the counseling. Counselors who keep in mind that clients' problems have usually developed long before they entered counseling and have been resistant to the client's independent efforts at self-change are better able to be patient with the client's rate of progress.

Finally, *feedback is presented for client consideration, not as indisputable truth*. Consider, for example, the case of a boy who repeatedly gets involved in fights with other boys on the playground. These incidents occur when other boys call him names or make remarks about his mother. The other children have learned that he responds excessively to their taunting and have made a game of antagonizing him. This feedback statement is quite interpretive: "You defend yourself and your mother at the drop of a hat. You seem to feel there is something wrong with your family." Although it might generate insight for the boy to consider this hypothesis, he may have trouble acknowledging it if he is sensitive about having a single mother with a live-in boyfriend. The hypothesis might be easier to contemplate if stated less bluntly and offered for consideration: "I wonder why you are so quick to become angry and to defend yourself and your mother. Could it be that you feel that your family is not as it should be?" This second statement, though still pursuing the hypothesis that the client is ashamed of his family, avoids a negative label and asks for the client's perceptions.

Research evidence (Lynn & Frauman, 1985) suggests that behavioral feedback, based on observation, is generally easier for clients to accept than inferential feedback. In the previous example, it would probably be easier for the client to accept that he responds with a short fuse to the taunting of other children (observation) than it would be for him to face what it is about his family that he feels he must defend (inference).

Because feedback is presented for client consideration, the counselor follows the feedback process with an assessment of whether the feedback was received and whether it proved useful to the client. Remember that even though the client may not appear to be receiving the feedback at the time it is given, the client may review the feedback and may bring it up again later after she or he has become used to the idea.

Importance of Feedback in the In-depth Exploration Stage

Feedback helps people grow and learn about themselves and their environment. As clients learn more about their present behaviors, they become clearer about their goals for change. But people tend to be in conflict about feedback; they want it for growth yet resist it at the same time.

The essential counselor work of the in-depth exploration stage is providing clients with feedback about themselves in such a way that it can be assimilated and used for growth. Because feedback often makes us uncomfortable, offering it is an art form. Working in line with the principles just developed will increase the chances of assimilation and use. The next sections discuss several modes of providing feedback: advanced empathy, immediacy, confrontation, interpretation, and role-playing.

ADVANCED EMPATHY

In Chapter 3, empathy was described as the "counselor's ability to enter the client's phenomenal world—to experience the client's world as if it were your own without ever losing the 'as if' quality" (Rogers, 1961, p. 284). Primary empathy, the level that is most appropriate for the initial counseling stage, was described as those responses that indicate the counselor has understood those themes that are readily apparent from the client's statements. Nonverbal communication and interchangeable responses were described as important modes of communicating primary empathy. The in-depth exploration stage is characterized by a deeper level of openness in the client—an increased readiness to explore significant themes and to become aware of the less obvious meanings behind those themes. Concomitantly, the counselor's level of empathy shifts to increasingly advanced empathy responses.

Advanced empathy includes the counselor sensing what the client has implied but perhaps not directly stated in his or her disclosures. Truax (1976) indicates that at an advanced empathy level the counselor "uncovers the most deeply shrouded of the client's feeling areas, voicing meanings in the client's experience of which the client is scarcely aware . . . [The counselor] moves into feelings and experiences that are only hinted at by the client and does so with sensitivity and accuracy" (p. 566).

Martin (2000) uses the term *evocative empathy* to indicate that at any stage of counseling the counselor should give voice to the client's *intended message*. However, he also indicates that "later in therapy the therapist can go a lot further and say much more emotionally poignant things—because the client intends the therapist to hear so much more then" (p. 6).

Advanced empathy is not to be confused with interpretation, in that empathy is always based on the client's frame of reference (Egan, 2002; Martin, 2000), though Cormier and Nurius (2002) point out that a purpose of advanced empathy is to "add to the client's frame of reference or to draw out implications of the issue" (p. 37). The empathic therapist sees the client as the source of the meaning and feeling. When conveying advanced empathy, the counselor uses statements whose purpose is to evoke the feeling and meaning that already reside in the client, even though the client may be barely aware of their existence. With interpretation, on the other hand, the assumption is that the counselor has an insight that is more perceptive than the client's and that should be shared.

Egan (2002) poses four questions that counselors should ask themselves to identify material for the additive statements that characterize advanced empathy:

- What is this person only half saying?
- What is this person hinting at?
- What is this person saying in a confused way?
- What messages do I hear behind the explicit messages? (p. 200)

The following example illustrates the difference between primary and advanced empathy and shows the differential impact of the two kinds of responses. The client was a 46-year-old European-American woman who was in an in-patient psychiatric unit to be treated for depression accompanied by suicidal ideation.

> CLIENT: My past caught up to me and really floored me. I've been trying to keep my past *in* the past.
> COUNSELOR 1: It's hard to talk about the past.
> COUNSELOR 2: Keeping the past bottled up hasn't worked. As difficult as it is to talk about it, you knew you had to do it.

The first counselor used a primary empathy response—restating the idea that it is difficult to talk about the past. This response serves some purposes. The client learns that the counselor understands that the process is emotionally sensitive. The client is also prompted to think again about how difficult it might be to talk and could possibly sense enough caring in the counselor to go on. The client feels some understanding from the counselor but has a lot of choices about how to continue, which is appropriate early in the counseling process.

The second counselor used an advanced empathy response. While recognizing the client's caution, the counselor sensed the client's intended message that it is time to get some of the past out on the table, however difficult it may be. This interaction took place a couple of days after the client was admitted to the unit and after considerable therapy had already taken place.

Following the advanced empathy response, the client proceeded to describe that she had been sexually abused many years ago by her brother. The incident that precipitated the suicidal depression and hospitalization at this time was the client's learning that this same brother had recently molested the client's 16-year-old daughter. She was suffering from guilt that she had never confronted the earlier attack and had thereby set the stage for her daughter's traumatic experience.

Note that the surface message in the client's statement was that talking about the problem is difficult and by implication she would prefer to let the past stay in the past. The real intended message at this stage of counseling, however, was that "it is important to me to deal with what I have been avoiding for so long."

Case: Colleen

Colleen was an adolescent with impaired vision whose parents were separated. She lived with her mother and occasionally visited her father at his apartment on weekends. She worked regularly with her counselor on a variety of themes. In one session, she appeared unusually depressed, which stimulated a discussion of her visit to her father on the previous weekend. The counselor first contacted emotions in her initial advanced empathy response: "Sounds like your visit with your father was very stressful for you." Colleen affirmed this observation and went on to explain that her father seemed withdrawn, distant, and uncommunicative. The counselor's advanced empathy response addressed the client's needs: "You need your father to communicate with you, and when he does not, that makes you wonder if he really wants you to be with him." Colleen nodded her head and showed signs of pain around her eyes and mouth. The counselor's next advanced empathy response identified an important need that Colleen had been holding inside for a long time: "I sense it's really important for you to know where you stand with your father." This brought agreement as well as tears.

When sufficient exploration had taken place, the counselor summarized: "What you want is to know how your father feels toward you. Let's see if we can figure out a way for you to find out." This introduced third-stage work into the counseling process. (The third stage is discussed in Chapter 5.) Some role-playing, including role reversal, was used to help Colleen learn how to ask her father about his feelings.

Colleen left the counselor's office appearing unsure, but she appeared happier the next week. She explained that she had visited her father and told him that she found it hard to know what to say to him when she visited. Her statement led to an intimate conversation in which her father acknowledged feeling cautious about what he said to her because he did not want to call attention to her vision limitations. He also said that he wanted to be a good father, but he simply didn't know what to say to her much of the time. Colleen reported that this made her feel relieved and that she knew what to say. Her response to her father, "Let me know that I'm important to you," appeared to mark an important transition in their relationship.

A key response in this episode was the clarification of Colleen's needs. This led to the establishment of a goal and strategies to fulfill the goal. She was able to identify a sense of personal power, which in later counseling was related to the sense of helplessness she felt because of her visual difficulties.

Questions for Further Thought

1. What problems in coping might you expect Colleen to have as a result of her impaired vision? What implications do your assessments have for the development of advanced empathy responses?
2. What constitutes a "healthy" adjustment to the separation of one's parents? A client's tears are a frequent part of the counseling experience, especially when the process reaches the second stage. What are your feelings when another person cries in your presence? How do your inner feelings influence how you respond? Would the gender of your client make a difference in your reactions? What should a counselor do when a client cries?

IMMEDIACY

"Immediacy refers to the current interaction of the therapist and the client in the relationship" (Patterson, 1974, p. 83). Thus, an immediacy response is a communication that provides feedback to the client about the therapist's inner experience of the relationship at a given moment. Egan (2002) discusses three kinds of immediacy responses: those that review the overall relationship with the client, those that explore changes in the client's demeanor as different issues arise in counseling, and those self-involving statements that reflect the counselor's affective responses to the client in the present moment.

Immediacy responses dealing with the overall relationship provide opportunities for the client and counselor to explore whether they are working effectively together as well as ways in which their relationship resembles or differs from the client's relationships outside of the counseling. Because many clients enter counseling in the first place because of relational difficulties (Egan, 2002), discussing the relationship affords opportunities for the counselor to identify effective relationship skills, to help the client examine his or her own relationship skills, and to draw attention to comparisons between the counseling relationship and the client's (often deficient) relationships with significant others outside of counseling.

Patterson (1974) emphasizes that "Concern with immediacy is significant because the client's behavior and functioning in the therapy relationship are indicative of his [or her] functioning in other interpersonal relationships" (p. 83). If, for example, the client exhibits unusual dependency in the counseling relationship, then it is likely that she or he may do the same with significant others. Helping the client to recognize, understand, and manage the dependency in the counseling relationship should generalize to the client's other relationships as well.

Immediacy responses can provide opportunities for the counselor to react to changes in client participation in the therapy—for example, changes in spontaneity or perhaps a sense that the counseling has "bogged down." These responses often take the form of "I" messages and are offered to stimulate exploration of some significant theme, not as criticism or punishment. Consider the following example of the use of immediacy responses with an adult male client whose progress in counseling has slowed. The initial statement came about 20 minutes into the session.

Example

COUNSELOR: Tom, for the past five minutes or so I have not been feeling comfortable about what is happening. To me it seems as though we are circling around the theme of you and your father without really getting into it. (Immediacy response indicating that progress in this session and related to this issue is different from the usual tone of the counseling.)

CLIENT: (Pause.) I think you are right. So what?

COUNSELOR: For the past two sessions I have felt as though we have circled without focusing. Today I decided I want to say something. (Immediacy response indicating that the blocking has been going on for a while and may signify something important.)

CLIENT: If that's how you have felt, why didn't you say something sooner?

COUNSELOR: I haven't been sure whether you would be open to hearing that message from me. (Immediacy response expressing concern that the client may not have been ready to go further.)

CLIENT: You must see me as pretty defensive.

COUNSELOR: All of us, including me, are defensive in some way. I can be excellent at intellectualizing. (Immediacy response that acknowledges counselor's human fallibility, giving client permission to be fallible as well.)

CLIENT: I've noticed that sometimes. But you seem to catch yourself and not let it get too much in the way.

COUNSELOR: Would you be willing to tell me about my defenses? (Immediacy response asking client to focus on counselor's behavior.)

CLIENT: Sure. Sometimes instead of getting me to talk more about what I've just said, you get into a big textbook explanation of how people react in general to situations like mine. (Thoughtful pause.) I guess I really do the same thing sometimes, don't I? Well, I guess what I've been trying to avoid talking about was that . . .

Sometimes the counselor's sense that the relationship is tense signals client discomfort with material being discussed. A self-involving statement identifying the counselor's feeling in the moment can often help the client to acknowledge discomfort and make a more conscious decision about how to proceed. Consider the following example of 25-year-old female client.

Example

COUNSELOR: Right now I am feeling very cautious. Part of me wants to explore how things are between you and your boyfriend, and part of me is holding back. I wonder if you may be having a similar experience. (Immediacy statement identifying the counselor's feelings.)

CLIENT: (Pause followed by slow speech.) Yes. This whole thing is so screwed up for me that sometimes I would just rather not think about it.

COUNSELOR: I get from that statement that you would feel more comfortable if we talked about something else. (Immediacy statement focusing on whether trust in the relationship is strong enough for the client to proceed.)

CLIENT: (Still slowly.) It would be safer, but I still need help sorting this all out.

COUNSELOR: I have a sense of how loaded this area is for you. Would it help you if I just listen while you talk? (Immediacy statement proposing a way to alleviate stress in the relationship at the moment.)

At this point the client inhaled and started to tell her story.

Immediacy statements are especially important in situations where the client and counselor are of different race, gender, ethnic background, sexual orientation, or are different in other ways: The client may fear that the counselor will lack the experience to truly understand his or her life situation, and open discussion of client–counselor differences will often clear the air and ease communication. Immediacy statements also allow the client the opportunity to explain the cultural influences on his or her reactions to the counselor and thereby reinforce the therapeutic alliance. Whenever issues of the client–counselor relationship that are experienced by the counselor as potentially disruptive are introduced for direct discussion, this is a form of immediacy response.

Our own experience as counselor educators, along with the clinical experience of other therapists (Egan, 2002; Jourard, 1971), leads us to believe that immediacy is one of the more challenging counseling skills to develop. First, immediacy communication is difficult because the counselor discloses his or her personal feelings and hunches about the relationship directly to the client. There is always the possibility that the client will reject the perceptions as erroneous or that the client will respond defensively. Immediacy responses place the counselor's perceptions directly on the line for another's reaction and with the clear possibility of rejection. This is a risky position, as it is in any human relationship. Egan (2002) states also that it is difficult "to be aware of what is happening in the relationship without becoming preoccupied and 'psyching out' the client" (p. 213). Finally, considerable social competence and verbal skill are required to formulate statements that are potent enough to achieve an impact and yet considerate and careful of the client's feelings.

To work on your immediacy skills you will need to identify your own possible sources of fear. The assistance of a supervisor or peers in group supervision can promote growth in your ability to use immediacy skills by providing feedback about opportunities for immediacy responses that are passed over.

CONFRONTATION

Confrontation is one of the more controversial counseling techniques, partly because the everyday use of the word often implies conflict or attack—for example, "Pro-life and pro-choice demonstrators confronted each other on the Capitol steps today." Implied are dimensions of anger, violence, struggles of power and control, and an adversarial rather than a cooperative relationship.

Confrontation as used in counseling is defined as a counseling intervention in which the counselor verbalizes the discrepancies, contradictions, and omissions expressed in the client's words or actions. Confrontation is done *for* and *with* the client, not *to* and *against* the client. In other words, the counselor does not confront to satisfy his or her own needs, to vent feelings of frustration with the counseling, or to punish the client. Instead, the counselor holds a sincere belief that the client will experience growth by paying attention to some discrepancy or incongruence he or she has revealed. Egan (2002) and Hill and O'Brien (1999) argue that the word *challenges* may more correctly describe the intent of responses that are commonly called confrontations. These confrontations or challenges may address behaviors, thoughts, or feelings and for that reason they take many forms discussed elsewhere in this text, including restatement, reflection, cognitive restructuring, or even interpretation.

The counselor's first step in the confrontation process is to identify the mixed messages, conflict, and incongruity in the client's statements and behaviors that require further attention through observation, questioning, and listening (Ivey & Ivey, 2003). In the sections that follow, we first describe some of the possible discrepancies, contradictions, or mixed messages that may be confronted (Dinkmeyer & Dinkmeyer 1985; Egan, 2002; George & Cristiani, 1995; Ivey & Ivey, 2003) and then consider the special sensitivities required to confront client defenses.

Discrepancies Between the Client's Perceptions and Accurate Information

People act on the basis of what they believe to be true, and when their beliefs are inaccurate, they act in ineffective ways. Helping a client correct misconceptions can lead to more rewarding behavior. For example, an adolescent female may express the belief that washing with soap and water after intercourse will eliminate the possibility of pregnancy. She is acting with serious misinformation; helping her understand her body more accurately may help her take more appropriate preventive actions. Her counselor may choose to confront her as follows: "Rina, it sounds as though you believe washing with soap and water will make sure you don't get pregnant. (Rina nods and has an anxious look.) There are several ways to prevent pregnancy but washing with soap and water is not one of them. Would you find it helpful for us to discuss the possible ways?"

Discrepancies Between Client Expectations and Likely Possibilities

Counselors help clients think rationally and sensibly about what is happening to them. A counselor who listens carefully will often hear statements that reflect irrational thinking (e.g., "I must be accepted and loved by everyone or I cannot be happy"). Such thinking is said to be irrational because common experience tells us that no one is loved by everyone, yet many people are able to achieve happiness. At other times, clients' beliefs are exaggerations of the negative consequences of their experience. For instance, a client might think, "I will lose all of my friends if I disclose my homosexuality." Although total rejection is possible, it is unlikely that every single person the client knows will reject him because of his sexual orientation. See Chapter 10 under the rational and cognitive therapies for further discussion of this kind of confrontation, also called cognitive restructuring.

Discrepancies Between Verbal and Body Messages

Perls (1969) has indicated that although it is relatively easy for people to use words to cover up internal truths, body messages provide more accurate information about what is happening within. Providing a client with feedback about body messages or discrepancies between verbal statements and body messages can lead to more honest communication. For example, a female client was speaking in a slow, labored, drawn-out fashion. The counselor asked the woman if talking about the particular theme was tolerable for her. While saying yes, the client crossed her arms and pressed them to her stomach. The counselor called her attention to her closed posture. "You say that you are comfortable with this but your arms are crossed in close to your body and you look tense." This led to some important exploration of the reasons why the theme was distressing for the client to talk about.

Sometimes, too, clients will try to hide their feelings about what they are saying by effecting a contradictory physical message. Perhaps the most frequent example of this is smiling while discussing or describing a distressing event. The true emotion may be fear, anger, or embarrassment, but the client presumes that the smile will make the message more acceptable. A simple observation like "Are you aware that you are smiling as you talk about this unpleasant topic?" will often elicit more honest and therefore more productive communication.

Discrepancies Between Behaviors and Stated Goals

Perhaps one of the most common manifestations of a discrepancy between behaviors and stated goals is seen in persons who seek to be accepted by others but whose behaviors make such acceptance unlikely. On the elementary school playground, this pattern is observed in the child whose goal is to gain the positive attention (friendship) of his peers. He or she seeks attention by tormenting his or her peers and consequently ends up without any friends. The case of Lionel presented later in the chapter illustrates a similar pattern of self-defeating behavior. Discrepancies between behaviors and stated goals are also seen in academic settings when students say they want to pass their courses but do not study.

Contradiction Between Statements and Actions

Consider the case of a woman who was trying to cope with a separation initiated by her husband. She described herself as a consistently good wife and expressed intense agitation and confusion about why her husband wanted a divorce. In a later session she told of having a recent affair. By presenting two pieces of information together in the same sentence, the counselor provided the client with feedback about the incongruence of her statement that she was a consistently good wife and her actions as seen by her husband: "You see yourself as a good wife and yet you also had an affair recently." This led to exploration about the client's concept of being a good wife, her standards of sexuality, and what the affair had meant to her husband, who had found out about it.

Mixed Messages

A mixed message is an incongruent message—one part of the message appears to contradict other parts of the message. Explore your own experience for mixed messages that you have received from others. One of the common kinds of mixed message is conditional love, "I love you when you do what I want." Such messages are commonly delivered by parents to children and by one spouse to another. The sender of the message is usually not aware that demands are being communicated along with the love statements and become confused when the receiver of the message does not feel loved. Confrontation with the demanding or negative part of the message creates fertile ground for further counseling work.

Omissions

At times, clients present incomplete information about their life experiences, leaving out details that are uncomfortable to discuss but that are crucial to resolving the problem. One example might be a mother who notes on her counseling intake form that she has three children, but who only discusses two during counseling. Or in situations when there is conflict between the client and another person the client may omit reference to his or her behaviors that provoke, exacerbate, or maintain the conflict. Sometimes people behave with passive aggression and are not fully aware of the aggressive motivation in their actions, whereas at other times they repress such an awareness. An example of passive–aggressive behavior came from a young man whose father had been pressing him to excel as a pitcher in baseball. A fleeting smile revealed the client's satisfaction when he told of pitching a ball to his dad so hard he broke his dad's hand. The client had omitted any verbal reference to his anger at his dad or to his satisfaction at the punishment he had meted out, but that anger became an important part of his counseling.

Obviously, counselors can only confront those omissions that they have discovered through listening carefully to the client or gathered from other sources. Sometimes, as in the first case, the omission may be discovered through records, statements of significant others, or clients' journals presented to the counselor. In other instances, there will be clues in the client's statements or behaviors (such as the smile) that the counselor observes and explores. If an apparent omission comes from a report of another person, the counselor must be cautious about its validity and recognize that the statement may include a bias on the part of the observer. School counselors often receive such information from parents and teachers and must be sensitive to the fact that clients often feel threatened if the counselor is discussing them with others. Confronting an omission in such instances demands attention to the primacy of the client as the focal person in the counseling experience and to his or her right to a confidential relationship.

Working with Client Defenses

Directly confronting a client's defenses is probably the most risky kind of confrontation, as such a frontal attack has a high possibility of raising the client's resistance. Consider the adolescent client with controlling parents who resists parental control by behaving in a surly and uncooperative manner. This regressive, childlike, and defiant behavior serves the purpose of demonstrating to the parents that they cannot control his behavior. It also has the side effect of keeping family life in a state of turmoil, and it delays the client's progress in developing better responses to the controlling behavior of the parents. For a more satisfactory relationship to be developed, the adolescent should come to understand the defense, but direct confrontation may not accomplish that end.

Skilled counselors recognize that a client's defenses may be longtime friends; often they have helped the client tolerate the stresses and pains of life over a long period (Clark, 1991). However, a person's defenses may also help him or her avoid the solution of problems and often result in self-defeat and misery. Even so, the client will resist giving up defenses. The counselor's task is to *work with* rather than to attack the client's resistances (Polster & Polster, 1973). Rather than demand that resistances be given up, the counselor must simply help the client to see and experience them with brighter clarity—to become familiar with his or her longtime friend. In the previous example, the counselor might tentatively test the client's ability to see his or her surly, uncooperative behavior as a defense: "Could it be that you act angrily so you won't feel so controlled?" "Do you see how behaviors that worked for you as a child are now getting in the way of your acting as an adult?" Working with defenses or resistances is only confrontational in the sense that the counselor's interventions are designed to provide the client with useful feedback. The effectiveness of the process is reduced and may even be counterproductive if there is any sense of attack involved.

Because resistance is often accompanied by physical responses such as tight muscles, constricted breathing, rigid posture, failed eye contact, and other signs of discomfort, drawing the client's attention to the physical manifestation can be helpful. This can be done by describing the client's activity, asking the client what the resisting muscles would say if they could talk, slightly exaggerating their behavior, or using one's own body to show the client what he or she is doing. To be effective with these interventions, the counselor will learn from experience with the client which kinds of approaches are most acceptable.

Guidelines for Constructive Confrontation

A serious risk in the confrontational process is that the client may be confused about whether the counselor is an ally or an adversary. When a counselor confronts a client, even with the noblest of motives, the client is not sure of the counselor's intent. Although the counselor may be an ally in the sense of wanting to encourage the client, he or she may come across as an enemy of the client's resistances. It is helpful if the counselor focuses on the fact that all confrontation is *for* and *with* the client, not *to* or *against* the client.

We suggest the following guidelines for confrontations:

- Remember that confrontation should not be the predominant mode of giving feedback to a client. Use it sparingly. Research shows that confrontation represents only 1 to 5% of counselor responses (Hill et al., 1988). It is one of the most powerful interventions a counselor can use, and if misused or overdone it can undo much of the therapeutic progress that has occurred (Miller, Benefield, & Tonigan, 1993). Counselors who use confrontation frequently may be underestimating the client's capacity for self-change and overestimating their role in enlightening the client about himself or herself.
- If you are feeling angry toward your client, you are at risk for misusing confrontation as a mask for anger. You won't help by punishing. If you are angry, you are probably reacting to one of your client's resistances. You can use your anger as a source of information to recognize your client's defense. If you have trouble resolving your anger, seek supervision or consultation with a trusted colleague.
- Be clear about your reasons for confronting. If you have a plan for what you are trying to accomplish with the client, it is more likely that the confrontation is based on the client's needs and not your own and it is more likely to be therapeutically appropriate. Research indicates that counselors view confrontation as a much more helpful mode of communication than clients who tend to see other modes as more useful (Hill et al., 1988).
- Be a total ally of the client, not an ally and an adversary. This means that confrontation should be a feedback experience and that it should not contain implied disapproval or manipulation. Feedback should be behavioral and not judgmental or categorical.

- Use direct and simple language. An inability to express the confrontation clearly should signal caution. Vague language implies that you are unclear about what client material you want to confront, unaware of your motives for confronting, or uncertain whether the client is ready to hear what you want to say. If any of these conditions exist, the time is not right for confrontation.
- Be prepared to admit that a confrontation may be wrong if the client denies its accuracy. Not all denial is resistance. Clients are experts on much of their own experience. After a client rejects a confrontation, the counselor needs to attend to the damage the confrontation may have done to the trusting relationship and to take action to repair the damage, often referred to as a therapeutic rupture.

Case of Lionel

Lionel was a college student seen by a male counselor in a college counseling center. His initial concern was a feeling of depression about being isolated from the other students on the campus. He reported having a few acquaintances but no friends, male or female. The pain of his isolation provided high motivation for him to work on the problem.

During the initial disclosure stage, Lionel and his counselor discussed how it was for him to be in college and what he noticed happening when he talked with fellow students. During these conversations, the counselor noticed a pattern of Lionel speaking disparagingly of others. He seemed to be quite cynical.

When this pattern continued, the counselor decided to confront. His confrontation was the critical moment that moved counseling into the second stage: "Lionel, often I have heard you make cynical statements about people in your classes. You say that you want to make friends, but you say things that are not friendly." This led to some intense exploration of how Lionel's cynicism might affect others with whom he wanted to develop relationships. It also opened up a pattern about which he previously had only a dim perception.

During the third stage, the counselor helped Lionel work on making more positive and supportive statements about others. Making this transition turned out to be difficult. The counselor concluded that Lionel was maintaining his cynicism because he was getting something from keeping it. Counseling moved back into the second stage, and further exploration disclosed that Lionel used his cynicism to maintain a safe distance in his relationship with his father. Lionel felt that if he let himself get too close to his father, he would be really devastated in case he learned, as he suspected, that he was low in his dad's priorities. He had unknowingly been holding on to this fear for a long time. Role-playing helped Lionel develop an important awareness of what was happening in his relationship with his father, what he wanted in the relationship that he was not getting, and what he feared losing. These awarenesses, although painful, helped Lionel conclude that the pattern of cynicism that he used to protect himself in his relationship with his father was not helping him in his peer relationships.

Moving again to Stage 3, Lionel and his counselor did some direct interpersonal communication training in which Lionel's task was to make honest and positive statements to the counselor. The counselor gave supportive feedback to Lionel's effective communications. Putting the principles into practice in his classes and in social situations, Lionel reported that he had made some friends and had two dates that went fairly smoothly. Counseling terminated when Lionel reported that he had been feeling much more comfortable in his peer relationships.

Questions for Further Thought

1. Stage 2 involves helping clients see something about themselves more clearly. What specific observations did Lionel see more clearly as a result of his counseling experience?
2. How do you think Lionel felt when he received the feedback he got from his counselor? How do you think the counselor felt about offering it?
3. During counseling, Lionel chose not to approach his father about their relationship. Do you think this was a good decision? What are the pros and cons?
4. How do you react to cynical people?

INTERPRETATION

Responses that promote in-depth exploration help the client add perspective to his or her conception of self in the environment. Advanced empathy is considered to be additive in the sense that the counselor includes in his or her response some material of which the client is only vaguely aware and that the client has only *implied* in previous statements. Confrontation is additive in the sense that the counselor pulls together elements of the client's story and in-session behaviors that are incongruent so that the client can integrate the inconsistencies. Interpretation is also a form of additive responding, the purpose of which is "to explain rather than merely describe a client's behavior and to change a client's frame of reference in a therapeutic direction" (Clark, 1995, p. 484).

Interpretation is often barely distinguishable from advanced empathy responses (Martin, 2000; Patterson, 1974). This is true because the counselor's listening is attuned by his or her theoretical frame of reference to focus on particular aspects of the client's story. With advanced empathy, the counselor stays with the client's frame of reference, regardless of how much she or he may extend the client's story through adding what is implied; with interpretation, the counselor introduces a new way of thinking about or accounting for the client's experience from the counselor's frame of reference. According to Ivey and Ivey (2003, p. 312), in using interpretation the counselor "provides the client with a new alternate way to consider the situation. . . . [I]nterpretation renames or redefines reality from a new point of view." Some therapists prefer to use the term *reframing* instead of *interpretation,* because it directly describes the introduction of a new *frame* for viewing the client's concern and may avoid some of the association with depth therapy carried by the term *interpretation.*

Constructing an interpretive response involves placing meaning on observational data using *theory* (Brammer, Abrego, & Shostrum, 1993). When interpreting, the counselor presents the client with hypotheses about relationships, meanings, or behaviors that emerge from his or her *theoretical* understandings of human personality. For example, consider Raynette, who lives with her mother, sister, and infant daughter. She reports feeling very "stuck," unhappy that her life is not going anywhere, and yet seemingly unable to take any steps to initiate change. An interpretive response might be, "In some ways you are still living much as you always have with your mother taking all the responsibility. I wonder if it is pretty scary to think of being responsible for not only yourself but also your daughter, and maybe that keeps you from taking any steps at all." Although this is not a strongly leading interpretation, it departs from the client's frame of reference that she just can't seem to get herself moving to the counselor's frame of reference that it is "scary"—and therefore immobilizing—to think of having all the supports of home removed. The counselor's view, based on his or her understanding of human personality, is that immobilization (like other human behavior) is not random; it has causes. Another hypothesis that may be applicable to Raynette is that she may be experiencing a clinical depression and that her mood contributes to her inability to take any action. Providing a label (from the counselor's frame of reference) for the behaviors, thoughts, and feelings identified as depression would open the possibility of talking about how people can manage depressed feelings and move beyond them.

The frequency with which a counselor uses interpretation and the nature of those interpretations depend on the theory or theories to which the counselor adheres, though research suggests that on average, interpretations account for 6 to 8% of counselor responses (Barkham & Shapiro, 1986; Hill et al., 1988). Person-centered counselors—that is, those who rely most heavily on the work of Carl Rogers—generate the fewest interpretations because they regard the client's frame of reference as the only one that matters and generally see interpretive responses as errors. In the psychoanalytic approach, interpretation is much more common, as it is seen as the essential process through which clients gain new insight into their symptoms and dynamics (Garske & Molteni, 1985). Psychoanalytic counseling "focuses on establishing causal relationships between past and current experiences" or between events in the present that the client has failed to connect (Clark, 1995, p. 485). On the other hand, a counselor with a cognitive theoretical orientation who sees client meanings, feelings, and behaviors as a function of thought processes would generate frequent hypotheses based on his or her observations about the client's faulty thinking. A behavioral counselor would use interpretation less commonly but may identify how a client's behaviors are self-defeating as seen from his or her frame of reference or may label some behaviors as "secondary reinforcers" to help explain why a behavior a client appears to find unrewarding has subtle reinforcers.

According to Frank and Frank (1991), interpretation is a valuable counseling intervention because it has the potential to bolster a client's sense of security and mastery. It offers a name to a set of experiences that had been confusing and overwhelming. As soon as it is named (assuming, of course, that the name makes sense to the client), the inexplicable becomes understandable and what is understood and identified loses the power to overwhelm. Properly used interpretation can increase hope and energy for change. Not surprisingly, then, accurate and well-timed interpretations appear to be viewed as strongly therapeutic by counselors and clients alike (Hill et al., 1988).

Most counselors agree, however, that interpretation is not therapeutic if used in the first stage of counseling. Precisely because it asks the client to think differently about the causes and sources of their problems, interpretation relies on both a strong, trusting relationship and a reasonably clear picture of the content and context of the client's problems. Premature interpretation backfires. It has the effect of making the counselor seem insensitive to the client's discomfort with disclosing negative material and of inducing the client to cling tightly to those defenses that have helped him or her construe reality in safe but ineffective terms. Interpretation should not be used at the close of a counseling session or in the termination stage of counseling so as to avoid opening issues that cannot be adequately integrated in the remaining time.

━━━━━━━━━━━━━━━━━━━━━ *Case of Michael* ━━━━━━━━━━━━━━━━━━━━━

Michael was a 24-year-old European-American male who presented for counseling with a history of having lost a half dozen jobs since graduating from college 3 years ago. In each instance, Michael described having been supervised very closely, treated like a child, and evaluated unfairly. In each case, he either quit or was fired after repeated squabbles with his supervisor. From Michael's frame of reference, the problem with each of the positions was his bad luck in having such ineffective supervisors.

Two weeks after starting yet another new job as manager of the photography department of a discount department store, Michael reported that the store manager was "on his back" about the time clock and was always "giving him orders" about maintaining the displays in neat order.

CLIENT: This guy is a real neat freak, and you'd think that 10 minutes in the morning would be the end of the world.
COUNSELOR: You really get ticked when a supervisor tells you what to do. (Simply a reflection of the reported affect.)
CLIENT: Yeah, and I sure seem to know how to pick 'em. Why do I always end up with such tight asses every time?
COUNSELOR: Have you thought about the ways in which all your relationships with supervisors are the same?
CLIENT: Well, none of them seem to trust me to do what is right. And when they start putting the pressure on, I just get angry and see what I can do to get back at them.

Although it is possible that Michael has had bad luck with supervisors, most counselors would consider the odds of finding a half dozen such poor situations unlikely and would begin looking for what the client may have contributed to the disputes that ensued. The preceding response is mildly confrontive, but by and large it stays with the client's frame of reference. However, in an earlier conversation the counselor had also learned that the client had a stormy relationship with his father during the growing-up years and continues to harbor anger toward his father.

COUNSELOR: "Do you see how similarly you seem to feel about your employers and the way your father always seemed to doubt your ability to do things right?"

CLIENT: (After a long pause.) Do you really think that I'm picking bosses who are just like my father?

This interpretation is based on the hypothesis that the client may be projecting elements of his relationship with a strict and controlling father onto his employers. Michael then moved into a discussion about how he hates to be told what to do, even though he knows that it is the supervisor's job to structure his work. He acknowledged that he sometimes even hears his father's voice coming from a supervisor and he just gets furious. From there, the counseling proceeded to the planning of some control and time-out strategies to help Michael deal more effectively with supervisors as a short-term goal while working toward a better understanding of his father as a long-term goal. The interpretation of the link between his job behavior and his reactions to a controlling father placed the employment problem in a new frame of reference and showed the way to some new goals and strategies for the counseling.

ROLE-PLAYING

Role-playing, also called behavior rehearsal, can be especially useful in solving interpersonal relationship difficulties and has its application in both the second and third stages. In the second stage, the focus is on increasing awareness of self and others and setting goals; in the next stage, action planning is the main agenda. In practice, the two stages often run together when role-playing is used.

The principal value of role-playing is that it can bring into the present events that have happened in the past or events that the client anticipates will be possible future encounters. Role-playing can be set up in various ways. Often the counselor will play one party to a conflict, perhaps the client's sibling, spouse, or parent, while the client plays himself or herself. The counselor can also play the client, freeing the client to play the other party. Or, with use of an empty chair, the client may take on both roles— himself or herself and the significant other—changing chairs between responses and delivering both person's lines.

Setting up the role-play is an important part of the activity. After carefully explaining how role-playing might help, the counselor will find it useful to give the client the role of drama director—that is, the client decides (with help) who plays which role, instructs the counselor on the characteristics of the person he or she is playing, and decides how to play his or her own role. The client should clarify details about the setting to achieve as much authenticity as possible. It may be useful to have several rehearsals to get all the details right and to portray personalities accurately. The rehearsals themselves deepen the client's understandings of the parties involved, while at the same time they inform the counselor.

During the role-playing, the counselor has several tasks: to play his or her own role accurately, to pay close attention to the client's behavior and emotions, and to pay close attention to his or her own inner experiencing. When the role-playing is completed, the client and the counselor discuss what has occurred. The counselor has a rich supply of information from the experience to offer as feedback to the client. The information can come from within oneself and be offered as immediacy communication ("As I played your wife I wanted to hear your ideas but was feeling talked down to and was hurt that you did not see me as an equal to you") or from the counselor's observations of the client ("As I asserted my ideas your muscles seemed to freeze"). The feedback helps the client clarify emotions, desires, beliefs about the other person, beliefs about himself or herself, and the impact of his or her behaviors. These new insights serve as the basis for developing action strategies in the third stage. Role-playing can have powerful emotional effects, and counselors should help clients sort through the affective components of role-playing as much as they attend to the insights gained in the process.

Case of Jack and Eve

Jack and Eve were a married couple in their mid-30s who had been married 8 years. Their one child, Tommy, was 6 years old. They came for counseling because, as Eve described it, "Our family is not a healthy place to live." Their relationship was characterized by disagreements over money, role assignments, and parenting practices. Jack felt stress at work and was short-tempered at home. Eve was primarily responsible for child care, managed the household affairs, and was not employed outside the home.

In one session, a recent episode in which Jack had yelled at Tommy was the focus of counseling. A role-playing session was established in which the counselor played the role of Tommy. The situation was as follows: Jack came home from work to find Tommy's room a mess. He hollered loudly for Tommy to come to his room immediately. Slowly and apprehensively, Tommy approached his room. Once Tommy was there, Jack proceeded to "read him the riot act." In the midst of Jack's diatribe, "Tommy" (the counselor) suddenly shut his eyes, held his hands over his ears, turned around, ran away, and hid under a piece of furniture in the next room. This infuriated Jack, who demanded in a loud voice that "Tommy" come back. In a quaking voice, "Tommy" said, "No, I'm afraid you might kill me."

The role-play ended. Jack was visibly shaken and waved his hand to stop the action. He sat down and held his head in his hands. He repeated several times, "I just never realized how frightening I am when angry." After a while the counselor asked Eve about her reactions to Jack's anger. Her statement, "Just like Tommy's. It terrifies me too," validated the feedback.

Until this experience, Jack had not taken seriously the effects of his own anger on others, rationalizing it away, disowning it, and arguing that other family members had to learn to accept his anger. The role-playing situation in which the counselor deliberately did what he thought Tommy wanted to do but was afraid to do helped Jack see and experience the effects of his anger. In a later session there was a follow-up exploration of what Jack would lose by controlling his anger. This led to discoveries related to his fear of losing power, fear of being the underdog, and the use of anger to intimidate. Over time, these insights seemed to help Jack reduce his expressed anger, show more patience, and express affection more easily.

Questions for Further Thought

1. What principles of role-playing did the counselor use with Jack and Eve? Were there other things he could have done?
2. From the information presented, how would you describe Jack? Do you see additional counseling work that may be needed?
3. What principles about giving feedback did the counselor use?
4. Have you ever received surprising feedback about how another saw you? How did you react when you received it? Did you change as a result?

SUMMARY

The second stage of counseling is a time for in-depth exploration of themes and issues related to the client's concerns. As exploration occurs, the counselor's task is to help the client develop deeper self-awareness and a fuller perspective on self and others that can lead to growth, more effective coping, and clarification of goals. Feedback is the primary vehicle through which awareness occurs. Communication modes such as advanced empathy, immediacy, confrontation, interpretation, and role-playing stimulate this process. Clients will be more likely to internalize feedback and use it to plan change if they feel safe and respected in the counseling relationship and if the counselor exerts every effort to continuously reinforce the message that she or he acts out of caring. Because these modes can disrupt the therapeutic alliance if overused or improperly implemented, counselors need to carefully monitor client responses to such statements and act quickly to repair any ruptures that occur.

≈≈≈ *DISCUSSION QUESTIONS* ≈≈≈

1. Research suggests that clients view interpretations more positively than they view confrontations in counseling. What do you think accounts for that difference when both modes of communication are somewhat anxiety provoking?
2. What is the difference between a mixed message and a straightforward message? What makes mixed messages so common in relationships?
3. Do you agree with the authors' position that insight alone is unlikely to result in meaningful therapeutic change? Why or why not?
4. What are the situations in which you think counselors would be particularly vulnerable to the misuse of immediacy and confrontation?
5. Because clients so often find confrontation anxiety provoking and threatening, should counselors simply avoid its use? What would be lost or gained?

REFERENCES

Barkham, M., & Shapiro, D. (1986). Counselor verbal response modes and experienced empathy. *Journal of Counseling Psychology, 33,* 3–10.

Brammer, L. M., Abrego, P. J., & Shostrum, E. L. (1993). *Therapeutic counseling and psychotherapy* (6th ed.). Englewood Cliffs, NJ: Prentice-Hall.

Clark, A. J. (1991). The identification and modification of defense mechanisms in counseling. *Journal of Counseling & Development, 69,* 231–236.

Clark, A. J. (1995). An examination of the technique of interpretation in counseling. *Journal of Counseling & Development, 73,* 483–490.

Cormier, S., & Nurius, P. S. (2002). *Interviewing strategies for helpers* (4th ed.). Pacific Grove, CA: Brooks/Cole.

Dinkmeyer, D., Dinkmeyer, D., Jr. (1985). Adlerian psychotherapy and counseling. In S. J. Lynn & J. P. Garske (Eds.), *Contemporary psychotherapies: Models and methods* (pp. 117–154). Columbus, OH: Merrill.

Egan, G. (2002). *The skilled helper: A problem-management and opportunity development approach to helping* (7th ed.). Pacific Grove, CA.: Brooks/Cole.

Frank, J. D., & Frank, J. B. (1991). *Persuasion and healing: A comparative study of psychotherapy* (3rd ed.). Baltimore: Johns Hopkins University Press.

Garske, J.P., & Molteni, A.L. (1985). Brief psychodynamic psychotherapy: An integrative approach. In S.J. Lynn & J.P. Garske (Eds.). *Contemporary psychotherapies: Models and methods* (pp. 69–116). Columbus, OH: Merrill.

George, R.L., & Cristiani, T.S. (1995). *Counseling theory and practice* (4th ed.). Boston: Allyn & Bacon.

Harrison, R. (1977). Defenses and the need to know. In R.T. Golembiewski & A. Blumberg (Eds.), *Sensitivity training and the laboratory approach: Readings about concepts and applications* (3rd ed., pp. 78–84). Itasca, IL: Peacock.

Hill, C.E., Helms, J.E., Tichenor, V., Spiegel, S.H., O'Grady, K.E., & Perry, E.S. (1988). The effects of therapist response modes in brief psychotherapy. *Journal of Counseling Psychology, 35,* 222–233.

Hill, C.E., & O'Brien, K.M. (1999). *Helping skills: Facilitating exploration, insight and action.* Washington, DC: American Psychological Association.

Ivey, A.E., & Ivey, M.B. (2003). *Intentional interviewing and counseling: Facilitating client development in a multicultural society* (5th ed.). Pacific Grove, CA: Brooks Cole.

Jourard, S.M. (1971). *The transparent self* (rev. ed.). New York: Van Nostrand Reinhold.

Lynn, S.J., & Frauman, D. (1985). Group psychotherapy. In S.J. Lynn & J.P. Garske (Eds.). *Contemporary psychotherapies* (pp. 419–458). Columbus, OH: Merrill.

Martin, D.G. (2000). *Counseling and therapy skills* (2nd ed.). Prospect Heights, IL: Waveland Press.

Miller, W.R., Benefield, R.G., & Tonigan, J.S. (1993). Enhancing motivation for change in problem drinking: A controlled comparison of two therapist styles. *Journal of Consulting and Clinical Psychology, 61,* 455–461.

Patterson, C.H. (1974). *Relationship counseling and psychotherapy.* New York: Prentice Hall.

Perls, F. (1969). *Gestalt therapy verbatim.* Moab, UT: Real People Press.

Polster, E., & Polster, M. (1973). *Gestalt therapy integrated: Contours of theory and practice.* New York: Brunner/Mazel.

Rogers, C.R. (1961). *On becoming a person.* Boston: Houghton Mifflin.

Truax, C.B. (1976). A scale for the rating of accurate empathy. In C.R. Rogers (Ed.) with E.T. Gendlin, D.J. Kiesler, & C.B. Truax (Eds.), *The therapeutic relationship and its impact: A study of psychotherapy with schizophrenics* (pp. 555–584). Westport, CT: Greenwood Press.

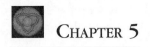

CHAPTER 5

COMMITMENT TO ACTION AND TERMINATION

The process of self-exploration and accurate assessment of problems with an empathic and perceptive counselor is sometimes sufficient to allow clients to identify what they need to do to solve problems and implement enduring change. This pattern is most common when the difficulties are short lived and circumscribed and clients have adequate coping skills and good support systems. At other times, particularly when the problems are chronic and personal resources limited, insight is insufficient to help clients make changes. In these situations, the activities inherent in the second stage of counseling bring the client to the point of understanding herself or himself better and more fully defining the problems that provoked entrance into counseling but do not clearly identify a preferred set of actions to resolve the concerns. The client is no longer so confused about the issues, has more insight into the sources and patterns of the problem, feels hopeful about success, and has experienced some release from emotional tension. However, the goals for change are still general, and the course of action to achieve them is still vague. Or the actions required for change are clear but entail risks that seem threatening to the client.

This chapter focuses on the third stage of the counseling process— commitment to action—and it describes procedures to bring counseling to a successful termination. It highlights the collaborative work of the counselor and the client to define specific outcome goals for counseling and use those goals to design action plans to achieve them. Also discussed are the counselor's and client's tasks while the interventions are being implemented, the need to evaluate the effectiveness of the interventions, and the counselor's responsibilities when the action plans are not implemented or don't work as intended. Finally, the process of ending counseling, referred to as termination, is described and options for ending the process on a positive note are examined.

THE PROCESS OF GOAL SETTING

The first task of the third stage of the counseling process is goal setting. At the end of the second stage, the counselor and the client have a clear assessment (or diagnosis) of the difficulties that brought the client to counseling and a good sense of the client's strengths and resources for coping with the problems. Consider the experience of the following client to better understand the transition from the second stage.

─────────────── *The Case of Bernard* ───────────────

At the end of the second stage, Bernard, a man who entered counseling because of loneliness and unsatisfying personal relationships, appreciates the way he seems to be distancing other people, the way he tends to misinterpret their desire for independence as rejection of him, and his propensity to think negative thoughts about himself and thereby heighten his feelings of loneliness and frustration. Bernard now sees how this pattern developed from his early relationships and how he acts to maintain that interpersonal style in current relationships. However, exactly what to do about this pattern or what he really wants from his relationships is not entirely clear yet. When asked, Bernard may respond that his goals are to get closer to people and feel less lonely and less self-critical. It is the job of the counselor at this point to help the client translate these general goals into more specific growth-oriented goals.

- Does he want a long-term intimate relationship with one person? Does he want to have more friends?
- Does he want to make new friends more easily? Does he want to know how to respond better to stressors and conflict in relationships?
- Does he want to be able to share his emotions and personal beliefs honestly and ask for support when he needs it?
- Does he want to be more giving to others and less self-interested? How will he know that he's not lonely anymore—that is, what internal and external markers will signal change?
- Does he want to learn how to substitute a realistic self-appraisal for his self-criticism?
- If he wants many of these things, which takes priority in his view? What first appears to be a clear goal may have a number of different meanings to the client.

───

The process of specifying growth-oriented goals ensures that both client and counselor know where they are headed in the third stage, enabling them to choose appropriate intervention strategies. Goal setting has been compared to identifying the route one is taking on a trip. A common expression is "If you don't know where you're headed, you may end up somewhere else." The most satisfying trips are usually carefully planned. The pretrip plan need not be rigidly adhered to, but a sense of the steps to the destination is not lost in the deviations from the plan. This is a fitting analogy for the task of counseling at the beginning of the third stage.

What are the signals that the timing is right for a transition from assessment and in-depth exploration to goal setting and commitment to action? The most important markers are that the problem(s) have been well defined, that a mutually agreeable assessment of the history and factors that have prevented change has been reached, and the process of self-exploration is no longer yielding new insights for the client. A client's responses change emphasis, indicating restlessness with the status quo and a need to change. If the person has entered counseling because of depressed feelings, the counselor may hear more comments that he or she is "tired of feeling this way" and is prepared to do what it takes to change even if risks are involved. There may be less hopelessness and more frustration, even irritability with the current state of affairs. The emotional release of sharing the pain with the counselor has become less rewarding for the client, and the need to focus on the future is stronger. Fear of change and resistance to change do not disappear, but a new sense that it is time to "get on with things" is added to those feelings.

At this point, counselors can shift their attention from problem assessment to goal setting. When a client has come to counseling to make a decision about an educational path or a career choice, the goals are fairly explicit from the start, and the transition to action planning is typically smooth. However, when a client comes with emotional pain or problem behaviors, the initial motivation for counseling is to stop feeling so bad or acting in such unproductive ways, and the goals are often vague. For example, a married couple may enter counseling because they want to stop arguing so much. This goal is entirely sufficient for the early stages of counseling; however, when exploration and diagnosis are complete, such a goal is unlikely to generate productive plans for change. The couple needs more clarity about what kind of relationship they want instead and how much less conflict will be defined as success. Plainly put, the question is "What else do you want to think and feel about each other besides anger, and what else do you want to do besides argue?" The counselor guides the transition to specific new patterns of thinking, feeling, and acting through the use of selective reflection, confrontation, and what Hackney and Cormier (2001) call "ability–potential responses" to clarify goals. Because the use of confrontation is described in detail in Chapter 4, the discussion here focuses on selective reflection and ability–potential responses. Confrontation when used in Stage 3 focuses on discrepancies between what the client has stated that his or her goals are and the actions that make those goals unlikely to be achieved.

Selective Reflection

When a counselor uses selective reflection, he or she chooses to respond more fully to the part of a client's statement that shows readiness or yearning for change. The focus is still on the affective message the client is sending, but the counselor responds to that message selectively. Here are some examples:

Interaction A

CLIENT: I really hate it when I yell so much at my daughter. I know it stems from the way I overidentify with her and worry that she will repeat the mistakes I've made in life. I know it's not healthy for either of us and it doesn't match with the way I want to relate to her.

COUNSELOR: Sounds like you are learning how your basic relationship problem with your daughter gets expressed in daily life. You also seem to have a picture in your mind of how you would like to act with her. I'd be interested to hear more about that picture.

Interaction B

CLIENT: I'm sick and tired of being alone in my room when I know other teenagers are out having fun. This fear I have of making a fool of myself is really self-defeating.

COUNSELOR: Sounds like you are fed up with the old pattern and are ready to do more of the things other people your age do. The other part of it may be that the fear doesn't seem so all consuming anymore and you feel stronger and better able to fight its negative effects in your life.

Interaction C

CLIENT: One thing has become clearer to me over the past few weeks in rehab. No matter how unfair it is that I'm stuck in this wheelchair or how angry or sad it makes me, I'm still going to be in this damn chair for the rest of my life.

COUNSELOR: You're becoming more aware now of the reality of your disability, and you seem to be looking for something else to fill your life besides rage and grief.

In each of these examples, the counselor reflected back affective content to the client, but the counselor's statements were centered on that portion of the feeling associated with readiness to change. These are, in essence, advanced-empathy responses as discussed in Chapter 4. If you look at Interaction A closely, you will see that the counselor responded to only one part of the emotion the client expressed; thus, the response is a selective reflection. The counselor offered no verbal response to the self-hate expressed in the opening phrase. An ordinary reflection would have attended to the anger at self implicit in the statement. It is important to note that this counselor is still reflecting the feelings expressed or implied by the client. No feelings are being suggested that are not at least at the edge of the client's awareness.

Selective reflection is used effectively when the client has progressed to the point of insight into self; clients who are pushed in this direction by their counselors usually respond with resistance. When the client feels he or she is not freely choosing a goal or action plan, the part of the self that fears change gains strength, and the counseling progress stops until the client feels in control again. Some clients may even drop out of counseling prematurely if they feel trapped into actions they do not wish to undertake. When clients feel distressed by a counselor's selective reflection, the counselor may wish to encourage the client to elaborate on that discomfort so that therapeutic progress is not interrupted. Clients are often uneasy about verbalizing negative reactions to their counselors who seem to be trying to help; as a result, the responsibility to monitor both verbal and nonverbal reactions to selective reflections and initiate open discussion of them lies with the counselor. Such a counselor response commonly takes the form of an immediacy statement, such as "I'm aware that you have begun fidgeting in your chair and your face looks more tense than it looked before. I'm wondering if you felt uncomfortable with my last comment."

In one way, most reflections of client feelings are selective regardless of the stage of counseling, because counselors choose how to respond to each client statement. Remember that in Chapter 4 selective reflection was used to increase the concreteness of counseling by electing to respond only to consequential material. Even so, a counselor does not choose to respond to every affective message conveyed by a client. If, for example, in Stage 2 a client expresses anger, hurt, and fear in the same comment, a counselor may elect to focus only on one of those emotions because that facilitates the process of self-exploration. Similarly, if a client hints at a feeling that may be difficult to discuss openly early in the counseling process, a counselor may decide not to reflect that feeling because of the fragile nature of the relationship at that point. Sometimes counselor reflections are selective because the counselor simply could not remember or attend to all the emotions expressed in a lengthy client statement. The deliberate use of selective reflection, though, is effective for facilitating a purposeful focus on goal setting and action planning in Stage 3.

━━━━━━━━━━━━━━━━━━━━━━━━━━ *Exercise* ━━━━━━━━━━━━━━━━━━━━━━━━━━

As an exercise, write selective reflections for the following client statements and share them with a partner for feedback.

1. I'm beginning to see that if I stay with my husband I'm likely to get hit again and again. He's not going to change. It's not so scary to accept that now.
2. Wow! I'm really enjoying this internship in biochemistry. It's so much more fun than the journalism internship I did 2 years ago. I can see this enjoyment of biochemistry lasting a long time too. (Statement of a college senior in career counseling.)
3. After the past few counseling sessions, I've been able to catch myself responding to my partner in passive–aggressive ways. The pattern is clearer and I'm tired of repeating it.
4. I guess that the only way I'm going to get free of the mindlessness of high school is to put up with the teachers and the homework and graduate. I don't want to drop out and end up in a dead-end job.

━━━

Ability-Potential Responses

Another way to clarify and specify goals is to use ability–potential responses. According to Hackney and Cormier (2001), an ability–potential response "allows the counselor to suggest that the client has the ability or potential to engage in a specified form of activity" (p. 105). Ability–potential responses may be used when the goals have been decided but the action plans to reach those goals are still under consideration. Consider the following examples in which the counselor gives an ability–potential response:

Interaction A

CLIENT: I could approach my professor about an extension to complete the course after my husband is out of the hospital, but this professor doesn't seem very understanding about the lives of students outside the classroom.

COUNSELOR: That's one good alternative. I can give you information about the college's procedures for getting course extensions. Let's use the next few minutes to think of other alternatives, and then you can choose the one you think best.

Interaction B

CLIENT: I'm sick of being alone. Next Friday I'm going to a bar to see if I can meet a woman there. I'm not likely to meet anyone if I stay in my apartment.

COUNSELOR: You're right. Putting yourself in a social situation where women are around is a first step to getting to know someone. Are there other social situations in addition to a bar that might also help you achieve this goal? Let's brainstorm about them, and then you can make the decision about which alternative you prefer.

Interaction C

CLIENT: I want to let my friend know how much she has hurt my feelings, but I'm afraid I'll use all the wrong words and risk the whole friendship.

COUNSELOR: I've noticed that in counseling you have been able to let me know when I have frustrated you and that you've done it without blaming me. How can you use your success with direct communication with me in your conversation with your friend?

The purpose of each of these counselor responses was either to help the client become aware of his or her capabilities or to expand the possible goals and choices generated by the client. When an ability–potential response is used to expand the available choices in a given situation, the client also learns a more adequate form of problem solving. All too often, what causes people pain and dysfunction is not so much the problems in living that they encounter but a constricted style of trying to solve those problems. The expectation is that the process of exploring a wide variety of alternatives and weighing the merits of each will help clients learn a new way of approaching difficulties that will generalize to other issues in their lives. In summary, the diagnostic and exploration processes help the counselor and the client assemble all necessary information. Confrontations and selective reflections further mobilize the client's readiness for change, and ability–potential responses structure the goal setting so that all possible alternative solutions to the problem are weighed.

What is involved in the process of weighing alternatives? It involves discussion of what the client sees as the likely outcomes of the possible alternatives and an evaluation of the degree of difficulty and desirability of each outcome. Schuerger and Watterson (1977) present one model for assessing the utility of each of several courses of action. They propose that two variables contribute to utility: (1) the probability that the course of action will result in success and (2) the value that the client assigns to succeeding with that alternative. In the end, what the client chooses should have both a high value to the client and a reasonably good chance of success.

Sometimes, ability–potential responses get confused with advice giving, a counselor response that is rarely useful. The underlying goal in giving advice is to get the other person to do what you think best. Advice giving often feels to clients as though the counselor is taking away some of their autonomy in decision making. It is important to keep in mind that clients have probably received lots of unhelpful advice from others before they sought counseling. In contrast, with ability–potential responses, there is no intent to compromise client autonomy or take on a parental role; rather, the counselor's motive is to respect the free choices of clients and enhance their innate capacity for effective problem solving.

One other aspect of ability–potential responses deserves mention. Implicit in an ability–potential response is an affirmation of the client's readiness to change and capacity to find a workable solution. The counselor is making an indirect statement of belief in the client's ability to resolve the problem. The affirming aspect of this type of counselor response is particularly apparent in Interaction B. Adler's term for this category of response is *encouragement* (Dinkmeyer, Dinkmeyer, & Sperry, 1987), and it refers to responses aimed at helping clients to affirm their own resources to reach their goals. Encouragement is also designed to help clients change their perceptions of traits they have been labeling as negative into traits that can be assets. For example, encouragement can help a client transform her perception of herself as stubborn into a perception of herself as persistent or tenacious. Then the client can begin to explore ways to use her persistence to help reach her goals.

Counselor Directiveness in Goal Setting

Counseling professionals debate about the degree of directiveness a counselor should show in goal setting and action planning. One part of the debate centers on whether a counselor ought to suggest goals and actions to a client. (No legitimate theory recommends giving advice in a paternalistic fashion.) One view is that counselors have a responsibility to share their expertise with clients and that failing to offer goals or alternative choices denies that expertise and is incongruent with an open and trusting relationship. The alternative position is that client goals or actions that come from others are not truly "owned" by the client and may meet with resistance. The resistance is sometimes shown by direct and open rejection of the suggestion and other times is expressed indirectly through "yes, but" comments about the suggestion. The following example illustrates a "yes, but" response. A counselor suggests that a client in career counseling may benefit from interviewing some people working in the careers the client is considering. The client's immediate response is to generate excuses about why such interviewing can't happen this week, or next week, and so on. When the counselor pursues other alternatives, a pattern of client responses beginning with "yes, but" occurs: "Yes, but that's my mother's birthday and I need to get the party ready that day," or "Yes, but I have a calculus test that week." In this situation, the client is feeling uncomfortable with the suggestion but is unable to express that discomfort directly. Indeed, sometimes clients who get into this pattern are unaware of their resistance to the counselor's proposal. When this happens, the counselor needs to redirect the discussion or gently confront the resistance.

The important factors in deciding whether to suggest a goal or alternative to a client are the depth of the trust in the relationship, the degree of the client's ambivalence about change, and the nature of the problem itself. In a trusting relationship with a client who is highly motivated to change, the presentation of a possible goal or alternative by the counselor has a reasonable probability of being fairly considered. For example, a client who has entered counseling devastated by his wife's breast cancer and feeling alone and fearful may welcome a suggestion that he consider attending a cancer support group for family members of patients. (Note how different this approach is from advising the client that he *ought to attend* such a support group.) In addition, when a client enters counseling with a skill or information deficit (as is often the case in educational or career counseling), the merit of suggesting a goal or alternative to a client is also strong because there is little likelihood that the client will independently generate such information. However, when trust is not deep, the fear of change is almost as strong as the desire for it, or the problem involves deep emotional distress or longstanding maladaptive thoughts and behaviors, the wiser course of action may be to elicit alternatives from the client. The case of the client who repeatedly offers "yes, but" responses illustrates the problems with suggesting goals when a client has some ambivalence about change and decision making.

Sometimes a process of brainstorming about all the possible approaches to resolving the problem can be used effectively. During brainstorming, the counselor and the client collaborate to generate a large pool of alternatives and then evaluate the merit of each possibility generated. Here too there is no expectation that any alternative the counselor has mentioned will be imposed on the client. In any case, the goals or alternatives suggested by the counselor need to derive from the assessment information gathered in Stage 2, with special attention to prior unsuccessful attempts to solve the problem. Suggesting an alternative that appears similar to a failed solution is obviously not likely to be acted upon by the client.

Whether to suggest goals or action plans to a client is also partially dependent on the theoretical orientation of the counselor. Humanistic counselors are reluctant to be directive, but cognitive and behavioral counselors view such activity as completely appropriate. Chapter 10 illustrates these differences more fully. Clearly, the counselor needs to avoid a pattern in which the client is attempting to guess at a goal or approach the counselor already has in mind. This way of interacting is artificial and unproductive from any theoretical perspective.

By including ability–potential responses, confrontations, and selective reflections in his or her repertoire of responses, the counselor can focus the client's attention on goals rather than problems and then, if necessary, divide the goals into achievable subgoals. The goals or subgoals then lead to action plans for change. Consider the following case.

Case: Dolores

Dolores was a 50-year-old widow when she came to a counselor to talk about her frustration with her 25-year-old son, who was still living at home. The son, the youngest of three children, had friends, a full-time job, a car, and other trappings that go with young adulthood. Dolores's problem was that her son would do nothing around the house and expected to be taken care of as a dependent child. He left his dirty clothes on the floor in his bedroom, did not assist in meal preparation or any other household chores, and spent his time at home working on his car or hanging around "underfoot." Dolores had repeatedly asked her son to take responsibility for his own things, to maintain his own room, and to help with the chores. She had refused to provide maid service for him, but the mess that accumulated was intolerable to her, so she eventually cleaned it up. Basically, Dolores wanted out of the "child" care business and felt that she had done her duty for all three children. She also realized that this arrangement was not healthy for her son either. The obvious solution was to tell her son that he would have to move, but that would be stressful because "a mother doesn't kick her own son out of the house, especially one who has lots of other good qualities." She felt hopeless about change.

The process of in-depth exploration and diagnosis by Dolores and her counselor resulted in a definition of the problem as a fear of confronting her son about his unacceptable behavior (the affective component), an exaggeration of the negative consequences if she took such an action (the cognitive component), and a lack of assertiveness with family members (the behavioral component). She was in good health, had reasonably good coping skills, and an adequate support network, in spite of the loss of her husband. Through in-depth exploration, she also came to appreciate more fully that she was doing her son no favor by letting him stay in a childlike role with her. She came to differentiate between her style of acting with family and her style with other people. Dolores saw that with coworkers or acquaintances she had little difficulty expressing her preferences and not acting in an overly submissive way. This healthy adult-to-adult style of interacting had not transferred to her relationship with her grown children or other relatives. In addition, in-depth exploration had also given her insight into the role her beliefs about mothering had played in her passivity with her son. Dolores modified these rather rigid beliefs to see the difference between promoting her son's welfare and simply submitting to his wishes. Through selective reflection, confrontation, and ability–potential responses, Dolores and her counselor generated these goals:

- To express to her son the need for a change in their living arrangements and her desire to have him find an apartment within 2 months without acting angry or sad while expressing this desire. (Dolores also examined two other alternatives before deciding on this goal. The first was to continue with the current situation while modifying her attitude toward it, and the second was to try to get her son to change his behavior at home. The first was quickly rejected, but the second was seriously considered. In the end though, Dolores concluded that it had a low probability of success and would cause even higher stress than asking him to leave.)
- To use positive self-statements while preparing for this conversation with her son and subsequent to it to remind herself that her desires are legitimate and probably better for her son in the long run.
- To generalize this assertive behavior with her son to her style of interacting with her parents, her other children, and her relatives.

If Dolores's case had been more complicated, with a larger set of problems or a wider range of alternative solutions, the use of a chart of apparent alternative goals with a listing of the pros and cons of each might have been helpful. The counselor and the client can work together to develop the chart, or the client can be assigned to work on the chart between counseling sessions. With this approach, the client learns a more constructive method of problem solving and gets the message that the counselor believes the client capable of change.

DESIGN AND IMPLEMENTATION OF ACTION PLANS

Once goals are agreed upon and the client has expressed a commitment to them, the next step in the counseling process is to decide on a set of action plans that will help achieve those goals. Just as the process of goal setting involves careful evaluation of alternative goals, the process of action planning includes a careful review of alternative actions to help the client reach a goal and then a mutual agreement to implement the chosen actions. An *action plan* is a specification of actions the client will take (with the help of the counselor) to reach a goal. An action plan is more than a set of activities; it is a carefully structured course of action that is clearly related to specific goals (Egan, 2002). This term implies change in visible behavior, but it is also used to describe strategies designed to facilitate changes in thinking or feeling. Action plans are typically initiated in the counseling session, but their implementation involves activities outside of counseling. After all, counseling amounts to no more than 1 or 2 hours each week. Real change requires more practice than is allowed within the sessions. In addition, the transfer of learning to other settings is critical if the counseling goals are to be achieved. Sometimes these structured outside activities are called *homework*. Research consistently demonstrates that well-planned homework assignments to which the client is committed result in better counseling outcomes. (See Kazantzis & Lampropoulos, 2002, for a comprehensive review of this literature.) Well-designed homework includes a coherent rationale for doing it, a clear connection between the task and the goals of counseling, a set of activities that are simple to understand and achievable, and a high probability of success. An action plan documentation or homework documentation chart can also be useful in fostering client success in implementing change and in clarifying which aspects of the tasks are most difficult (Razzhavaikina, Scheel, Allen-Portsche, Shamburg, & Bonsi, 2002). When these features are absent, client compliance with homework decreases and ultimately their success in reaching their goals can be compromised (Kazantzis & Lampropoulos, 2002).

In Dolores's case, the action plans were (1) an assertive discussion with her son about her decision, (2) the development and use of positive self-statements when she felt self-doubts, and (3) the use of assertive statements with other relatives when appropriate. To implement these action plans, Dolores needed information about assertiveness, practice in acting assertively, a set of positive self-statements that she believed in and was prepared to use, and guidelines for timing the use of the positive self-statements. The agenda of the third stage of counseling focused on these tasks. The counselor had choices about how he would help Dolores become more assertive. Dolores could join an assertiveness training class, read books on assertiveness, or allow her counselor to guide her in learning assertive behavior. The counselor introduced the alternative methods to Dolores, and together they decided which approach best fit her situation.

A counselor has a responsibility to discuss available options for intervention with a client, explaining how each plan could be carried out, the possible merit and drawbacks of each, and the probable time involved in implementing each. If the counselor believes one plan is superior to the others, he or she should share that judgment with the client. However, unless the client chooses a path the counselor sees as harmful or counterproductive, the counselor should accept the alternative the client selects. Because Dolores seemed to demonstrate appropriate assertiveness with people outside her family, she did not think an assertiveness training class was necessary. Similarly, she found reading a book on assertiveness with family members relatively unappealing because she didn't like to read much. The alternative of practicing assertive behavior in-session with the counselor, who would be able to role-play family members and anticipate especially challenging situations during role-playing, appeared to have the most merit. Then a homework plan was set up for Dolores to practice assertive action with other family members between sessions and report her success or difficulties to the counselor. Once she had succeeded in behaving assertively with other relatives, she would be able to discuss her son's living arrangement with him. Because the client believed this plan would help, they implemented it.

Action planning requires the counselor to possess both sound clinical judgment and practical skills to help implement plans. Judgment involves differentiating between workable and unworkable plans, and skill involves knowledge and experience in using designated methods to carry plans out. A counselor who has only one of these attributes is unlikely to be able to help the client make significant change. One of the authors remembers a powerful experience from counseling practicum in graduate school. Supervision of her counseling was taking place through an audio connection in an adjoining room. The counselor spent a difficult session using a person-centered counseling approach to a client's career indecision and sense of hopelessness about resolving this dilemma. In this hour, the counselor showed unconditional positive regard, empathy, and respect for the client. Her reflections of feeling were concrete and right on target, it seemed. As she entered the "debriefing" with the supervisor after the session, the supervisor opened with this comment: "That was skillful Rogerian counseling with your client. Unfortunately, in my judgment, Rogerian counseling was not what that client needed at this time." The supervisor went on to explain his view and made an excellent case for an alternative approach to career counseling. This example epitomizes the need for both skill in carrying out interventions and judgment in selecting wisely among the wide variety of interventions available. At this stage in training, the counselor had plenty of the former but not enough of the latter.

In the case of Dolores, the counselor needed to use professional judgment to determine whether the goals chosen by Dolores were realistic and likely to be helpful. Professional judgment also comes into play in deciding what kind of assertiveness-training method would be most suitable for Dolores. Finally, the counselor needs skill in conducting assertiveness training and in tailoring positive self-statements to Dolores's needs.

Beginning counselors may find the variety of intervention strategies available to them overwhelming. Hill and O'Brien (1999) refer to this phase of counseling as the most daunting for the novice counselor. One helpful way to organize action planning is by using the template offered by Brammer, Abrego, & Shostrum (1993), who divide action planning into three categories: "(1) strategies for restructuring client self-perceptions; (2) strategies for reducing physiological and emotional distress; and (3) strategies for behavior change" (p. 172). The counselor's theoretical orientation influences the degree to which counselors rely on strategies from each of these three categories, but most counselors use some combination of interventions from each category.

Strategies for changing self-perceptions can be viewed as interventions that help modify a client's thinking about self. In the case of Dolores, the action plan that involved increasing the use of positive self-statements was a strategy to change her view of herself. Consciously telling herself accurate positive things would help to counteract the destructive and untrue negative messages that were part of her prior learning. In essence, one could view the whole in-depth exploration stage of the counseling process as a plan to change self-perceptions. What is distinctive about this intervention in the third stage of counseling is the explicit focus on changing self-perceptions as a goal of counseling. In the second stage, such changes often occur, but they tend to emerge from the exploration and diagnostic process rather than in response to explicit goal setting. Clients may also seek change in their perceptions of others. For instance, a young woman who experienced date rape may have decided that all men will take advantage of her if given the opportunity. Because she has come to recognize that this generalization is untrue and compromises the quality of her life, one of her goals for counseling is to help her change her thinking about men.

Another goal of this young woman may be to reduce her emotional distress over her sexual assault. An action plan aimed at this goal avoids minimizing the seriousness of the assault and helps her learn strategies to cope with the powerful negative emotions those memories engender. Her counselor may teach her a deep-breathing technique to use when fearful feelings emerge or may help her to develop ways to work off her anger without hurting herself or others. If she feels depressed, her plan may be to seek out contacts with friends or to substitute positive statements for the negative ones the depressive affect produces.

Strategies for reducing emotional distress are not as directly applicable to Dolores's case, because she is not highly fearful or angry about the confrontation with her son. Such strategies are applicable to assisting a client who suffers from panic attacks, for example. Relaxation techniques or biofeedback procedures fall into this category, as do strategies that involve expanding the client's support network or, in the case of severe anxieties or depression, using anti-anxiety or antidepressant medications.

Interventions for behavior change are apparent in the assertiveness-training plans Dolores and her counselor developed. She intended to change her verbal behavior by applying the assertiveness skills she used in other situations to her family interactions. In the case of the person who suffers from panic attacks, possible interventions include contracts with the client to gradually engage in feared activities, the initiation of pleasurable activities such as exercising to distract from the obsessive worry about whether a panic attack will occur, and the design of a plan for self-reward as each small change is accomplished.

The counselor and the client also make a mutual decision about whether involving other people in the action plan would be helpful. If Dolores's son agreed to come to counseling with her, would such an activity have merit? Would it be better than the other alternatives chosen? Still other intervention strategies could have been useful to Dolores.

Exercise

Try brainstorming with a partner about other intervention strategies that might have been useful with Dolores. After you have developed at least three such strategies, role-play a session in which one person takes the role of the counselor and the other plays the role of Dolores. The role-play should last at least 10 to 15 minutes. In that session, the task is to discuss the three possible action plans and come to some agreement about their merits and limitations. The goal of this exercise is to gain some insight into how alternatives are generated and how the collaboration process proceeds in this stage of counseling. When the role-play finishes, discuss the experience.

Evaluate Outcomes

In the final analysis, the quality of an action plan depends on the satisfaction that its implementation brings to the client. Only after the fact can the counselor know whether his or her hypotheses were sound and whether the decision-making process took into account all the important factors. In counseling about the management of interpersonal affairs, a counselor often has the opportunity to help a client evaluate choices by reviewing events that occur between counseling sessions as the client implements his or her decisions. In matters requiring long-term planning, implementation may occur over a period of years, and evaluation will be a prolonged process. A client who has experienced effective counseling is likely to have the resources to analyze progress and likely to seek the help of another counselor if new problems he or she faces are complex.

To return again to Dolores, she did ask her son to leave. He was not at all upset and, in fact, seemed almost to have been waiting to be "pushed out of the nest." He liked his new independence, and he checked from time to time to see how his mother was getting along. Dolores enjoyed the freedom of not struggling with her son about mundane things, but she was still not fully satisfied with her living situation.

Repeat the Process

If, after evaluating the outcomes of a choice or course of action, a client still experiences stress or dissatisfaction, the whole process must be repeated. It is possible that the lack of success resulted from oversights somewhere along the line. The problem may not have been defined properly, or the decision about which problem was of greatest importance may have been wrong. Perhaps there was insufficient attention to information about the client's preferences or skills. Some of the hypotheses about the likelihood of success or the value attached to certain successes may have been in error. The choice may have been made impulsively or implemented poorly. Perhaps everything worked as predicted, but the solution of one problem produced another.

Dolores's case provides a good illustration. Because she still seemed somewhat dissatisfied with her living situation, she returned to the counselor about 6 weeks after her son moved. A review of the decision-making process indicated that a good outcome had been achieved. Dolores had gained what she wanted and had not had to suffer the negative consequences that she had anticipated. The fact that her son so readily accepted the move and seemed happy with his new lifestyle affirmed Dolores's decision and alleviated any concerns she had about not being a good mother. In fact, she had more "good mother" feelings after having asked him to move than she had before.

However, Dolores had not anticipated that she would be lonely when her son left, even though this possibility was addressed in the original counseling. She now described her life as dull. It no longer mattered to her whether or not the house was in order, because people visited her infrequently and she was so lonely that she didn't care how it looked herself. A whole new problem existed, and a new set of goals and action steps had to be considered. In a sense, one could say that a bit of information was overlooked in making the original decision, in that she did not anticipate that she would feel so lonely and sad. On the other hand, the favorable consequences of the decision regarding her son affirmed its basic soundness (in spite of her current difficulties, Dolores never regretted her son's departure). Final resolution of the new problem came for Dolores when she decided to take in a housemate to share her home and add variety to her life. In the process of making this decision, she considered the prospects of moving to a place where there were some group activities, living with relatives, and other options. If she had been involved in a romantic relationship that had the possibility of leading to a long-term commitment, this factor would have been weighed into her goal setting. In the end, she decided that her new goal was to find a housemate because this action plan called for the fewest changes in her life—retaining the things she valued and providing company. The action plan involved helping her structure her search for a housemate so that it would maximize her chances of finding someone with whom she felt compatible.

Obstacles to Implementing Action Plans

It would be easy to conclude from the preceding discussion that clients who are helped through the systematic problem-solving approach move easily from making plans within counseling sessions to actions in real-life outside counseling. Unfortunately, the change process is not that easy for many clients. There are two major reasons why people have trouble implementing behavior that they have helped to decide on: (1) any new course of action feels unfamiliar and includes the risk of failure, no matter how logically it has been derived; and (2) old familiar behaviors frequently have rewards as well as difficulties. Even though change may reduce the adversity, it may also reduce the rewards. These rewards are also referred to as *secondary gains.*

Dolores's case again illustrates each of these points. First, there was the prospect of failure when she confronted her son with the decision that he must leave. She did not know if he would become angry and unreasonable. She was not even sure that he would leave if she asked him to do so. If he refused to leave and she could not convince him to do so, there was the potential for the situation to become even more intolerable. The potential for an intervention to backfire also presents an obstacle to implementing action plans. No matter how carefully thought out an intervention is, unintended consequences may ensue. In this respect, clients' caution about change is fully appropriate.

Second, Dolores had adapted her lifestyle to accommodate the behavior of her son. Even though she objected on one level to serving as caretaker to an adult son, her life had a predictable quality. She had a daily routine that obviously would change markedly if she asked her son to leave. This predictability was a secondary gain from the status quo. Another major deterrent to action for Dolores was the secondary gain she experienced from being able to think of herself as a "good mother." A good mother takes care of her "child" and gains a measure of self-identity through the process of being a good caregiver. A final reward of the status quo that did not become obvious to Dolores or her counselor until after it was removed was the fact that she enjoyed having another person in the house for companionship. Failure to understand that secondary gain led to the need for further counseling and probably some delay in establishing a satisfactory long-term living situation.

This analysis can be extended to Dolores's decision to seek a housemate. This decision brought up the question of how well she would get along with a stranger living in her house. The housemate could have personality attributes or personal habits as objectionable as those of Dolores's son. Furthermore, the rewards of living alone included privacy and the freedom to do whatever she wanted whenever she wanted to do it. These secondary gains would be sacrificed if someone came to live in her home.

Supporting a Client's Action Plan

Because it is challenging for many clients to change behaviors in ways they think will improve their lives, counselors frequently find that they must lend support to a client's decision to act. This happens initially within the counseling session when the goal is translated into an action plan, but it must be repeated in subsequent sessions with each homework task and each action plan.

Support for a client's action plan can take several forms. The counselor may focus attention on the benefits the client will derive from acting and achieving desired outcomes, feeling in control of his or her own life, or eliminating unwanted hassles. The counselor may also work on reducing the client's fear of acting by reviewing the potential negative outcomes and helping the client to minimize their likelihood of happening or see that such outcomes might not be so difficult to handle. Clearly, ability–potential responses, selective reflections, and confrontations also bolster the client's energy for implementing the action plan.

The counselor might ask the client to actually picture himself or herself employing some new behavior and describing the scene. By examining such imagery (mental pictures), both client and counselor can gain insight into the client's needs, aspirations, and fears concerning the specific situation. Picturing anticipated outcomes of a new behavior provides an opportunity to rehearse the behavior itself and ways to handle the responses of significant others. Sometimes unexpected responses of significant others can be major interferences with the success of a plan. For example, a spouse accustomed to one set of household routines may express frustration or sadness at the disruption of those routines when a client gets a new job or otherwise changes the daily schedule. These negative reactions can cause a client to retreat from the new behavior or get discouraged about the merits of change. The counselor may choose to bring some scenes to life through role-playing and give the client practice in dealing with anticipated reactions of significant others. At times involving loved ones in the counseling process at this stage can help garner their support for the client's plan.

Support-for-action principles can be applied to Dolores's case. The counselor validated Dolores's wish to be free of unwanted maid duties. He also emphasized her right to assert control over her own life and to establish a desirable lifestyle in her own home. Dolores was asked to picture the worst possible outcome of asking her son to move out. She saw him stalking out of the house angrily, returning the next day for his belongings, and then avoiding contact with Dolores for weeks. After some thought, she concluded that he would not become permanently estranged and that, undesirable as the scene was, she could stand his temporary hostility and absence if she had to. She thought it unlikely that her son would refuse to move, and she felt that other people, especially her son's friends, could be called on to reestablish contact if need be. With clients like Dolores, who have a history of coping effectively with life's difficulties, minimal levels of honest encouragement are usually sufficient to produce action.

With clients who find the solution to a problem to be rather painful or who have a history of being ineffective under stress, the process of mobilizing energy for constructive action may take longer. Frequently, such a client will leave a counseling session having decided on a course of action only to return to the next session having failed to act. In some cases, feeling embarrassed about failing to act, the client will interrupt counseling rather than face the counselor again. The possibility of such a negative outcome reminds counselors how important it is to design action plans and homework tasks carefully and to be alert to signs that the client may not be ready to implement them. Counselors should emphasize that it is normal for some plans to be unsuccessful so that the client feels permission to return to counseling even if he or she could not implement the planned change.

In still other cases, a client may have acted, only to find that stress was still at a high level and the problem had become worse. Consider what might have happened in Dolores's case if her son had refused to move and had increased his demands for caretaking. As mentioned previously, such behavior would not have been unusual; a client's family will often react to changes in his or her behavior by trying to maintain the status quo. Dolores's son could have responded to her request for freedom with an insistence that she maintain her present role. If that had occurred, different strategies and substantially more encouragement would have been needed.

When a client returns to counseling (or is sought out by the counselor) after having failed to carry out the action plan, a reexamination of the plan is in order. The counselor might ask the client to consider what it was about the plan that made it seem so problematical to carry out. Sometimes small changes are indicated, whereas at other times a completely different, more feasible plan may have to be devised. When a client has difficulty coping with stress or is facing a complex situation resistant to change, the counselor needs to help design action plans that are *successive approximations* to the goal. In other words, together with the client, the counselor must design a series of interventions, each of which brings the client one step closer to the goal. For example, if a client's goal is to express anger more appropriately when in conflict with her mother, a successive approximation to the goal is to use the skills learned in counseling with siblings or friends first. The client is more likely to achieve success in such situations and more likely to cope with small failures with these people. The successes and difficulties with these less threatening people can be examined in subsequent sessions, and the client's conflict management skills can be reinforced or modified. When confidence and skills are built, the client will have maximized her chances of handling conflict with her mother appropriately.

Direct Intervention

If a client's stress levels are high and careful implementation of disclosure, exploration, goal setting, and problem solving fails to reduce the stress or produce any promising plan of action for the client, a counselor may decide to take steps to change some condition of the client's life.

There are a variety of possible situations in which a counselor may conclude that a client's present resources are inadequate to his or her circumstances and in which intervention will require manipulation of the environment. It is a heavy responsibility for a counselor to reach such a conclusion because direct intervention is likely to create a feeling in the client that he or she is in need of being taken care of and that other people will always step in to "fix" things when they go wrong. In short, a counselor's failure to help a client exhaust all of his or her own resources can cause the client to become dependent on others and fail to try to cope when the going gets rough.

Nevertheless, there are times when a counselor must step in to avoid unnecessary harm to a client. Situations in which professionals or caregivers act destructively represent one such circumstance and are more common than most people suspect. There are also instances when depressed clients are self-destructive in their behavior and unable to judge for themselves what is best for them. Other clients may be so angry and out of control that the safety of other people is at stake unless the client is placed in a safe environment, such as a hospital. These examples illustrate the kinds of dead-end situations in which a counselor must choose to act in the client's behalf. Unfortunately, aside from the situation in which the client or other people are in imminent danger, there are no easy rules as to when such intervention is required. The counselor must judge that the client is incapable of effective action and that failure to make some kind of change will result in significant harm to the client or other people.

Counselors frequently enlist the help of parents, spouse, teachers, and other significant people in the client's life to assist and support the client. Of course, unless there is real danger, this involvement takes place only with the consent of the client. Environmental support capitalizes on the caring and competence of these people. The usual role of the significant others is to reinforce the change process by carrying out plans that are developed by the client in consultation with the counselor and the significant others. This approach is used frequently with children and is a mainstay of the work of the elementary school counselor (see Chapter 13). Nevertheless, it is essential to involve the client in the planning and to give him or her as much responsibility for change as possible. In this way, the client develops coping skills and confidence in his or her ability that cannot be developed by having others do things.

The Organizational Context of Goal Setting and Action Planning

The model we have presented thus far assumes that the decision about the course of counseling is in the hands of the persons involved. Unfortunately, such control and freedom are not always available. Counselors in community agencies operate under reimbursement constraints that often shorten both the diagnostic and intervention stages of counseling. Similarly, counselors in educational settings are often responsible for large numbers of students as well as having other job responsibilities, so the time for counseling is limited. Even counselors in university settings, who are often free of concerns about insurance or other administrative tasks, experience budget pressures that can limit the number of sessions with any individual client.

In the long run, counselors need to get politically active to modify policies that restrict individual access to counseling. In the meantime, counselors need to be clear in communicating to their clients the constraints that are operating, to focus their attention on the issues of most concern to the client, and work to hone their counseling skills so that the available time is used with maximum effectiveness.

TERMINATION

Ending counseling on a positive note is the final task of Stage 3 of the counseling process. Ideally, termination occurs by mutual agreement when the goals set out by the client are achieved to the satisfaction of the counselor and the client. The client has grown in the ways he or she wanted, often in unexpected yet desirable ways. In addition, in the process of solving the current problem, the client has deepened his or her self-understanding and broadened his or her coping skills; thus, other difficulties that arise will not seem so overwhelming. In other words, the client is better able to transfer learning from this situation to other problems. A positive termination process can provide another important kind of learning for the client—it can instruct clients on how to leave relationships with a sense of "mastery and fulfillment" (Kleinke, 1994, p. 225).

There is another aspect of termination that is important for counselors to recognize in some counseling situations. When the counseling relationship has been intense or prolonged, termination also means dealing with the issue of loss (Ward, 1984). Readiness for termination (which will be discussed in more detail later in this section) is primarily a function of the achievement of outcome goals and secondarily a function of these relationship issues.

We recognize that termination also occurs because of an independent decision by the client, because of the unavailability of the counselor, or because of institutional factors unrelated to either party, such as the end of insurance reimbursement or the end of the academic year. Sometimes counseling is interrupted because of an illness or long absence on the part of the counselor. (An article by Seligman, 1984, deals with this kind of temporary termination and is a helpful resource in such situations.) Under these circumstances, the principles we will describe do apply, although implementing them often requires ingenuity and persistence. Because clients often drop out of counseling or are forced by outside factors to go through termination, the counselor ought to be continually aware of the possibility of a premature end to the relationship and intermittently focus with the client on what has been accomplished thus far in counseling. When premature termination is a possibility, counselors and clients who think in terms of short-range and long-range goals will be more likely to feel some satisfaction and closure when counseling ends, even if the termination date is artificially imposed. Research suggests that when clients voluntarily end counseling prematurely, they do so for one of two reasons: they believe they have accomplished what they set out to do (even if the counselors view that differently) or they feel dissatisfied with the counselor or counseling relationship and want to explore other options for solving their problems (Renk & Dinger, 2002; Todd, Deane, & Bragdon, 2003). These studies highlight the need for active collaboration with a client and an open discussion of client reactions to counseling even when nearing the end of the counseling process.

Readiness for Termination

It is time to terminate counseling when the client has achieved what he or she wants from the experience—that is, when designated goals are attained and desired changes have been sufficiently internalized to be maintained independently. Signs of readiness include positive and identifiable changes in the client's behavior, positive and pervasive changes in the client's mood, consistent reports of improved ability to cope with stress, and clear expressions of commitment to verbalized plans for the future. Important but less obvious signs include a sense of relief and an increase in energy. These signs of readiness for termination begin to appear before the final session, and counselors need to prepare clients for termination before the last appointment. How much preparation is required is largely dependent on the intensity and length of the counseling relationship. For long-term clients, termination should be discussed weeks in advance of the last session. For example, Shulman (1984) recommends that termination from long-term counseling should constitute about one-sixth of the counseling process, and Ward (1984) suggests that termination from counseling takes on special importance when the issues the client brought to counseling deal with dependency and separation from significant others. Regardless of the exact length of time devoted to termination, it is best to conceive of it as a process rather than a single event or session.

With many clients, readiness for termination is not difficult to assess. The client reports changes that have occurred, indicates a clear sense of having acquired what she or he wanted from the experience, and shows clear signs of being ready to end counseling. The changes the client reports are consistent with the counselor's observations. At this point, either the counselor or the client may bring up the idea of termination. In circumstances such as these, the final counseling session is usually devoted to three tasks: looking back, looking forward, and saying goodbye (Marx & Gelso, 1987; Ward, 1984). Looking back involves reviewing the major themes, changes, and critical moments that have occurred during counseling. One of the counselor's goals in termination is to help clients gain deeper insight into just how far down the road of change they have traveled. The counselor offers honest expressions of support to encourage the client to maintain the changes he or she has implemented. Then the counselor helps the client prepare for future developments (i.e., look ahead) and cope with the unavoidable stress and minor regressions that may occur. Counselors need to normalize "setbacks" in progress so that clients can mobilize their newly developed resources to respond effectively to them. Giving clients clear markers for recognizing when they are likely to be able to handle setbacks independently and when they may need a booster session is a wise idea as well. As Martin (2000) notes, quitting counseling is not an "all or none decision" (p. 232) or an irrevocable choice. In fact, the idea that people may need various doses of counseling at several points in their lives is becoming well accepted among mental health professionals. The stresses of 21st century life and the differing needs of people at different life stages (in addition to external limits on access to long-term counseling) have made such an intermittent approach both practical and clinically sensible (Budman & Gurman, 1988; Cummings, 2001).

With other clients, readiness for termination may not be so easy to determine. The client wanting to overcome depression may be depressed less often but may still get mildly depressed occasionally, or the client wanting to behave more assertively may be able to respond assertively to some situations but may still have difficulty under more challenging conditions. Under these conditions, the general principle is that if a client shows strong signs of insecurity about being able to maintain desired changes, he or she is probably not ready to terminate counseling. These conditions may suggest that other themes need exploring as part of second-stage work or that the client needs more practice with interventions as part of third-stage work. Many counselors move to a less frequent schedule of counseling sessions to help the client become more self-reliant and self-confident.

When real change has been accomplished but a client expresses feelings of insecurity in the final session, the insecurity may be more related to difficulty handling the loss of the counseling relationship (i.e., saying good-bye). The counselor and the client need to work together to sort out the source of this insecurity. Sometimes it is simply an indirect expression of the loss of the regular contact with the counselor. When this pattern emerges, it is important to frame the end of counseling as a step forward in client growth rather than a trauma (Pate, 1982, p. 188). Scheduling a follow-up session some time in the future may relieve some of the client's fears about handling the world independently.

When a counselor has a cognitive or behavioral theoretical orientation, the time for termination may be apparent from the beginning of counseling. Many counselors using these frameworks contract with clients for a specific number of counseling sessions. Contracts, of course, are always open to renegotiation as new information emerges, but the time-limited nature of the counseling relationship is apparent from the start in these cases. Those who operate from a humanistic or psychoanalytic tradition typically leave the process more open ended. Thus, no specific ending date is obvious from the start of counseling.

Client Responses to Termination

Research by Marx and Gelso (1987) suggests that clients experience positive feelings about termination—such as calmness, health, and satisfaction—more commonly than negative feelings. Still, sometimes termination can be an emotional experience, even when the client has acquired what he or she wanted from counseling. This can be especially true when a high level of intimacy has been established or when the client's problems are related to dependency, intimacy issues, or traumatic loss. In this circumstance, the experience of separation may be a reminder of past experiences (Goodyear, 1981; Hackney & Cormier, 2001; Weinberg, 1984). To the client, the counselor may have become an anchor and a source of security in a life of stress. The experience of being cared for and prized by the counselor, the feelings of relief and restoration of hope, and the discovery of new sources of personal strength and new capacities may all create strong attachment bonds (Lowenstein, 1979; Weiss, 1973). Letting go under these conditions may cause the client to feel a sense of loss.

Occasionally, clients who have made significant progress in counseling feel insecure about ending and try to prolong counseling by reverting back to problematic patterns or initiating entirely new counseling goals. When any of these symptoms of resistance appear, counselors need to get clients to focus on the source of these feelings and behaviors. Then they can decide together whether the concerns are legitimate reasons for extending counseling beyond the agreed upon termination date.

To prepare clients for termination, counselors ought to raise the topic well in advance of the end of counseling and not encourage too great a dependency on the counselor. Counselors should be especially cognizant of their role as anchor and work to help clients establish close friendships and support systems before counseling is ended, as these will ease the sense of loss of contact with the counselor. A counselor who has not helped a lonely and isolated client develop friendships has not really attended to a fundamental counseling issue for that client.

Quintana (1993) cautions mental health professionals that it is an error to conceive of termination as a crisis for most clients. Although some clients may experience feelings of loss and worries about coping after counseling is concluded, the majority manage the transition well, and few allow those feelings to overwhelm the progress they have attained. In fact, he suggests that when clients express strong and persistent resistance to termination, counselors should look first at the accuracy of their evaluation of the effectiveness of counseling. When clients have such strong emotional reactions to termination, they may be signaling that outcome goals have not been realized or that the counselor is mismanaging the termination process.

Counselor Responses to Termination

According to Nystul, "the ultimate goal in counseling is for counselors to become obsolete and unnecessary to their clients" (2003, p. 64). Counselors who are rewarded by helping others and who come to cherish their clients may forget this basic concept. Thus, resistance to separation may also come from the counselor. Ward (1984) suggests that the relative scarcity of published material on the counselor's resistance to termination reflects the profession's discomfort with open discussion of this topic. He argues that ending is often a difficult issue for counselors to talk about. The writings of Kovacs (1965), Mueller and Kell (1972), and White (1973) suggested that people who choose counseling as a career may be especially high in needs for intimacy, for giving nurturance, for gaining acceptance, and for receiving acknowledgment of their competence. Keeping a counseling relationship going provides an opportunity for these needs to be satisfied. Ending a counseling relationship risks the loss of satisfaction. The very needs that motivate people to become counselors may create barriers when it is time to let go. Goodyear (1981) suggests eight conditions under which letting go may be especially challenging for the counselor:

1. When termination signals the end of the significant relationship
2. When termination arouses the counselor's anxieties about the client's ability to function independently
3. When termination arouses guilt in the counselor about not having been more effective with the client

4. When the counselor's professional self-concept is threatened by a client who leaves abruptly and angrily
5. When termination signals the end of a learning experience for the counselor
6. When termination signals the end of a particularly exciting experience of living vicariously through the adventures of a client
7. When termination becomes a symbolic recapitulation of other farewells in the counselor's life
8. When termination arouses in the counselor conflicts about his or her own individuation (p. 348).

Psychoanalytic counselors argue that termination of counseling can symbolize early loss for both the counselor and the client. It is also possible that the positive counseling relationship that is about to end has been a particularly important source of gratification for the counselor during a period of stress and pain in his or her own life. Under such circumstances, relinquishing a rewarding experience can be difficult regardless of early life experiences.

It is not appropriate for counselors to postpone termination in order to continue having their needs met. This stance violates the basic ethical principles of the profession—to do good and avoid harm. Counselors who repeatedly experience intense feelings of loss when terminating counseling or who foster dependency rather than independence in clients should seek counseling to clarify and resolve their resistance to separation.

Ending in a Positive Way

As mentioned earlier, in intensive and long-range counseling, preparation for termination begins well before the last counseling session. As the signs of a client's change become more evident, the issue of termination emerges quite naturally. In this context, it is appropriate for the counselor to share his or her honest assessment of the client's growth. As the signs of completion become apparent, counselors should schedule one or two more sessions that concentrate on follow-up work and helping the client apply what he or she has learned. Then, when the last session arrives, both the client and the counselor will be prepared, termination will be easier, and the focus will be on the gains achieved.

The principles we have developed in this chapter lead to some important guidelines for ending an intense counseling experience in a positive way:

- Be aware of the client's needs and desires and allow the client time to express them. Client expressions of gratitude for the counselor's help should be graciously accepted and not

minimized, but the ultimate credit for change belongs to
the client.

- Review the major events of the counseling experience and
  bring the review into the present. This focus helps the client
  affirm that growth and change are part of life and gain greater
  perspective on his or her changes. Seeing self over time helps
  create closure. Using "I" messages ("I remember when we first
  started" or "Some moments that seemed especially important
  to me are . . .") helps to personalize the summing up.
- Supportively acknowledge the changes the client has made.
  Implementing changes and using new behaviors is never easy,
  natural, or automatic. Maintaining changes requires affirmation
  and encouragement. When a client has chosen not to
  implement action plans for other issues that emerged during
  the in-depth exploration phase of counseling, the process of
  termination should also include an inventory of those issues,
  and the client and the counselor should discuss the option of
  future counseling if the client ever wants it.
- Request follow-up contact. This request not only provides the
  counselor with information about the long-term effectiveness
  of the counseling strategies used, but it also demonstrates a
  sense of respect and caring for the client. Follow-up contact
  can be accomplished in person, over the telephone, or
  through correspondence. The knowledge that follow-up will
  occur also acts as an additional incentive for the client to
  maintain the changes that counseling has produced. The
  timing of follow-up varies with the client's circumstances,
  but 3 to 6 months after termination is typical. A second
  follow-up may be conducted a year after termination.

SUMMARY

The counselor promotes commitment to action in the first part of the
third stage of the counseling process. Sometimes the sharing of concerns
during the disclosure and exploration stages of counseling will have reduced
tension and suggested obvious goals and actions that the client has already
begun to undertake. In such cases, the third stage may be brief or nonexis-
tent. Frequently, though, the client does not spontaneously solve his or her
problems during the earlier stages of counseling, and specific goals and
action plans must be developed and reinforced during the final stage. Three
types of counselor responses are especially helpful in defining specific goals
and action plans. The first is selective reflection, attending to the affective
message that suggests a client's readiness to change. The second is confrontation, pointing out the discrepancies between current circumstances

and the client's goals. The third is the ability–potential response, a counselor response that helps the client generate alternatives to current behavior and offers reinforcement for readiness to initiate real change.

Clients are fearful of change, even desired change, and they usually require encouragement to act on their plans. Ability–potential responses offer this encouragement. The counselor supports the decision to act and helps the client to rehearse new behaviors. Sometimes the client may be in a position in which no solution appears to exist, or it may appear that the client can do some things independently but would make more rapid progress if significant others assisted. In such cases, the counselor may influence the client's environment by securing the intervention of other people, assuming the client agrees.

Some courses of action bring relatively quick success. In other cases, goals and action plans must be reviewed and refined. In still other cases, the results of action plans will not be known until the client has lived with the decision for a period of years. Nevertheless, changes in a client's thinking, feeling, and behavior are important goals of counseling, and the effectiveness of the client in mobilizing resources to accomplish his or her goals is a tangible measure of success for both client and counselor.

Termination constitutes the second part of the third stage of the counseling process, and it is a critical point in that process. Effective termination provides a positive closure to the experience and encourages the client to continue using his or her new learning by reviewing all that has been accomplished and preparing for what lies ahead in the client's life. Because termination is an experience of separation after an intense relationship, feelings of loss can sometimes emerge for both counselor and client. The counselor should try to be aware of his or her emotions as well as those of the client and to communicate honestly about present emotions. Offering a personalized review of the overall counseling experience is often helpful. Guidelines for helping the client work through resistance to referral include giving support, presenting the idea at the proper time, and having reliable information about the resource involved.

≈≈≈ *DISCUSSION QUESTIONS* ≈≈≈

1. Sometimes a client may ask a counselor to "tell me what I should do." This request appears to violate the authors' perspective on advice giving. In light of your own experience and the content of this chapter, how do you think you ought to respond to a client who is asking to be told what to do? What do you think underlies that request?

2. Selective reflections and ability–potential responses seem more directive and less genuine in some ways than empathic responding. On one hand, they could be viewed as manipulative; on the other hand, they could be

seen as encouraging the client to go in a direction he or she really wants to take. Under what conditions do you think selective reflections and ability–potential responses would be interpreted positively or negatively by clients?

3. The use of the term *homework* makes counseling sound like being enrolled in a course. Is that term appropriate—that is, do you see counseling as an educational process, at least partly? Is there another term for the between-session tasks that you would prefer?

4. What environmental conditions do you think are ideal for making action plans succeed? What kind of support of family, friends or others is essential? How can you help clients whose loved ones are ambivalent about the changes the clients really want and need to make in their lives?

5. When clients terminate counseling prematurely (i.e., before the counselor has judged counseling to be nearing completion), should counselors attempt to contact them to discuss the reasons for their decision to end counseling? Under what conditions do you think counselors should ask the client to return for at least one more session?

6. Now that e-mail and other forms of electronic communication are widely available, should counselors use these methods to follow up with clients about their progress after counseling ends? What are the advantages and disadvantages of this approach?

REFERENCES

Brammer, L.M., Abrego, P.J., & Shostrum, E.L. (1993). *Therapeutic counseling and psychotherapy* (6th ed.). Englewood Cliffs, NJ: Prentice Hall.

Budman, S.H., & Gurman, A.S. (1988). *Theory and practice of brief therapy*. New York: Guilford Press.

Cummings, N.A. (2001). Interruption not termination: The model from focused intermittent psychotherapy throughout the life cycle. *Journal of Psychotherapy in Independent Practice, 2,* 3–18.

Dinkmeyer, D.C., Dinkmeyer, D.C., Jr., & Sperry, L. (1987). *Adlerian counseling and psychotherapy*. Columbus, OH: Merrill/Prentice-Hall.

Egan, G. (2002). The skilled helper: A problem approach to counseling (7th ed.). Pacific Grove, CA: Brooks/Cole.

Goodyear, R.J. (1981). Termination as a loss experience for the counselor. *Personnel and Guidance Journal, 59,* 347–350.

Hackney, H., & Cormier, L.S. (2001). *The professional counselor: A process guide to helping* (4th ed.). Boston: Allyn & Bacon.

Hill, C.E., & O'Brien, K.M. (1999). *Helping skills: Facilitating exploration, insight and action*. Washington, DC: American Psychological Association.

Kazantzis, N., & Lampropoulos, G.K. (2002). Reflecting on homework in psychotherapy: What can we conclude from research and experience? *Journal of Clinical Psychology, 58,* 577–585.

Kleinke, C. (1994). *Common principles of psychotherapy*. Pacific Grove: Brooks/Cole.

Kovacs, A.L. (1965). The intimate relationship: A therapeutic paradox. *Psychotherapy: Theory, Research and Practice, 2,* 97–103.

Loewenstein, S.F. (1979). Helping family members cope with divorce. In S. Eisenberg & L.E. Patterson (Eds.), *Helping clients with special concerns* (pp. 193–217). Boston: Houghton Mifflin. Reissued (1990). Prospect Heights, IL: Waveland Press.

Martin, D.G. (2000). *Counseling and therapy skills* (2nd ed.). Prospect Heights, IL: Waveland Press.

Marx, J.A., & Gelso, C.J. (1987). Termination of individual counseling in a university counseling context. *Journal of Counseling Psychology, 34,* 3–9.

Mueller, W.J., & Kell, B.J. (1972). *Coping with conflict: Supervising counselors and psychotherapists.* Englewood Cliffs, NJ: Prentice-Hall.

Nystul, M.S. (2003). *The art and science of counseling and psychotherapy* (2nd ed.). New York: Macmillan.

Pate, R.H. (1982). Termination: End or beginning? In W.H. VanHoose & M.R. Worth (Eds.), *Counseling adults: A developmental approach* (pp. 188–195). Pacific Grove, CA: Brooks/Cole.

Quintana, S.M. (1993). Toward an expanded and updated conceptualization of termination: Implications for short-term individual psychotherapy. *Professional Psychology: Research and Practice, 24,* 426–432.

Razzhavaikina, T.I., Scheel, M.J., Allen-Portsche, S.M., Shamburg, B.S., & Bonsi, E.E. (2002, August). *The therapeutic value of client experiences with homework.* Paper presented at the annual meeting of the American Psychological Association, Chicago.

Renk, K., & Dinger, T.M. (2002). Reasons for therapy termination in a university psychotherapy clinic. *Journal of Clinical Psychology, 58,* 1173–1181.

Schuerger, J., & Watterson, D. (1977). *Using tests and other information in counseling.* Champaign, IL: Institute for Personality and Ability Testing.

Seligman, L. (1984). Temporary termination. *Journal of Counseling and Development, 63,* 43–44.

Shulman, L. (1984). *The skills of helping* (2nd ed.). Itasca, IL: Peacock.

Todd, D.M., Deane, F.P., & Bragdon, R.A. (2003). Client and therapist reasons for termination: A conceptualization and preliminary validation. *Journal of Clinical Psychology, 59,* 133–147.

Ward, D.W. (1984). Termination of individual counseling: Concepts and strategies. *Journal of Counseling and Development, 63,* 21–26.

Weinberg, G. (1984). *The heart of psychotherapy.* New York: St. Martin's Press.

Weiss, R.S. (Ed.). (1973). *Loneliness.* Cambridge, MA: MIT Press.

White, R.W. (1973). The concept of healthy personality: What do we really mean? *The Counseling Psychologist, 4,* 3–12.

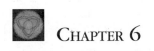 CHAPTER 6

ETHICS IN COUNSELING

As earlier chapters have demonstrated, effective counseling requires that a client be capable of self-disclosure and self-exploration and feel motivated to change attitudes and behaviors. Successful counseling also demands a skilled, empathic, and trustworthy counselor to guide and support the client through the change process. Counselors who violate their clients' trust, are insensitive to clients' needs and values, use their power exploitatively, or experiment with counseling interventions for which they have no training or experience are acting unethically. In each of these situations, the counselor is not fostering the best interests of the client and is instead serving some other purpose—usually self-interest. Whenever this happens, the counselor's behavior is defined as unethical. For example, suppose a counselor called Linda shares confidential information from Joe's counseling session with friends at a party because "it makes such a funny story." Linda is putting her own needs to impress her friends ahead of Joe's welfare. One partygoer may recognize the client's name and decide not to offer the client a job, or another may repeat the story so that eventually Joe hears it from some stranger and feels betrayed by the counselor he trusted. Joe may even resolve never to visit another helping professional again, regardless of his distress. In several ways, then, negative effects may come to a client when the counselor's self-interest is placed above the client's welfare.

Counselors have two other broad ethical obligations: to be loyal to the institution that employs them and to promote the good reputation of the counseling profession. Linda, the talkative counselor, not only violated the interests of her client, she also tarnished the reputation of the counseling profession and violated the rules of the counseling service for which she worked. Others who heard her story at the party may conclude that this is typical behavior for professional counselors in general or for those who work at that agency. As a result, they too may be reluctant to seek counseling for themselves or recommend it to others. This example represents an obvious breach of ethics that all responsible helping professionals would condemn, but other counselor behaviors are not so easily defined as ethical or unethical.

The following cases illustrate more complicated dilemmas that require more than good intentions and good sense to resolve ethically:

- A counselor's spouse's boss asks that the counselor see her college-aged son in counseling because he is confused and lonely. The spouse is being considered for a promotion. The counselor works at the college the son attends.
- The parents of a 10th grader see a school counselor because they want her to counsel their son, who is dating a girl of another race. They say they're old-fashioned and believe that "people should stay with their own kind."
- A 79-year-old man sees a counselor because he wants to maintain his own home, but his children and neighbors insist that he can no longer care for it properly. He threatens suicide if he loses his home, but he admits to having some problems with independent living.
- A colleague at a counseling agency routinely uses diagnostic categories more severe than the client's actual difficulties suggest in order to get the "most insurance reimbursement possible and give clients the full benefit of counseling."
- A counseling session with an adult client ends at dinnertime. This client came to the counselor because of difficulties in social assertiveness. He asks the counselor to join him for dinner at his parents' restaurant.

In each of these dilemmas, it is not easy to discern what really promotes the welfare of the client, the employer, or the profession. The counselor who fudges diagnoses for insurance purposes appears to be attempting to promote the welfare of her clients. But is she really? The person who counsels the boss's son may truly help him in his life choices. Should the personal connection with this young man stop the counseling from taking place? After all, the connection to this young man comes only through the counselor's spouse. Would accepting the client's dinner invitation facilitate trust in counseling and reward the client's social assertiveness, thereby helping the client, or would it jeopardize the counselor's objectivity and therefore risk harm to the client? This chapter sorts out these and other ethical dilemmas by discussing the ethical standards and principles that underlie the counseling profession and make counselors better equipped to act responsibly in such situations.

CODES OF PROFESSIONAL ETHICS

When most people think of professional ethics, they think of written codes of conduct that identify one set of behaviors that is expected of all professionals (e.g., keeping counseling records confidential) and another set of behaviors that is prohibited to all members (e.g., inaccurately advertising one's credentials). Codes of ethics also include a set of aspirational principles that professionals can use to guide their actions. One example of these aspirational statements comes from the "Ethical Principles" of the American Psychological Association (2002): "Psychologists respect the dignity and worth of all people, and the rights of individuals to privacy, confidentiality, and self-determination (p. 1063)." Every helping profession has a code of ethics, and some have special codes of ethics for particular kinds of counseling, such as group counseling. You will find the codes of ethics of the American Counseling Association (ACA) (1995) and the American Psychological Association (2002) in Appendixes A and B of this book. Each member of these professional associations is expected to read the code thoroughly and to abide by its contents.

Becoming familiar with a code of ethics is one way a counselor-in-training can be sensitized to situations that may be ethically problematic. Sensitivity to ethics is important because no client, colleague, or supervisor ever announces in advance that he or she is about to present an ethical dilemma to the counselor. Usually, the other party is oblivious to the ethical dimensions of the situation. Thus, the counselor must be able to independently identify an ethical dilemma as soon as it arises. Ethics scholars argue that counselors who are ethically sensitive are less likely to inadvertently choose inappropriate alternatives (Pope & Vasquez, 1998; Welfel, 2002). Please review the codes in Appendixes A and B before you continue with this chapter.

Note that a good deal of the content of the codes overlaps, although the organization of that content differs somewhat. Each code includes a discussion of how the helping professional ought to relate to clients, to colleagues, to employers, and to the public, emphasizing the responsibility to promote client welfare as the main goal. Each also includes statements describing the client's rights to privacy, accurate assessment of needs, freedom of choice, and fair and competent treatment or referral. Both codes define the responsibilities of helping professionals to present their training and experience honestly, to be direct and fair in assigning fees for services, to keep current with changes in practice, to conduct research responsibly, and to train competent future professionals. They elaborate on how professionals ought to balance their professional responsibilities to clients and to employers, and they explicitly prohibit certain behaviors such as sexual intimacies with clients, claiming titles or degrees not earned, and using psychological tests inappropriately. Each code recognizes the relationship between ethical standards and the law and advises practitioners to abide by the laws of their jurisdiction. These ethical standards are also fairly explicit about counselors' responsibilities to and for other counseling professionals. For example, each code addresses the responsibility of a counselor when he or she witnesses or learns of a colleague's unethical conduct. Although the wording differs somewhat, the essence is that each helping professional has an ethical responsibility to try to right any wrong he or she knows of and to see to it that the colleague works to correct the problem. In the case of a serious breach of ethics, the codes demand that the colleague's misbehavior be reported to the appropriate ethics committee or licensing board. In other words, the ethics codes obligate counselors not only to act ethically in their own interactions, but also to intervene at some level in known ethical violations of colleagues.

Ethical standards not only sensitize a professional to the kinds of ethical issues likely to arise in practice, they also act as a first resource when such a counselor is faced with a dilemma about what really promotes the client's well-being. To illustrate, when trying to decide whether to counsel the boss's son in the previous example, the counselor can refer to Section A of the Code of Ethics of the American Counseling Association (1995). Two subsections of the ACA code address this issue. Section A.5 states, "In the counseling relationship, counselors are aware of the intimacy and responsibilities inherent in the counseling relationship, maintain respect for clients, and avoid actions that seek to meet their own personal needs at the expense of clients." Section A.6 goes on to say,

> Counselors are aware of their influential positions with respect to clients, and they avoid exploiting the trust and dependency of clients. Counselors make every effort to avoid dual relationships with clients that could impair professional judgment or increase the risk of harm to clients. (Examples of such relationships include, but are not limited to familial, social, financial, business, or close personal relationships with clients.)

Although these sections do not specifically identify the relatives of a spouse's boss as an inappropriate client, they strongly advise against counseling people with whom the counselor has another relationship, especially if that relationship might impair objectivity. The existence of two ways of relating to the client is what the code refers to as a *dual relationship*. The counselor has a dual relationship with the young man because he would be both a client and a relative of a significant person in the counselor's spouse's life. Another example of a dual relationship is if the same person were both a client and a student. The language in the ACA code unequivocally prohibits such a relationship (ACA Code of Ethics, Section A.6b). This dual relationship is unethical because the counselor is in an evaluative relationship with the prospective client. As a teacher, that professional must evaluate the quality of the student's work. Not all dual relationships are automatically problematic. As the quote from the ACA code indicates, dual relationships in which the objectivity or professional judgment of the counselor may be compromised are unethical. The careful reader of the code can then surmise that accepting the son of a spouse's boss as a client is unethical because the counselor may not be able to be objective about the client's needs. For instance, the counselor might hesitate to recommend a course of action to the client with which the boss is likely to disagree because of the possible repercussions on the spouse. The counselor in this case has another reason to see the client other than the client's well-being (i.e., impressing the boss and getting the spouse promoted). When self-interest becomes a prominent motivation, accepting a client becomes unethical. It is worthwhile to note that accepting this client may not really be in the best interests of the counselor either. The counseling may fail and the spouse would be worse off, or the counseling may succeed from the client's perspective but fail in the boss's view and the spouse may still suffer harm. The boss may also expect the counselor to reveal confidential information to her, putting the counselor at risk of betraying the client's trust.

Similarly, in the case of the counselor who reports more extreme diagnoses to insurance agencies in order to "beat the bureaucracy" and get what she sees as a full measure of reimbursement for needed counseling time, Section 6.06 of the *Ethical Principles* of the American Psychological Association (2002) provides the following guidance: "In their reports to payors for services or sources for research funding, psychologists take reasonable steps to ensure the accurate reporting of the nature of the service provided or research conducted, the fees, charges, or payments, and where applicable, the identity of the provider, the findings and the diagnosis." Misrepresenting a diagnosis is also prohibited because it is probably illegal and may represent fraud. Although insurers sometimes have standards for care with which counselors disagree, disagreement about what is appropriate for the client does not justify lying to the insurance company. The counselor may ethically assist the client in appealing an insurance denial, complain to the insurer about its rules, or ask the professional association to lobby the insurance industry and legislative bodies for more appropriate standards for care. However, the counselor who knowingly falsifies a diagnosis is subject to both ethical and legal penalties. In this case, a careful reading of the code gives the counselor the answer to this ethical dilemma.

To illustrate the usefulness of the code further, if Linda, the loquacious counselor in the initial example in this chapter, had examined either of these codes of ethics she would have known that sharing confidential information from clients in a social setting is also clearly prohibited (ACA Code of Ethics, Section B.1.a, and APA *Ethical Principles,* Section 4.05). In other words, in a number of situations faced by counselors in their daily work, the codes provide the information necessary to make responsible ethical decisions. Thus, it is critical for all counselors and therapists to be thoroughly knowledgeable about the current code of conduct for their profession. Many licensing and certification standards include assessment of ethical knowledge for this very reason.

In at least three other types of situations, the codes are less clear or even mute. First, the changing nature of the helping professions limits the usefulness of codes. Counseling practice changes rapidly, and new intervention strategies are developed with great frequency. In this pluralistic society, counselors serve increasingly diverse populations of clients, whose needs, values, and beliefs may differ substantially from those of more traditional populations. New populations often require new counseling approaches. However, codes of ethics can never be fully current because the process of updating a code is cumbersome and professional associations usually take several years to revise any code. In the case of innovations in practice, only the general aspirational statements from the code may apply. Thus, counselors cannot rely on codes of ethics to clearly identify the ethical choice under such circumstances.

Even when the codes of ethics make good faith efforts to respond to new issues, in practice their efforts are not always fully successful. One example is the section of the ACA code that discusses the responsibilities of the counselor when a client has a contagious fatal disease (Section B.1.d). This section allows counselors to break confidentiality to inform others who may be at risk for infection. This provision was written primarily to assist counselors providing services to persons infected with the HIV virus. At the time it was published, HIV still was considered a fatal and contagious disease. With recent medical advances in treating HIV disorders, it is no longer clear whether HIV is necessarily a fatal disease. Medical science is not even entirely clear at this point about whether HIV is communicable when medication reduces the level of the virus in the bloodstream to "undetectable." Thus, the capacity of this section of the code to answer the questions of a counselor debating the issue of risk to a third party from an HIV-infected client has been diminished greatly in just a few years. Here too, the responsible counselor needs to look beyond the code to resolve this dilemma.

One resource, of course, is the growing body of literature in professional journals and professional conferences on this and other emerging ethical issues (e.g., Anderson & Barret, 2002; Melchert & Patterson, 1999). In essence, the literature suggests that counselors faced with this dilemma should balance the client's right to privacy with the danger to a specific individual. If a client who is HIV-positive is having unprotected sexual contact with a specific partner who has no knowledge of the person's HIV status and the client shows little concern about the well-being of the partner, then the responsibility to break confidentiality is strong. On the other hand, the rights of the client also need consideration, and the implications of breaking confidentiality should be weighed carefully. Breaking confidentiality is likely to terminate counseling, and the client who needed assistance from a professional may now refuse to engage in the counseling process with any counselor. In addition, the potential to get the client to change his or her behavior toward sexual partners through counseling is also gone, and the counselor will have no impact whatsoever over the client's sexual behavior in the future. In any case, the counselor's decision about confidentiality should not be based on irrational fears about AIDS or any generalization that HIV-positive clients automatically have no rights to privacy and confidentiality because of their health status. The central issue should be a known danger to an identifiable victim.

The second limitation of codes of ethics is that no code can address every complicated situation a counselor will encounter. Codes of conduct are not blueprints for action but rather are signposts that identify the most obvious and frequently occurring ethical problems. The best interests of the client may not be clear, and some good and some bad may happen no matter what choice the counselor makes. The case of the 79-year-old man illustrates such a dilemma. Supporting the man in what he wants may not be in his best interest in the long run. At the same time, if the family's desires take priority, the man may indeed become depressed and lose his motivation for living, an outcome that would also be clearly detrimental to him. (The next section of this chapter provides a strategy for trying to resolve such a complicated issue.)

Finally, there is a third way in which codes of ethics are an incomplete resource. If a counselor is a member of more than one professional association or is licensed by more than one licensing body, it is possible that the statements in the codes will conflict with each other. The counselor then has to choose between codes. The standards of licensing boards generally take priority over professional organizations, because they carry legal authority as well.

Obviously, then, a code of ethics cannot be the counselor's only resource in sorting out ethical dilemmas. No written standards can ever substitute for the judgment of the individual practitioner. Wrestling with complicated ethical dilemmas is as much a part of the counseling profession as building trust or choosing intervention strategies. The next section describes the ethical principles underlying the codes, which are the counselor's next resource should the codes be inadequate to resolve a dilemma.

ETHICAL PRINCIPLES

Kitchener (1984, 2000) identified five ethical principles as fundamental to the ethics of counseling. These principles are respect for autonomy, beneficence (doing good), nonmaleficence (avoiding harm), justice (or fairness), and fidelity (or promise keeping). Kitchener argues that these five principles provide the primary rationale for the contents of codes of ethics for helping professions. Ethics codes inform professionals as to *what* behaviors are ethical or unethical; ethical principles explain *why* behaviors have been so labeled. Kitchener states that counselors need to turn to the broader principles when written codes fail to provide clear guidance for action. Taken together, these principles encompass the primary values shared by the profession and, in essence, its reasons for existence. This section defines each ethical principle and demonstrates how it can be used in reasoning about ethical dilemmas.

Respect for Autonomy

The first ethical principle is respect for autonomy, an individual's right to self-determination. Individuals have a right to think as they wish, even if others disagree. They also have the right to act freely even if others don't like their choices. Autonomy must be respected, with two restrictions. First, the rights of the individual end where others' rights begin. In other words, a person has the freedom to act as long as others' rights are not limited. Second, respect for autonomy assumes that individuals are capable of understanding the implications and consequences of the choices they make. This ability to comprehend the meaning of choices is called competence. Society gives little autonomy to children because, at their developmental level, they are unlikely to understand the implications of their choices. Similarly, the autonomy of people with severe organic brain damage or those who are in the midst of psychotic episodes and not oriented to reality can also be restricted because these individuals are at least temporarily unaware of the meaning and consequences of their choices.

Let us return to the example of the aging man presented at the beginning of the chapter to illustrate the role of respect for autonomy in resolving ethical dilemmas. The autonomy principle suggests that the older man has the freedom to choose where he wants to live if he understands the meaning of that choice. His choice need not be logical or even in his ultimate best interest as long as he understands its meaning. In this case then, the principle of autonomy obligates the counselor to first evaluate the man's competence to make autonomous choices. If the man is competent, then the counselor must respect his choice as a priority, even if the counselor doesn't approve of it. The issue is not whether the counselor should decide for him what is best, but rather how the counselor can help him to live the way he wishes with the least possible risk to him and help him resolve the conflicts with those worried about him. Counselors need to avoid acting paternalistically—that is, in the role of a parent who knows better than the adult client. This is sometimes difficult because client values conflict with the values of their counselors. Potential conflicts are in the areas of women's rights, abortion rights, and social justice. A client may believe that wives should be submissive to their husbands in all things, and the counselor may believe in equality between marital partners. The principle of autonomy means that counselors cannot ethically impose their values on clients or use their influence to get clients to "see things the right way." Client beliefs and values can and do change during counseling. The issue is not whether the counselor helps the client explore beliefs that are troubling, but rather whose agenda it is to explore those beliefs. If the client freely chooses to focus on values and is free to come to an independent decision based on the exploration, the counselor can ethically explore these delicate subjects.

Beneficence

The second ethical principle—beneficence—is at the core of the profession. As members of a profession whose justification for existence is to do good for others, counselors have deeper ethical responsibilities than ordinary friends or confidants who receive no payment for their trust and do not purport to have any special training in counseling. Counselors publicize themselves as expert helpers, and people therefore come to see them precisely at those moments when they think the support of loved ones won't be sufficient to help or when they're desperate to get out of a situation they can't cope with. Counselors must do all they can to help. Moreover, counselors' status as paid professional helpers means that leaving clients at the end of counseling in the same place as they began is also inconsistent with counselors' role. Without commitment and skills to help their clients, counselors are guilty of a kind of false advertising of their services. Of course, there are times when counseling has negative outcomes. What is important in these cases is whether the counselor did all within his or her control to assist the client. Thus, one additional criterion for evaluating whether a particular course of action is ethical or not is to ask, "Is this course of action likely to benefit the client?"

Nonmaleficence

The responsibility not to make the client worse by intention, reckless action, or incompetence is the third ethical principle, also called the principle of nonmaleficence. This principle is also at the foundation of biomedical ethics (Beauchamp & Childress, 1994). Some have argued that it is the most fundamental ethical principle guiding all human service professions. Precisely because counselors profess to be helping professionals, they have a duty not to make a client worse if this outcome is avoidable. In the past, scholars thought that counseling was not a risky activity; they admitted that it did not always help but suggested that it could not really hurt a client either (Eysenck, 1952). More recent evidence has overwhelmingly contradicted that perception (Hubble, Duncan, & Miller, 1999; Lambert & Barley, 2002; Seligman, 1995). Counseling and therapy can be powerful tools and can be used to a client's significant advantage or disadvantage. Thus, the burden on the counselor to assess client problems accurately, choose counseling strategies wisely, and monitor the impact of counseling on each client is great. It is this ethical principle that underlies the statements in the ethics codes about practicing within the "limits of one's competence"—that is, dealing with client problems with which one has been trained and using counseling strategies with which one is skilled unless under supervision. This ethical principle is also at the core of the requirement that clients not be exposed to research or experimental treatments with high risk and little hope of real benefit. Thus, when evaluating whether a course of action is ethical, the counselor must also ask whether the client is at risk for harm. If the answer is yes, then alternative courses of action are usually more ethical.

Justice

The fourth ethical principle is justice, or fairness. Justice is a value at the core of democratic societies, and it demands that people be treated equally and that judgment about counseling goals and strategies must be based on the individual characteristics of the client and not on discriminatory attitudes toward groups. Stereotyping and bias are unethical because they are unjust, regardless of whether the discriminatory attitudes are conscious or not. Justice demands that no person be given better or worse treatment in counseling based on his or her status in society. Thus, when evaluating whether an action is ethical or not, a counselor needs to ask whether that action is based on any factor other than the unique needs of the individual.

The principle of justice also helps guide the counselor in responding to the parents of the 10th grader who don't want their son dating a girl of a different race, one of the examples presented at the beginning of this chapter. If the counselor learns that the only attribute of the young woman the parents find offensive is her race, then justice demands that the counselor refrain from involving himself in the situation in the way they want. Counselors cannot allow themselves to be put into the service of discrimination. The counselor may work with the family to foster communication and help resolve the conflict, but to agree to try to dissuade the boy from dating the girl on the basis of her race is unethical. Justice also demands that counselors display respectful and unbiased attitudes when counseling clients who are different in culture, background, lifestyle, or gender. This principle also requires counselors to use counseling strategies appropriate to the culture of the client. Three documents are especially helpful in assisting counselors in responding sensitively to diverse clients: *Principles Concerning the Counseling Psychotherapy of Women* (Fitzgerald & Nutt, 1986), *Operationalization of the Multicultural Counseling Competencies* (Arrendondo et al., 1996), and *Guidelines for Providers of Psychological Services to Ethnic, Linguistic and Culturally Diverse Populations* (American Psychological Association, 1993).

Fidelity

The fifth ethical principle is fidelity. One helpful way to think about the principle of fidelity is to use of the term *promise keeping*. Counseling professionals are taught attitudes and skills that help build the client's trust and encourage his or her self-disclosure. Promoting trust is the counselor's main goal in initial counseling sessions because self-disclosure and trust are critical to the success of the counseling process. Once the counselor has gained the client's trust, he or she becomes a powerful person who can do harm to the client. Because the counselor engages in a set of actions designed for the sole purpose of promoting trust, it is particularly despicable when that trust is betrayed. When counseling begins, counselors implicitly promise not to divulge what a client tells them unless there is some overwhelming reason that is ultimately in the client's or society's best interests. Research suggests that most clients assume that everything they tell a counselor will be kept confidential (Miller & Thelen, 1986). However, confidentiality is limited in some circumstances, and it is important for counselors to explain those limits to clients before self-disclosure begins. For example, ethical and legal standards demand that confidentiality be broken if the counselor learns of ongoing child or elder abuse or if the client is at great risk to harm self or others. In addition, if a court orders a counselor to testify about a client, confidentiality cannot be maintained. Thus, before clients disclose such information, they need to know the consequences of their disclosure. (For a fuller discussion of the limits of confidentiality, see Welfel, 2002.)

Another way to think of fidelity is to use the word *loyalty.* The principle of fidelity demands that counselors be loyal to clients, to employers, and to the profession. Thus, current ethical standards prohibit the abandonment of a client in the midst of counseling. Clearly, there are good reasons why a counselor may need to terminate counseling before the client is finished. However, the principle of fidelity requires that the counselor must provide the client with an appropriate referral to be faithful to the initial promise to provide help. The principle of fidelity is also the reason why the codes of ethics include statements about responsibilities to employers and fellow professionals. To be ethical, counselors must be faithful to the mission of their employer, unless that mission interferes with the best interests of the clients. After all, counselors accept salaries and other benefits from their employer with the implied promise to do what the employer expects. Similarly, counselors enjoy the benefits of their professional status, so they must be loyal to the profession as well. Thus, when trying to decide on the ethics of an action, the counselor must ask, "Is this choice in keeping with the promises I have made, either implied or explicit?"

Using the ethical principles, think about the following case:

━━━━━━━━━━━━━━━ *The Case of Millie* ━━━━━━━━━━━━━━━

Millie is a 59-year-old executive with a sporting goods company who has lived a full and rewarding life. She won medals in track in three Olympic competitions, established a foundation to help child refugees from war-torn countries, and adopted and successfully raised three orphans from Somalia. She was recently diagnosed with advanced cancer for which treatment is rarely successful. Therefore she has decided to forego treatment and live the fullest quality of life she can in the months available to her. She has come to counseling not because of worries about herself, but because of concerns about how her grown children and other family members will cope with her impending death. In the course of the conversation she reveals to her counselor that she intends to end her own life when the pain becomes intolerable and she becomes a burden to her children. She wants to save her family from watching her suffer even more than she wants to avoid the suffering herself. She asks the counselor to help her family adjust to her illness and her choice about the end of her life.

Questions for Further Thought

1. Based on these facts, how do you think the counselor should respond to Millie's request for service under the circumstances?
2. How can the ethical principles and ethics codes help the counselor decide what to do?
3. What emotions do you think the counselor will experience as he or she wrestles with this request?
4. Discuss your responses with a fellow student to compare the factors each of you found most salient and most difficult in this case.

ETHICAL THEORY

Sometimes the five ethical principles are insufficient for resolving an ethical dilemma. The principle of beneficence, for example, sometimes conflicts with the principle of autonomy. In the example of the aging man who wishes to live alone, the conflict is apparent: the actions that may help the man most may also contradict his wishes. How is such a conflict resolved? Many scholars say that the most fundamental ethical principle is avoiding harm and that one must examine the alternatives and decide on the basis of which one risks the least harm. It is still possible, however, that an ethical dilemma will remain unsolved because the greater harm is not apparent. In these situations, Kitchener (1984, 2000) suggests that even broader ethical theories need to be consulted. These theories are broad frameworks that ethicists use for examining good and evil; examples are utilitarianism (the greatest good for the greatest number) and the moral law tradition (the definition of certain rules for human behavior as absolute). These ethical theories act as the ultimate criteria in resolving a professional ethical dilemma. For a more detailed discussion of ethical theories, see Kitchener (1984).

Other resources are available for counselors who are agonizing over an ethical dilemma. Over the past two decades, the literature on professional ethics has expanded rapidly. There are several published models of ethical decision making (e.g., Cottone & Claus, 2000; Welfel, 2002), casebooks that give counselors practice in resolving ethical issues (Fisher, 2003; Herlihy & Corey, 1996), and a large body of articles that examine a range of specific ethical issues, such as confidentiality in counseling children and adolescents (Gustafson & McNamara, 1987; Koocher & Keith-Spiegel, 1990; Taylor & Adelman, 2001), the ethics of group therapy (Corey & Corey, 2001), counseling supervision (Bernard & Goodyear, 2004; Vasquez, 1992), and the ethical responsibilities of researchers and faculty (Keith-Spiegel et al., 1993; Sieber, 1992; Welfel, 1992). The reference list at the end of this chapter is a good introduction to this body of scholarship. In addition, professional conferences often include panel discussions about ethics and presentations of research findings on professional ethics. Finally, professional associations have ethics committees that can advise members about troublesome ethical dilemmas. In short, no counselor needs to feel that ethical decisions must be made in isolation and without consultation. Abundant resources are available to assist counselors in the difficult ethical decision-making process.

THE RELATIONSHIP BETWEEN ETHICS AND THE LAW

Ethical standards are internal guidelines developed by a profession to govern the activities of its membership. In fact, the existence of enforceable ethical standards is what distinguishes a profession from a trade. In contrast, the state laws regarding counseling practice are determined by the statutes passed by legislatures and the case law determined by court rulings. These laws vary widely from state to state. All 50 states now have a statute regarding mandated reporting of child abuse, for example, but exactly what behaviors are defined as abusive, which professionals are covered by the statutes, and the penalties that exist for failure to report differ somewhat from state to state. Thus, counselors must educate themselves about the statutes within each state where they practice.

In addition, case law from litigation involving therapists has come to influence the current contents of ethics codes. The most famous example is the Tarasoff case from California (Tarasoff, 1976). The court's ruling in this case established what is called the "duty to warn" a potential victim when a client makes a threat to cause harm to a particular person. In this case, the victim's parents sued the therapist for failing to notify the victim that the client had made serious threats against her life. The victim's family won the case with the judge arguing that the therapist's duty in this case went beyond notifying the police (as had been done) of the client's murderous intent. The court asserted that the duty of the therapist was to break confidentiality and warn the intended victim. The court held that "the protective privilege ends where the public peril begins" (Tarasoff, p. 347). Subsequent to that ruling, the ethics codes of counseling, psychology, and social work were revised to include a duty to warn and protect.

Most often, counselors are defendants in court cases because they have been sued for professional negligence, also called malpractice. In recent years, civil suits against mental health professionals have multiplied, and counselors have become increasingly concerned about how to avoid malpractice claims. At conferences and workshops, presentations about avoiding malpractice are often filled to capacity. The primary message about avoiding malpractice is to abide by the ethics code of the profession (Swensen, 1997). Counseling is a risky profession, and even responsible and skilled professionals are sometimes sued for malpractice. Those who abide by their profession's ethics code, understand the ethical principles underlying the code, and keep current with the literature about emerging ethical issues are as well protected as one can be against such lawsuits.

COMMON ETHICAL VIOLATIONS
BY MENTAL HEALTH PROFESSIONALS

Over the past two decades, much information has been gathered regarding the ethical practice of mental health professionals. Research has been conducted, and licensing boards and ethics committees have published summaries of the complaints presented to them each year. Taken together, these data provide a fairly clear picture of the kinds of ethical difficulties most frequently encountered by helping professionals.

Ethics committees deal overwhelmingly with one type of ethics violation: dual relationships with clients, especially sexual intimacies with current or former clients. This violation is particularly troubling because of the clear evidence of harm coming to clients who have been sexually exploited by their counselors (Bouhoutsos, Holroyd, Lerman, Forer, & Greenberg, 1983). This kind of behavior has been termed a form of sexual assault and has been compared to incest in its devastating effects on clients (Pope, 1994). (In fact, sexual exploitation of a client carries criminal penalties in some states. See Haspel, Jorgenson, Wincze, & Parsons, 1997, for a state-by-state review of these laws.) The personal difficulties that brought these clients to counseling in the first place are not helped; in fact, they are often worsened. Moreover, such clients often become averse to getting the therapy they need because of their victimization by a counselor. So troubling are the consequences of sexual exploitation by mental health professionals that the American Psychological Association has published a brochure intended to help clients learn about their rights (Committee on Women in Psychology, 1989).

Because counselors are human, it is not surprising that they sometimes feel sexual attraction toward a client. Experiencing such attraction is not unethical in itself. What is unethical is acting on it. The first step for a counselor who experiences sexual feelings for a client is to consult with a supervisor or colleague to discuss the case and decide on an appropriate course of action. The frank discussion about the attraction is often sufficient to help the counselor attend to the client's concerns. If the consultation does not refocus the counselor's attention, referring the client to another counselor is usually the wisest choice. If sexual attraction to clients happens persistently and frequently, the counselor should seek counseling to better understand the personal issues that may be provoking this reaction. Obviously, a counselor who is having persistent sexual thoughts about a client is likely to be distracted from the client's needs and concerns. Sometimes counselors have responded to their attraction to a client by terminating the counseling relationship, referring the client to another professional, and then beginning a social relationship with that former client. This "solution" to the problem of sexual attraction to a client is unethical. The fact that counseling has officially ended does not immediately change the client's perception of the counselor as a professional or diminish the problems that provoked that client to seek counseling in the first place. Counselors need to base their working life on the assumption that clients will never be a population from which they will obtain friends or lovers. The risk of harm to clients is too great.

Nonsexual dual relationships account for another large category of misconduct. Counselors who borrow money from clients, employ their clients in their practices, or begin a close personal relationship with a current client have all been found guilty of misconduct. In such cases the counselor jeopardized the client's welfare by embarking on the additional personal contact with the client.

Other breaches of ethics that commonly come to the attention of licensing boards include other forms of unprofessional conduct (such as using counseling sessions to discuss the counselor's problems), unethical billing practices, incompetent practice, fraudulent application for license, violations of confidentiality, misrepresentation of competence, and violations relating to reporting of child abuse (Welfel, 2002). Pope and Vetter (1992) surveyed psychologists about the kinds of ethical issues they encountered in their work. Those who responded to the survey reported more ethical dilemmas about confidentiality than about any other issue. They expressed concerns about how and when to disclose confidential information about minors and how to respond when one client has several caregivers or the same professional has clients who know each other. In addition, they also described ethical dilemmas about the definition of dual relationships that are not sexual and about payment, insurance, and the like. It is interesting to note that although confidentiality was the issue mentioned most frequently by the respondents in this survey, confidentiality violations are seldom reported to ethics committees. A national survey of certified counselors revealed that the overwhelming majority saw sexual exploitation of clients and violations of informed consent, confidentiality, and voluntary participation in counseling as unethical. Counselors were more uncertain about the ethics of charging and collecting fees for counseling and the ethics of non-sexual dual relationships (Gibson & Pope, 1993).

Which counselors commit these ethical violations? No particular demographic characteristics have been associated with unethical practice. Experience, gender, type of degree, and similar characteristics do not predict who will act unethically, with one exception. Complaints about dual relationships with clients, especially sexual intimacies with clients or former clients, have been largely made against male mental health professionals. The usual pattern is of an older male therapist and a younger female client. However, cases against women therapists have also been reported.

Some counselors blunder into unethical actions because they just don't think about the ethical issues or they are not familiar with the code of ethics of the profession. Given the needs to establish a trusting relationship, to assess the client's concerns, and to develop appropriate strategies to assist the client, it is not altogether surprising that counselors become distracted from otherwise obvious ethical issues. However, counselors must maintain their attention to ethical issues even while attending to therapeutic concerns if they are to merit the title of professional.

Other counselors act unethically because their primary motivation is self-interest or because they think codes of ethics are for professionals who are less experienced or gifted than they are. Such grandiose thinking has led to serious ethical violations and puts a counselor at risk for a pattern of unethical behavior with a number of clients. Although most helping professionals are dedicated to serving their clients, some seem to show interest in nothing but self-gratification.

Professionals sometimes act unethically because they are distracted by personal difficulties or are made especially needy by a personal crisis. A counselor who is lonely and sad after a difficult divorce may step over the boundaries of the counseling relationship because of those personal needs. Such cases have come before ethics committees and licensing boards on numerous occasions. The codes of ethics all address this kind of circumstance, putting the responsibility to be aware of personal limitations on the counselor. If unable to attend to the client's needs because of personal difficulties, the responsible counselor must not attempt counseling until the personal issues are resolved. The power of the counselor to do harm is too great to allow this distortion of the counseling process to occur or continue. In this type of situation, counseling for the counselor is the best solution. Some professional associations are beginning to develop resources to assist distressed professionals in recovering their equilibrium.

SUMMARY

A counselor is in a position of power and trust and has a duty to be respectful of that special status. Counselors who act irresponsibly cause real harm to their clients, their employers, and the reputation of the profession. The most fundamental ethical imperative is to act in the best interests of the client and avoid actions that risk harm to him or her.

Professional codes of ethics provide statements of the specific ethical duties of professionals and the aspirational principles that are endorsed by the profession. These codes should not just be read; they should be digested so that professionals will know how to respond as soon as an ethical issue arises. Familiarity with a code of ethics also assists the counselor in recognizing an issue as an ethical problem. Some counselors act unethically because they failed to see the ethical dimensions of a situation until too late.

Codes of ethics cannot resolve every ethical dilemma. Some issues are too new to be included in a code, and some situations are too complicated to be resolved by reference to any written standards. To deal with these situations, the counselor must understand the five major ethical principles underlying the code: autonomy, beneficence, avoidance of harm, justice, and fidelity. These principles can guide a counselor's ethical decision making when the relevant code does not provide clear direction. The responsibility for ethical behavior rests with the individual practitioner. No code of ethics can substitute for the judgment of the individual professional.

≈≈≈ *DISCUSSION QUESTIONS* ≈≈≈

1. When you face your first ethical dilemma as a practicing counselor, what do you think will be the most difficult part of acting responsibly?
2. Licensing boards and ethics committees sometimes mandate that professionals convicted of unethical behavior enroll in ethics courses if they wish to regain their right to practice independently. What are the benefits and liabilities of this idea? How helpful do you think it really is in preventing further episodes of unethical behavior?
3. Some scholars have argued that relying on understanding the codes and the ethical principles alone makes ethical decision making too intellectual and leaves out issues related to the character and motivation of the professional. They argue that ethics education should instead focus on the virtues that the profession values, such as honesty and integrity. What do you think of this viewpoint?
4. Do you agree that avoiding harm is the most fundamental ethical principle? Can you imagine any circumstances in which the other ethical principles might take priority over this one?
5. In addition to educating students about the ethics codes, principles, and research, what other steps should training programs in counseling take to

ensure that their students will act ethically after graduation? Is there anything else they can do?

REFERENCES

American Counseling Association. (1995). *Code of ethics and standards of practice.* Alexandria, VA: Author.

American Psychological Association. (1993). *Guidelines for providers of psychological services to ethnic, linguistic and culturally diverse populations.* Washington, DC: Author.

American Psychological Association. (2002). Ethical principles of psychologists and code of conduct. *American Psychologist, 57,* 1060–1075.

Anderson, J. R., & Barret, R. L. (Eds.). (2002). *Ethical issues in HIV-related mental health practice: A casebook and resource manual.* Washington, DC: American Psychological Association.

Arrendondo, P., Toporek, R., Brown, S. P., Jones, J., Locke, D., Sanchez, J., & Stadler, H. (1996). Operationalization of the multicultural counseling competencies. *Journal of Multicultural Counseling and Development, 24,* 42–78.

Beauchamp, T. L., & Childress, J. F. (1994). *Principles of biomedical ethics* (4th ed.). Oxford, England: Oxford University Press.

Bernard, J. M., & Goodyear, R. K. (2004). *Fundamentals of clinical supervision* (2nd ed.). Boston: Allyn & Bacon.

Bouhoutsos, J. C., Holroyd, J., Lerman, H., Forer, B., & Greenberg, M. (1983). Sexual intimacy between psychotherapists and patients. *Professional Psychology: Research and Practice, 20,* 112–115.

Committee on Women in Psychology. (1989). If sex enters into the psychotherapy relationship. *Professional Psychology: Research and Practice, 20,* 112–115.

Corey, M. S., & Corey, G. (2001). *Groups: Process and practice* (6th ed.). Pacific Grove, CA: Brooks/Cole.

Cottone, R. R., & Claus, R. E. (2000). Ethical decision-making models: A review of the literature. *Journal of Counseling and Development, 78,* 275–283.

Eysenck, H. J. (1952). The effectiveness of psychotherapy: An evaluation. *Journal of Consulting Psychology, 16,* 319–324.

Fisher, C. B. (2003). *Decoding the ethics code: A practical guide for psychologists.* Thousand Oaks, CA: Sage.

Fitzgerald, L. F., & Nutt, R. (1986). The Division 17 principles concerning the counseling/psychotherapy of women: Rationale and implementation. *The Counseling Psychologist, 14,* 180–216.

Gibson, W. T., & Pope, K. S. (1993). The ethics of counseling: A national survey of certified counselors. *Journal of Counseling and Development, 71,* 330–336.

Gustafson, K. E., & McNamara, J. R. (1987). Confidentiality with minor clients: Issues and guidelines for therapists. *Professional Psychology: Research and Practice, 17,* 111–114.

Haspel, K. C., Jorgenson, L. M., Wincze, J. P., & Parsons, J. P. (1997). Legislative intervention regarding therapist sexual misconduct: An overview. *Professional Psychology: Research and Practice, 28,* 63–72.

Herlihy, B., & Corey, G. (1996). *Ethical standards casebook* (5th ed.). Alexandria, VA: American Counseling Association.

Hubble, M. A., Duncan, B. D., & Miller, S. D. (Eds.). (1999). *The heart and soul of change: What works in therapy.* Washington, DC: American Psychological Association.

Keith-Spiegel, P., Wittig, A. F., Perkins, D. V., Balogh, D. W., & Whitley, B. E., Jr. (1993). *The ethics of teaching: A casebook.* Muncie, IN: Ball State University.

Kitchener, K. S. (1984). Intuition, critical evaluation and ethical principles: The foundation for ethical decisions in counseling psychology. *The Counseling Psychologist, 12,* 43–55.

Kitchener, K. S. (2000). *Foundations of ethical practice, research and teaching in psychology.* Mahwah, NJ: Erlbaum.

Koocher, G., & Keith-Spiegel, P. S. (1990). *Children, ethics and the law.* Lincoln, NE: University of Nebraska Press.

Lambert, M. J., & Barley, D. E. (2002). Research summary on the therapeutic relationship and psychotherapy outcome. In J. C. Norcross (Ed.), *Psychotherapy relationships that* work (pp. 17–32). New York: Oxford.

Melchert, T. P., & Patterson, M. M. (1999). Duty to warn and interventions with HIV positive clients. *Professional Psychology: Research and Practice, 30,* 180–186.

Miller, D. J., & Thelen, M. H. (1986). Knowledge and beliefs about confidentiality in psychotherapy. *Professional Psychology: Research and Practice, 17,* 15–19.

Pope, K. S. (1994). *Sexual involvement with therapists: Patient assessment, subsequent therapy, forensics.* Washington, DC: American Psychological Association.

Pope, K. S., & Vasquez, M. J. T. (1998). *Ethics in psychotherapy and counseling* (2nd ed.). San Francisco: Jossey-Bass.

Pope, K. S., & Vetter, V. A. (1992). Ethical dilemmas encountered by the members of the American Psychological Association: A national survey. *American Psychologist, 47,* 397–411.

Seligman, M. E. P. (1995). The effectiveness of psychotherapy: The *Consumer Reports* study. *American Psychologist, 50,* 965–974.

Sieber, J. E. (1992). *Planning ethically responsible research: A guide for students and internal review boards.* Newbury Park, CA: Sage.

Swensen, L. (1997). *Psychology and the law for the helping professions* (2nd ed.). Pacific Grove, CA: Brooks/Cole.

Tarasoff v. Regents of University of California, 551 P2d 334 (Cal, 1976).

Taylor, L., & Adelman, H. S. (2001). Enlisting appropriate parental cooperation and involvement in children's mental health treatment. In E. R. Welfel & R. E. Ingersoll (Eds.), *The mental health desk reference* (pp. 219–225). New York: Wiley.

Vasquez, M. J. T. (1992). Psychologist as clinical supervisor: Promoting ethical practice. *Professional Psychology: Research and Practice, 23,* 196–202.

Welfel, E. R. (1992). Psychologist as ethics educator: Successes, failures and unanswered questions. *Professional Psychology: Research and Practice, 23,* 182–189.

Welfel, E. R. (2002). *Ethics in counseling and psychotherapy: Standards, research, and emerging issues* (2nd ed.). Pacific Grove, CA: Brooks/Cole.

PART TWO

COUNSELING STRATEGIES AND TECHNIQUES

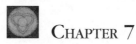 CHAPTER 7

ASSESSMENT AND DIAGNOSIS IN COUNSELING

Assessment is a collaborative process in which the client and counselor work together to gather information that will clarify the problem(s) the client brings to counseling and to decide whether counseling is an appropriate intervention for the client to use to resolve them. The counselor and client test hypotheses about the nature and sources of the problems the client is experiencing and the strengths the client possesses to resolve them. Assessment continues until both the client and the counselor agree to a tentative conclusion about the nature of the problem. This tentative conclusion is called the *diagnosis,* the mutually agreed upon name for the problem(s) that provoked the counseling. This is a critical step in the counseling process, because decisions about action plans and change strategies are built on assessment and diagnosis. If the assessment process is flawed, an accurate diagnosis cannot be determined, and plans designed to address the problem have little chance of success. Critics contend that diagnosis can be used as a pejorative way of labeling the client as sick, losing sight of his or her individuality, or reinforcing gender or racial bias (e.g., Stiver, 1986). Others see it as a potential distraction from the client's human needs (Gladding, 2000). For this reason, some counselors avoid the term *diagnosis* altogether. In addition, Shaffer (1986) cautions that unless diagnosis is tied to treatment, it is a futile process. Our position is that if a clear understanding of exactly what is troubling the client is brought forth in counseling, the whole counseling process is more productive and goal oriented. Assessment and diagnosis done poorly, incompletely, or without the engagement of the client can indeed lead to the ills cited by these critics.

This chapter presents a frame of reference for understanding assessment in counseling, a description of the components of assessment and the tools available to help counselors make accurate diagnoses, and a discussion of the relationship of assessment to the trusting relationship between counselor and client. We believe that this model helps prevent the problems with diagnosis so often cited by its critics.

A FRAME OF REFERENCE FOR UNDERSTANDING ASSESSMENT AND DIAGNOSIS

Diagnosis is a term borrowed from the medical lexicon, where it refers to the identification of a disease or dysfunction that is compromising a person's health. Its use in the counseling literature has become commonplace, but real parallels to the medical definition are limited. The primary parallel is that diagnosis in counseling also involves problem definition and the use of that definition of the problem to decide on the appropriate goals and interventions. However, there are several important ways in which diagnosis in counseling differs from the process in medicine. In medical diagnosis, there is usually a physically identifiable cause for the disease, such as the presence of cancerous cells, the fracture of a bone, or the dysfunction of a kidney. In counseling, the causes of a person's sadness, anger, or poor interpersonal skills may be almost entirely outside that individual (such as a physically abusive parent or a sexually harassing boss) or may stem from a range of factors too numerous or too far in the past to identify specifically. Certain difficulties may also be a function of the developmental stage of the individual and thus normal rather than dysfunctional. The fear of strangers in the toddler or the adolescent's worry about attractiveness to others are examples of normal developmental difficulties. In other words, problems in living simply don't lend themselves to a clear diagnostic classification as easily as medical problems. (For a perceptive and comprehensive analysis of the differences between medical diagnosis and psychological diagnosis, see Bohart and Tallman, 1999.)

The next major difference in the assessment process in counseling lies in the role and activity level of the counselor and the client. In medicine, the usual procedure is for the physician to ask the patient a series of questions about symptoms, conduct a physical examination, order relevant medical tests, and then make a diagnosis once all the information is available. Implied here is a highly active role for the physician and a rather passive role for the patient. The patient's primary responsibility is to fill in the blanks, to be compliant and cooperative with the medical experts. Once the diagnosis is made, the patient becomes more active, asking questions about the diagnosis and deciding whether to undertake the recommended treatment. In counseling, however, the assessment process is a joint enterprise in which a partnership develops. The counselor actively seeks the client's input about the nature of the problem, and the diagnosis itself is a product of their work and not a conclusion the counselor comes to independently. Part of this difference stems from the philosophical roots of counseling, which lie in humanistic psychology and the writings of Carl Rogers (1951). Rogers rejected the notion that problems in living were like sicknesses that needed the intervention of health professionals. Instead, he posited that psychological pain and dysfunction are best resolved by a partnership with a committed counselor that allows the client to come to his or her own assessment of the difficulties and to choose actions to resolve them. As discussed in Chapter 10, humanistic psychologists like Rogers believe that humans are inherently self-actualizing—that is, motivated to become healthier and solve their problems. Our model of the counseling process amends Rogers's approach by making the counselor equally active with the client in defining the problems to be solved.

Although assessment is a bilateral activity, counselors and clients do not always become aware of the likely diagnosis at exactly the same point in the counseling process. Because the issues clients bring to counseling usually provoke feelings of pain and anxiety, clients sometimes block full awareness of the difficulties or their causes. When this happens, the client is said to be well defended, or to have strong defenses against the painful material. Defenses protect the psyche from content that appears to be overwhelming or threatening to psychological survival. To illustrate, the client who describes several sources of evidence he has uncovered that his spouse is having an affair may be unable to "connect the dots" because he is well defended against this overwhelming event. In a clear trail of motel receipts, phone messages, evenings away from home, and long nights chatting on the Internet, this otherwise intelligent and perceptive man may deny, minimize, or intellectualize about what he sees.

When the client's defenses appear to be delaying awareness of the diagnosis, the counselor's role is to help the client feel safe enough to explore the difficulty so that the client's defenses can be lowered and the counselor can discuss the full dimensions of the problem with the client. The counselor ought not to announce his or her diagnosis to the client as soon as a plausible one becomes apparent, nor should the counselor initiate action planning until the client's defenses are lowered. There are several reasons for this prohibition. First, the counselor could be in error and would then pursue an inappropriate intervention. It is important to remember that clients have the fullest knowledge of their own experience and that the process of exploring all components of assessment takes time and trust. Second, even if the counselor's diagnosis is accurate, when the client's defenses are heightened, the client may reject that definition, resist the recommended plan for change, or even prematurely end counseling. In this situation, the mistiming of the counselor's discussion of the diagnosis can be as great an error as a faulty diagnosis. Third, the presentation of the diagnosis by the counselor to the client implies that solving the problem is the counselor's rather than the client's responsibility. Thus, a unilateral diagnosis by the counselor can undermine the partnership essential to the effectiveness of the entire counseling process. It is important to remember that research consistently shows that the client's engagement in counseling is the single most important variable in determining a good outcome (Bohart & Tallman, 1999; Lambert & Barley, 2002). Whenever counselors pressure clients to think or act in ways they find inconsistent with their self-understanding or too threatening to entertain, clients' commitment to the work of counseling diminishes.

Diagnosis in counseling differs from medical diagnosis in a third important way in that it often entails discussing several other significant people in the client's world. In fact, it may be that the person who makes the appointment to see a counselor is not the primary client at all. The person sitting in the counseling office could be a parent, friend, or partner of the one suffering the most distress. (Of course, the person in the office may still benefit from counseling; the point is that counselors cannot assume that he or she has the greatest need for counseling.) Even when the person at the appointment is the one in difficulty, the cause of the problem may be outside that individual. For example, a gifted Latino middle school student may be seeing a school counselor because of frustrations at school and dislike of his teacher. The process of exploring the situation may lead to the conclusion that a large part of the problem is the teacher's prejudice against persons of Mexican background. After the available evidence has been gathered, the assessment may be that the teacher's bias, more than any other factor, has resulted in the student's dislike of that teacher and his placement in the wrong ability group. Although the student may benefit from counseling in dealing with his negative feelings and acquiring better ways of addressing his problems with this teacher and other prejudiced individuals he may encounter in his life, effective diagnosis in this case mandates that the counselor attend to the teacher's behavior and her misplacement of this student. Perhaps the counselor may need to have the student transferred to another class. In other words, a counselor who assumes that the current client is the only potential client and has caused or can solve the problem is risking a diagnostic error.

Assessment and diagnosis in counseling are also dependent on the theoretical orientation of the counselor. Along with presenting a system for intervening to help clients cope better, counseling theories provide models for defining normal and abnormal behavior and for describing how and why dysfunctions develop. A counselor whose theoretical orientation rests in the behavior therapy tradition will define the problem the client presents differently than will a humanistic or cognitive counselor. The behavioral counselor will also tend to use substantially different counseling interventions than will a humanistic or cognitive counselor. As Brammer, Abrego, and Shostrom (1993) suggest, "theories act as 'templates' that indicate the client behaviors they consider most important" (p. 149). During the counseling process, counselors receive an overwhelming amount of information (both verbal and nonverbal) from the client. Theories help to organize that information and make it sensible. The process of deciding what theoretical orientation or combination of theories provides the most adequate representation of human development and dysfunction is a long and complicated one for a beginning counselor. Clarity about one's theory of counseling comes with education and practice with real clients under supervision. Beginning counselors ought to test out different theories of counseling and approaches to assessment in order to judge for themselves the adequacy of each model and its appropriateness for particular clients. Supervision by a licensed mental health professional during this period provides a safeguard that clients' concerns are competently evaluated and that they are receiving needed support and assistance. Of course, given the evolving nature of theories and the research evidence regarding their veracity and effectiveness, the process of defining a theory of diagnosis and interventions must continue throughout a counselor's career.

COMPONENTS OF EFFECTIVE ASSESSMENT

There are five components to the information-gathering and hypothesis-testing process of assessment. Taken together, these components flesh out the problem(s) and give the counselor and the client the fullest insight into the circumstances that provoked the client to seek help.

The first component is *an understanding of the boundaries of the problem*—that is, the scope and limits of each difficulty the client is experiencing. Attaining clarity about the scope of the problem involves understanding its boundaries in current functioning as well as its history and duration. For example, if a client enters counseling because of feelings of loneliness and social isolation, identifying the boundaries of the problem means exploring exactly how socially isolated the person is and how limited his or her close connections with others are. For one person, lonely feelings can arise when a rich and extended social life has been temporarily reduced to a fairly ordinary number of social contacts because of a new living situation; for another, such feelings can be the result of an entire life of social distance and trouble with intimacy. In the first situation, the boundaries of the problem are limited and its solution fairly straightforward. The second situation has wide boundaries, making its solution more complicated and time-consuming.

The second component of assessment is *the mutual understanding of the pattern and intensity of the problem*. It is unusual for a difficulty to be experienced at a uniform level at all times. The discomfort is worse at some times, better at other times, and does not appear at all at still other times. The aim of assessment is to understand whether there is a pattern to these variations and to identify jointly the factors associated with them. Recognizing the pattern of the problem also helps the client to view the situation as less overwhelming and more manageable. There is reassurance in the discovery that the difficulty is not randomly occurring, and the pattern makes its causation clearer. For example, a college student who feels shy and socially uncomfortable may come to notice that the feelings of shyness are worse in unstructured social situations than in structured academic or athletic situations where her role is fairly well defined. She may also come to see a pattern of greater shyness after visits home to her critical and demanding parents or when she is with people in whom she has a romantic interest. Taken together, this information helps the client and the counselor better define action plans to resolve the episodes of shyness. Through understanding the pattern of the problem, the client may also gain better control of her feelings of helplessness.

Understanding the intensity of the feelings surrounding the difficulty is the other side of this component of assessment. For example, when a client talks of feeling angry and frustrated with his disabled child, the goal is to identify the feelings involved and get a clear sense of the dimensions of those feelings and the associated behaviors. Does the father feel impatient and then withdraw from the child, or does he experience deep rage that makes him want to strike out at the child? Knowing the intensity of the feelings is important to the client's self-understanding and to the choice of appropriate counseling approaches. When clients enter counseling because of affective difficulties such as feelings of sadness, anger, anxiety, or emptiness, the exploration of the intensity of these feelings is a natural part of the first stages of counseling. However, when a client seeks problem-solving skills, assistance with career decision making, or help in stopping habitual behavior, discussion of the intensity of the feelings surrounding the issue may be neglected. However, knowledge of the intensity of feelings is also important in these cases because it can affect the commitment to change and the difficulty of relinquishing old patterns.

The next component of assessment is *an understanding of the degree to which the presenting problem influences functioning in other parts of the client's life*. The aim here is to ascertain how circumscribed or diffuse the difficulty is and to clarify the degree to which it compromises other parts of the client's experience. For instance, if a woman comes to counseling because of worry about her future and a sense of emptiness and dissatisfaction with her current life choices, it is important for her and the counselor to explore the effects of these concerns on her daily living and her relationships. Has this worry caused her to avoid friends, defer important financial planning, act angrily with her partner, drink more alcohol, and otherwise show a pattern of fairly wide disruption in her life activities? Or is her concern more limited, perhaps causing some sleepless nights or loss of interest in some activities but little observable change in behavior or social relationships? By exploring the broader pattern of functioning, both the client and the counselor get a clearer picture of the nature and seriousness of the problem.

The fourth component of assessment is *an exploration of the ways of solving the problem that the client has already tried before entering counseling*. In many cultures, counseling is often a last resort for people who have tried all of the other alternatives they could identify. Typically, clients have attempted a number of strategies on their own, and usually these solutions have failed or their success has been short lived. The following situation illustrates this point. The parents of a toddler who wakes up several times during the night have attempted to let the child cry it out (in an effort to teach her that nights are for sleeping) but then have given in and taken her into bed with them when she continues crying. Their sleep is further interrupted with the child in their bed, and they worry that they are not helping their 2-year-old to develop in a healthy way. They have read a self-help book on the subject and sought the advice of their pediatrician to break the cycles. Only the failure of all of these strategies causes them to seek counseling. The counselor and the client need to examine any prior attempts to cope so that fruitless strategies are not resurrected and so that the counselor can get a sense of the determination (or desperateness) of the client to get help. Some of the prior strategies may also have made the problem even harder to solve. In this case, attempting to let a toddler "cry it out" and then giving in and picking her up has reinforced the child's learning that crying works, in that it gets a parent to take her out of her crib at night. Thus, stopping the nighttime waking is more difficult than it would have been had this strategy never been attempted. When counselors and clients understand the impact of the problem's history on the current status of the problem, strategies for change can be selected more prudently, and clients can be better prepared for the obstacles they may meet as they pursue these interventions.

The last component of assessment is *an understanding of the strengths and coping skills of the client.* Some of this information is revealed as the other four components are explored, but too often client strengths are not clearly identified. Knowing the strengths and coping skills of the client is important because it provides both the counselor and the client with a balanced perspective. Even though the current difficulty is painful, the client does have resources to bring about its resolution and deliberately focusing on them prevents a distorted view that the dysfunction represents the whole person. Because of their distress, clients often lose track of their positive characteristics and thereby may feel more overwhelmed by their problems than they really are. In addition, evaluating strengths also reminds the counselor that the client can take responsibility for herself or himself and should not be treated paternalistically. Finally, when several possible intervention strategies might be effective for a particular dysfunction, knowledge of the client's strengths and coping skills can help the counselor and client choose wisely. Related to a knowledge of personal strengths and coping skills is the need to be familiar with the support system available to the client. The central question is this: What significant others who are capable of positive interaction with the client are available during this stressful period? Clients without supportive persons in their lives may have substantially more difficulty resolving their problems. In fact, in itself, the lack of such supports can be seen as a problem that may need to be addressed before the other counseling issues can be tackled.

Exploring all components is important because typically two or three possible hypotheses about the client's discomfort emerge in the first and second stages of the counseling process. For example, a person's high anxiety in social situations may be related to low self-esteem, poor communication skills, a history of being demeaned by a parent or spouse, or a combination of these factors. By discussing all five components, the counselor and the client begin to test out the accuracy of the possible explanations and rule out some and agree on others. Attending to each component also helps the counselor avoid the mistake of deciding on a diagnosis too quickly and with too little data.

Counselors who work in community agencies are usually required to use the most recent edition of diagnostic system developed by the American Psychiatric Association published in the *Diagnostic and Statistical Manual of Mental Disorders,* abbreviated as the DSM-IV-TR (American Psychiatric Association, 2000). A discussion of the strengths and weaknesses of this system is beyond the scope of this chapter. It is important to note, however, that the approach to assessment and diagnosis we present is not incompatible with the use of this system. Counselors using the DSM-IV-TR can still attend to all five components of the diagnostic process and work to make the hypothesis-testing and information-gathering process a joint enterprise.

Several other models for structuring the assessment process have been presented in the professional literature (e.g., Lazarus, 1976; Leitner, Faidley, & Celentana, 2000; Seay, 1978; Swenson, 1968). The model offered by Leitner and colleagues is representative of attempts to assess client issues without reference to medical terminology. It presents a taxonomy of life problems and categories of optimal functioning rather than psychological disorders. Arnold Lazarus (1976) published one of the best-known of these assessment models, which is labeled with the acronym BASIC ID. In his view, good diagnosis includes attention to behavior, affect, sensation, imagery, cognition, interpersonal relationships, and drugs. Lazarus contends that only with attention to all these client domains can the counselor accurately assess the problems and plan effective interventions. Family counselors often eschew the medical terminology and the language from individual psychotherapy and use an entirely different set of diagnostic terms for family problems based on a systems perspective (Sporakowski, Prouty, & Habben, 2001). We encourage you to explore the views of these writers in greater detail to learn about other taxonomies of diagnosis.

TOOLS FOR EFFECTIVE DIAGNOSIS

Counselors rely heavily on verbal discussion with the client to arrive at a diagnosis. The process of facilitating self-disclosure and in-depth exploration, discussed in Chapters 3 and 4, implies that verbal communication is the primary mode of analyzing and solving problems. However, counselors and clients have other tools available to help them understand the presenting problems. These include standardized tests, behavior rating measures, observations of the client in the natural setting, input from significant others, and role-playing exercises. Art, music, or play media may sometimes give the counselor and the client a deeper understanding of the issues. Art and play therapy techniques are standard assessment tools with children, but they also have application with adolescents and adults. This section briefly describes the array of tools available to assist in the assessment process. We encourage you to read sources such as Anastasi and Urbina (1997) to acquire a fuller understanding of the use of these tools.

Counselors who are trained in the responsible use of standardized tests can find them a valuable resource for understanding clients, especially clients who present with complicated issues, who are not adept at verbal exploration of difficulties, or whose concerns are highly specific. Clients who have difficulty initiating conversation about embarrassing aspects of a problem may be more comfortable discussing these issues in the context of a seemingly more objective information such as the results of testing. Similarly, tests can reveal dimensions of a problem that a client never thought to bring up because he or she didn't see the connection to the presenting issue. Of course, no test is infallible, and all test data must be supplemented with supporting evidence before any credibility can be given to the findings. When used responsibly, however, standardized tests can clarify confusing or hidden aspects of a problem. Professional guidelines for the responsible use of tests have been published by the American Educational Research Association (2000) in conjunction with the American Counseling Association, the American Psychological Association, and other educational and mental health organizations. In a now famous publication, Paul Meehl (1973) makes a compelling argument that standardized tests provide more reliable assessments of client attributes when compared to clinical interviews alone.

Personality tests can be useful when a client's concerns are longstanding or relate to negative feelings about self or difficulties in interpersonal relationships. These tests compare the responses of the client to the responses of a norm group on a variety of dimensions of personality. Many personality inventories broadly assess intrapsychic functioning and attitudes toward others and thus help clarify the boundaries of the problem, the intensity of the feelings, and the personal resources of the client. The most commonly used personality inventory in mental health settings is the *MMPI-2* (Butcher, Dahlstrom, Graham, Tellegen, & Kaemmer, 1989). Many other tests also examine multiple dimensions of personality. Some focus on identifying significant psychological dysfunction; others, such as the *Revised NEO Personality Inventory* (Costa & McCrane, 1992), the *California Personality Inventory* (Gough, 1987), or the *Sixteen Personality Factor Questionnaire* (Cattell, Cattell, & Cattell, 1993) attend to personality style or the functioning of psychologically "normal" individuals experiencing situational problems. For those who function in settings where the DSM-IV system is used, the *Millon Clinical Multiaxial Inventory-III* (Millon, 1994) is a useful instrument for clarifying appropriate diagnostic categories within that classification. Those with extensive, specialized training may find projective personality tests, such as the *Thematic Apperception Test* (Murray, 1943) or the *Rorschach* (Rorschach, 1942), helpful in exploring client feelings and attitudes not fully available in conscious thought.

There are also tests that center on a particular issue such as self-esteem, anxiety, or depression. These measures are appropriate when the general nature of the problem is fairly clear, but its seriousness or specific definition is hidden from the client and the counselor. One of the best known of such instruments is the *Beck Depression Inventory-II* (Beck, Steer, & Brown, 1996), which examines the intensity of sad and hopeless feelings and can clarify depressed feelings that are obscured by anxiety or blocked from awareness by defenses. This instrument can also help determine the intensity of depression in a client who is not comfortable conversing about such painful material. When examining self-esteem, for example, the *Tennessee Self-Concept Inventory Revised* (Roid & Fitts, 1988) is widely used to explore more deeply the client's view of the self. If used at intervals throughout the counseling process, these kinds of tests can mark the client's progress in specific domains.

When the client presents with a career or educational decision-making issue, interest inventories such as the *Strong Interest Inventory* (Harmon, Hansen, Borgen, & Hammer, 1997) or Holland's *Self-Directed Search* (Holland, 1994) may be appropriate. They articulate occupational and educational interests with a detail usually not possible through the interview process and compare the client's pattern of interests with others in the same occupation. Interest inventories also familiarize clients with a broader range of occupational choices than they might be able to produce on their own.

Still other tools are available to help clients and counselors make accurate assessments. Included among these are observational checklists that involve either self-observation by the client or observation by someone else in the situations that provoke the problem. When the observation is of self, this procedure is also called self-monitoring. Structured checklists have been developed for special problems, such as school misbehavior, but individually developed models for self-observation or observation by others are commonly used in counseling as well. The critical component of these tools is a system for collecting data about the client's behavior that the person gathering the information will easily understand. When the data are internal to the client, such as the number of self-depreciating thoughts, obviously only self-monitoring will be effective. Observational checklists and self-monitoring activities bring objectivity and specificity to client reports about negative experiences. Checklists are especially valuable when the difficulties seem centered on interpersonal interactions. For example, a client who finds himself getting into arguments with people in social situations but who doesn't understand the dynamics that lead to the disagreements may find it revealing to gather observational data to document the sequence of events. Similarly, when someone seeking a new job experiences repeated rejections after face-to-face job interviews, observation of interview behavior may unearth the problems better than any other diagnostic tool. (Practicality may dictate that observation be of a simulated interview rather than an actual one.) Also included on the list of useful tools are methods that involve input from significant others about client behavior. The value of such a tool is most apparent when a child is having difficulty, either in the classroom or at home. Because children do not have the cognitive or emotional maturity to observe their own behavior, feedback from a teacher or parent can be particularly helpful to the client and the counselor in diagnosing what's wrong. The most widely used instrument for the behavioral observation of children is Achenbach's *Child Behavior Checklist* (Achenbach, 1991). When input from significant others is included in the diagnostic data gathering, the counselor needs to be cautious about its interpretation, however. Most significant others will have difficulty being objective about the client and may inadvertently distort the data because of their personal relationship. Therefore, data from significant others should be supplemented with other, more objective information before a diagnosis is reached. Direct observation by the counselor is often helpful if it can be arranged.

Journals or diaries kept by clients can be another resource for defining the problem and for understanding the variations in the intensity of the problem from day to day. A journal may be a routine part of the client's life before counseling or can be "assigned" by the counselor for homework between sessions. (For a detailed description of the use of journals as a counseling assignment to assist self-exploration and reflection, see Burnett and Mecham, 2002.) In either case, the client must be completely willing to share such private writings with the counselor. For a client who is not interested in writing down thoughts and feelings, a tape-recorded journal may serve the same purpose.

Counseling techniques usually used for intervention purposes can also be useful to assess the presenting problem(s). As mentioned in Chapter 4, one of the most important of these tools is role-playing during the counseling session. For example, a client who complains about not knowing how to make friends may be asked to role-play with the counselor a contact with a new person he or she wants to get to know better. The counselor takes the role of the potential friend, and the client assumes his or her usual role. In this interaction, skill problems or negative feelings may come to the surface and be more readily discussed in the session. Later on, role-plays can be used to test the degree to which the client has learned new social skills or overcome negative feelings during such encounters.

PLACEMENT OF ASSESSMENT IN THE COUNSELING PROCESS: RISKS AND OPPORTUNITIES

Essentially, the assessment process begins with the first contact between the counselor and the client. A client's fundamental motivation for seeking counseling is to get help in figuring out what is wrong, why independent efforts to change have not been successful, and to solve the problem. Thus, the appraisal of problems starts during the first session to some degree, but a concentrated focus on assessment at the beginning of counseling is a risky and often counterproductive strategy. Its risk is tied to the nature of the content to be discussed and the client's fears about how the counselor will respond. Specifically, because accurate assessment involves both revelation of highly personal and painful information and attention to aspects of the situation that the client would rather avoid, it requires a trusting relationship between the counselor and the client. Research evidence demonstrates that clients are reluctant to reveal painful information. They tend to leave some relevant aspects of their experience undisclosed even in long-term therapy either because they are embarrassed by the content or because they are afraid that they or their therapists can not handle the disclosure (Hill, Thompson, Cogar, & Denman, 1993; Kelly, 1998). These findings highlight the client's need to know that counseling is a safe environment where respect, caring, and understanding will be communicated. Only in such an atmosphere will the client be able to undertake the process of self-exploration essential to diagnostic accuracy. Counselors who focus immediately on assessment are vulnerable to getting faulty or incomplete answers from clients to their questions. It is important to keep in mind that clients often fear that counselors will ridicule or judge them for their feelings and behaviors or will label them as sick or evil. Even if a client gives a counselor the benefit of the doubt about such harsh judgments, that client probably still needs to be reassured that his or her individual experience will be heard. A client often fears that he or she will be treated as "just another depressive" or a "typical example of an uncontrollable student" or labeled in some other way that diminishes uniqueness. The counselor needs to allay these fears before clients will feel free to divulge intimate information about their experience. Without time to establish trust, clients are more likely to be well defended and unable to process their own experience fully.

Assessment, then, clearly fits into the second stage of the counseling process as we define it. It is a focused and structured activity within the deeper self-exploration of this stage, and like all self-exploration, it can be threatening to the client. With full discussion of the problems inherent in covering all five components of diagnosis comes a confrontation with the reality that the client faces. Often that reality means an acknowledgment of the client's own role in the problem and a putting aside of the denials, rationalizations, or easy explanations that have made living with the situation more bearable in the short run, but are not compatible with real change. This deeper understanding is threatening because the old ways of thinking about the problem are relinquished before new ways of understanding it and coping with it are fully established. Clients sometimes drop out of counseling at this stage because the threat is too great. There is an old Irish proverb that helps explain this phenomenon: "The devil you know is better than the devil you don't know." In other words, however painful the current situation, there is almost always a way it could be worse. When clients commit to the deep exploration of the second stage and the assessment process, they are risking the banishment of the devil they know without any certainty that the path they choose will be better. Counselors who understand the threat will support the client's exploration in a way that acknowledges the risk and reminds the client of the possible gains from counseling.

The assessment process also presents an opportunity for the counselor to model effective problem solving. Clients often feel that their problems are insoluble and hopeless. During the days that preceded counseling, they probably experienced concision and frustration whenever they tried to think clearly about their problems. Clients often feel demoralized. The methodical process of exploring each aspect of the problem and the client's life situation will help bring clarity to the client. It also teaches the client another way to examine the issues. Furthermore, in watching the counselor proceed with the assumption that things can be improved or made easier to tolerate, the client gains hope that counseling will result in change.

INTAKE INTERVIEWS

In many college counseling centers, mental health agencies, and private counseling practices, a tentative diagnosis is reached during a separate intake interview conducted by an intake counselor. The intake interview usually involves a single meeting in which a counselor works with a client to gather information about the client's presenting problem, general life situation, history, and interpersonal functioning (Sommers-Flanagan & Sommers-Flanagan, 2003). The counselor and the client both understand that this session is separate from the regular counseling, and it is usually conducted by a person different from the regular counselor. One structure frequently used in intake interviews with people who have serious mental illnesses is called the mental status examination. The mental status examination is a structured interview format that assesses current behavior and cognitive functioning. In this kind of intake interview, the counselor covers nine specific categories of information: client appearance, behavior/psychomotor activity, attitude toward the counselor, affect and mood, speech and thought, perceptual disturbances, orientation (to reality) and consciousness, memory and intelligence, and reliability and judgment (Sommers-Flanagan & Sommers-Flanagan, 2003).

The intake interview has become common because it can result in a more efficient use of staff resources and a better match between counselors and clients. When conducting intake interviews, counselors cover the same five components of diagnosis as they do in regular counseling sessions, but their attention must be highly focused. By necessity, intake interviews are more structured and directed by the counselor than are ordinary sessions. The use of an intake interview has its limitations, the most important of which is the need to discuss sensitive and painful information without time for trust and partnership between the participants to develop. (The difficulties with an immediate focus on diagnosis were discussed in detail earlier in this chapter.) In addition, clients can be taken aback by the possibility that they may have to tell their story again once a regular counselor is assigned. Even when the counselor permanently assigned to a client reads the intake report before the initial session with the client, there are likely to be aspects of the report that the counselor will want to explore further. Thus, this worry has some basis in fact.

The intake interview has one other limitation. A directive intake procedure can leave clients with the impression that their proper role is to be passive, waiting for the counselor to ask questions and guide discussion. In other words, they may "learn" that counseling is a process akin to an appointment with a physician and thus take on the role of the patient. The client passivity that may result can undermine an effective partnership for problem solving. As a result, in an intake system, counselors have an added responsibility to educate the client about the mutuality of effective counseling and encourage the client's active involvement in the process. During intake interviews, counselors also have a duty to make the client as comfortable as possible by attending to feelings and nonverbal behavior and using the active listening skills appropriate for the first stage of counseling. The questions and specific probes often required in the intake procedure must be built on a foundation of these listening skills. (For a detailed discussion of methods for improving the effectiveness of intake interviews, see Sommers-Flanagan & Sommers-Flanagan, 2003.)

Because the data collected in an intake interview may not be complete or accurate, counselors assigned for subsequent sessions ought to reexamine the content areas discussed in that interview once trust has been established and the client's self-exploration has begun. The diagnosis reached in an intake interview is always tentative, because the session is brief and the reliability of the information is unknown.

MISTAKES COUNSELORS MAKE IN THE ASSESSMENT PROCESS

Counselors frequently make three errors during the assessment process. The first is the assumption that the difficulties the client is experiencing are caused by psychological, interpersonal, or social factors. Clients sometimes experience distress because of medical dysfunctions, or their psychological pain is complicated by medical problems. In these cases, the sadness, irritability, or anxiety can only be treated properly if the physical condition is remedied. As a routine part of the assessment process, counselors need to explore the client's medical history. Clients who have not had a physical examination by their medical doctor since the onset of their distress should be encouraged to schedule an appointment. The need for a medical checkup is especially important when the distress is persistent, severe, or of sudden onset. A client's distress may be related to a medication that has been prescribed for an unrelated medical problem. Clients who are not familiar with the side effects of their medication ought to discuss this possibility with their physician. Most of the time, of course, the sadness or irritability a client is experiencing is not related to any medical problem, and counseling interventions will be necessary to help the client change. However, because the medical problems that can cause emotional changes are often serious and sometimes life threatening, counselors should encourage all clients to see their physician to rule out physiological explanations for their difficulties.

The second mistake counselors sometimes make is thinking that there is only one diagnosis for a client's problems. Typically, clients come to counseling with more than one difficulty or more than one domain in which their functioning is somewhat compromised. Consider the following case.

The Case of Howard

Howard, a 54-year-old computer analyst who has been married for 31 years, enters counseling with the statement that "he's at his wit's end." Exploration of the problem reveals that he has been laid off from work, that his 27-year-old son (his only child) has been diagnosed as HIV-positive, and that he is having frequent panic attacks and is becoming afraid to leave his home. Howard goes on to say that he and his wife have been unable to give each other support in their distress about their son's illness, that they have been arguing often, and that he has lost interest in sex. He finds himself procrastinating in his job search and sometimes spending money foolishly.

Questions for Further Thought

1. Imagine yourself in Howard's situation. How would you feel and what might you expect from your counselor? Share your response with a partner.
2. With the same partner, identify several diagnostic possibilities for this case.

3. Referring to the five components of diagnosis, identify other diagnostic information you would need to assess Howard's counseling needs accurately.

In this case, each difficulty ought to be explored as fully as time allows, and the relationship between the problems should be examined. Real grief about his son may be underlying Howard's anxiety and distance from his wife. Financial worries may be preventing him from attending to his grief, his partner, or his job search. His loss of interest in sex may be a consequence of the decline in emotional closeness with his wife or may be a symptom of an unrelated medical condition.

No single diagnosis is likely to account for all of Howard's concerns. Counselors who believe that there can be one, overriding diagnosis for complex situations such as this one risk oversimplifying the situation and thereby neglecting intervention in some important aspects of the problem.

The third mistake counselors may make is treating a diagnosis as though it were unchangeable and absolute when, of course, a diagnosis is always tentative to some degree and always open to new information. The process of exploring and making changes in one area may bring into the client's awareness other issues that he or she had little memory of before that point. These forgotten issues may be highly painful, such as a history of physical abuse, an instance of date rape, or a highly disturbing combat experience. This painful information becomes available to the client when trust in the counselor has been tested out a number of times and when the client begins to feel stronger in other ways. Sometimes clients have kept pertinent information secret from the counselor for many sessions out of embarrassment or fear. When that information is finally revealed, it may also change the diagnosis. When new disclosures are made, the counselor and the client need to reassess the diagnosis and amend it if necessary. If counseling is at the third stage and plans for change have been implemented, then both parties need to decide whether those plans are still appropriate. Often, additional interventions are needed.

SUMMARY

Assessment and diagnosis in counseling are the activities of systematically defining the difficulties that caused the client to seek counseling. Neither assessment nor diagnosis is something the counselor does to the client, but rather an information-gathering and hypothesis-testing process carried out in collaboration with the client. Both assessment (the process of identifying the problem) and diagnosis (the formal name the counselor and the client give to the problem) can be somewhat threatening to the client because they necessarily include deep exploration of sensitive material and imply risking change. Consequently, assessment is best conducted only after a trusting relationship is well under way and the client understands the mutuality of the counseling process. Counselors can anticipate some resistance to both assessment and diagnosis from clients, because of the confrontation with sensitive material. When resistance occurs, attention to empathic understanding and active listening skills will usually diminish it.

There are five components to an effective assessment process: a definition of the boundaries of the problem, a mutual understanding of the factors that maintain and lessen the problem and their intensity, a definition of the degree to which the presenting problem is affecting functioning in other parts of the client's life, an exploration of the attempts to solve the problem undertaken prior to counseling, and an identification of the strengths and coping skills of the client.

When there are multiple problems, a counselor explores each difficulty with the same thoroughness. The counselor should also be open to the possibility that counseling is not the best intervention or that the client needs a different counselor. In these cases, the client should be referred to other helping professionals better equipped to address the client's concerns.

≈≈≈ *DISCUSSION QUESTIONS* ≈≈≈

1. The medical model (DSM) of diagnosis has acquired dominance in community agency practice. Discuss ways that a more humanistically oriented counselor can meet his or her own standards while fulfilling agency (and insurance) demands.
2. Psychological testing is vulnerable to misuse, especially with diverse populations and by untrained people. Funding for testing is also limited. Given these problems, under what circumstances do you think testing may be productive in the setting in which you plan to work?
3. The authors emphasize the importance of assessing client strengths and resources as part of diagnosis. Discuss how you might go about collecting information on strengths and resources. What do you think this process may accomplish for a client?
4. The model of assessment and diagnosis presented in this chapter requires time and possibly multiple meetings before any conclusion is reached. It also relies on the partnership of the client and the counselor in determining a diagnosis. What are the strengths and weaknesses of this approach in both school and community counseling settings?

REFERENCES

Achenbach, T. M. (1991). *Manual for the Child Behavior Checklist*. Burlington: University of Vermont Press.

American Educational Research Association. (2000). *Standards for educational and psychological tests*. Washington, DC: Author.

American Psychiatric Association. (2000). *Diagnostic and statistical manual of mental disorders* (4th ed. text revision). Washington, DC: Author.

Anastasi, A., & Urbina, S. (1997). *Psychological testing* (7th ed.). New York: Prentice-Hall.

Beck, A. T., Steer, R. A., & Brown, G. K. (1996). *Manual for the Beck Depression Inventory-II.* San Antonio, TX: Psychological Corporation.

Bohart, A. C., & Tallman, K. (1999). *How clients make therapy work.* Washington, DC: American Psychological Association.

Brammer, L. M., Abrego, R. J., & Shostrom, E. L. (1993). *Therapeutic psychology: Fundamentals of counseling and psychotherapy* (6th ed.). Englewood Cliffs, NJ: Prentice-Hall.

Burnett, P. C., & Mecham, D. (2002). Learning journals as a counseling strategy. *Journal of Counseling and Development, 80,* 410–415.

Butcher, J. N., Dahlstrom, W. C., Graham, J. R., Tellegen, A., & Kaemmer, B. (1989). *MMPI-2 manual for administration and scoring.* Minneapolis, MN: University of Minnesota Press.

Cattell, R. B., Cattell, A. K., & Cattell, H. E. (1993). *Sixteen Personality Factor Questionnaire* (5th ed). Champaign, IL: Institute for Personality and Ability Testing.

Costa, P. T., & McCrane, R. R. (1992). *Revised NEO Personality Inventory: Professional manual.* Odessa, FL: Psychological Assessment Resources.

Gladding, S. (2000). *Counseling: A comprehensive* profession (4th ed.). New York: Macmillan.

Gough, H. G. (1987). *California Personality Inventory administrator's guide.* Palo Alto, CA: CPP.

Harmon, L., Hansen, J., Borgen, F., & Hammer, A. (1997). *Strong Interest Inventory: Applications and technical guide.* Stanford, CA: Stanford University Press.

Hill, C. E., Thompson, B. J., Cogar, M. M., & Denman, D. W. (1993). Beneath the surface of long-term therapy: Client and therapist report of their own and each other's covert processes. *Journal of Counseling Psychology, 40,* 278–288.

Holland, J. L. (1994). *The self-directed search professional manual.* Odessa, FL: Psychological Assessment Resources.

Kelly, A. F. (1998). Client secret keeping in outpatient therapy. *Journal of Counseling Psychology, 45,* 50–57.

Lambert, M. J., & Barley, D. E. (2002). Research summary on the therapeutic relationship and psychotherapy outcome. In J. C. Norcross (Ed.), *Psychotherapy relationships that* work (pp. 17–32). New York: Oxford.

Lazarus, A. A. (1976). *Multimodal behavior therapy.* New York: Springer.

Leitner, L. M., Faidley, A. J., & Celentana, M. A. (2000). Diagnosing human meaning making: An experimental constructivist approach. In R. A. Neimeyer & J. Raskin (Eds.), *Constructions of disorder: Meaning making frameworks for psychotherapy* (pp. 175–203). Washington, DC: American Psychological Association.

Meehl, P. E. (1973). *Psychodiagnosis: Selected papers.* Minneapolis, MN: University of Minnesota Press.

Millon, T. (1994). *Millon Clinical Multiaxial Inventory-III.* Minneapolis, MN: National Computer Systems.

Murray, H. A. (1943). *Thematic Apperception Test.* Cambridge, MA: Harvard University Press.

Rogers, C. R. (1951). *Client-centered psychotherapy.* Boston: Houghton Mifflin.

Roid, G. H., & Fitts, W. H. (1988). *Tennessee Self-Concept Inventory Revised: Manual.* Los Angeles: Western Psychological Services.

Rorschach, H. (1942). *Psychodiagnostics: A diagnostic test based on perception.* New York: Grune & Stratton. Originally published in 1921.

Seay, T. A. (1978). *Systematic eclectic therapy.* Jonesboro, TN: Pilgrimage Press.

Shaffer, W.R. (1986). Diagnosis as a sham and a reality. *Journal of Counseling and Development, 64,* 612–613.

Sommers-Flanagan, J., & Sommers-Flanagan, R. (2003). *Clinical interviewing.* New York: Wiley.

Sporakowski, M.J., Prouty, A.M., & Habben, C. (2001). Assessment in couple and family counseling. In E.R. Welfel & R.E. Ingersoll (Eds.), *The mental health desk reference* (pp. 372–378). New York: Wiley.

Stiver, I. (1986). The meaning of care: Reframing treatment models for women. *Psychotherapy, 2,* 221–226.

Swenson, C.H. (1968). *An approach to case conceptualization.* Boston: Houghton Mifflin.

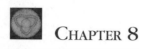 **CHAPTER 8**

STRUCTURING, LEADING,
AND QUESTIONING TECHNIQUES

The process of counseling has been described in previous chapters as a sequence of stages in which the focus shifts from initial disclosure of concerns to deeper exploration to plans of action. These stages may all occur within a single session, but more commonly the process develops over two or more sessions. We have urged the counselor to pay special attention to building a good relationship with the client early in the counseling process. Later, because of continuity of this positive relationship, its maintenance will require less attention, and the trust that has been built can make it easier for the client to explore deeper and more threatening issues. Commitment to action may require the counselor to plan actively with the client to implement change and to reinforce the client's efforts to change.

This chapter considers the moment-to-moment decisions that a counselor makes each time he or she responds to a client. In the instant just after a client has completed a communication to the counselor (verbally or otherwise), the counselor has a whole universe of possible responses available. In a few seconds, the counselor formulates a response and, in so doing, influences the subsequent response of the client and ultimately the direction counseling will take. However, as Ivey and Ivey (2003) have stated, there is no one correct response at any given instant, but rather many alternative responses that may move the client toward a sense of capability.

A similar-appearing process occurs in ordinary conversation, of course. However, because counseling is a dialogue with a purpose and the counselor is responsible for facilitating positive progress, individual responses are more significant. To improve counseling skills, it is often necessary to study the timing, content, and effect of specific responses. Supervised practice in counseling provides counselors-in-training with feedback on how specific responses contributed to or interrupted a client's progress. This chapter will help you to formulate specific counseling responses and provide a basis for analyzing the counseling process bit by bit.

STRUCTURING

Structuring describes any statement by the counselor that lets the client know what to expect of the process and outcomes of counseling. It may address "the nature, conditions, limits, and goals" of counseling (Brammer, Abrego, & Shostrum, 1993, p. 123). It refers to counselor communications that address the process as a whole and comments that structure discussion within a session. Structuring helps to keep the process focused on the client's goals and keep current conversation purposeful. According to Corey (2001), "All the approaches (to counseling) are in basic agreement on the need for some type of structure in the counseling experience, although they disagree over its nature and degree" (p. 433).

Many clients arrive at a counselor's office with no idea what to expect of counseling. Others arrive with unreasonable or inappropriate expectations. Patterson (1974) has observed that many clients not experienced with counseling think of counselors as experts who will give them advice and solve their problems. Some of a counselor's earliest statements to a client will suggest how the client might participate and what the counselor will contribute to the conversation. These comments can serve as part of the process of obtaining informed consent for counseling from the client. When clients lose momentum during counseling, they need help in maintaining the motivation to work on their concerns or to move to a new stage. Therefore, it may be necessary for the counselor to return to structuring at various times throughout counseling. At its most fundamental level, structuring acts as a message to the client that he or she is respected and is a partner—not a subordinate—in the counseling process. It lets the client know that the counselor wants the client to be comfortable with the process and that the client has a right to know what to expect.

The counselor must decide how much structuring to use and when to use it. Too little structuring contributes to the possibility of rambling, unfocused interaction that lacks concreteness and is unproductive; another possible outcome is that the client will present an initial concern and then withdraw to await the counselor's solution. Too much structuring distracts from discussion of the client's concerns and feelings, sounds preachy, and may seem condescending and controlling to the client. It is also possible, especially with clients who have previously experienced counseling, that poorly timed efforts at structuring may interrupt important client thought processes. Formative statements that refocus the working agenda when necessary are better than protracted speeches that describe the counseling process. These formative statements are timed so as to set the initial working agenda or to maintain the momentum of the client's work on his or her concerns.

Structuring at the Beginning of Counseling

The initial sessions determine how the client and counselor will work together. With adolescent and adult clients, the counselor usually initiates specific discussion about confidentiality, length and frequency of counseling sessions, projected duration of counseling, client and counselor responsibilities, and possible outcomes, with the intent of obtaining the client's consent to the process. With children, there is discussion of action limits as well (e.g., "You may not break the equipment or hit the counselor"). Also, wording of the other elements of structure must be adjusted to the client's ability to comprehend.

Confidentiality frees clients to talk about personal material without the fear that what they say will be repeated to others who might use the information against them or think less well of them as a result. Discussing confidentiality early in the counseling process and any other time it is introduced by the client is therefore important. With a client who is known to have experienced counseling previously, the counselor may begin by asking about the client's understanding of confidentiality and then elaborating as necessary. With younger clients and those who may not have had previous exposure, the counselor can make a statement worded something like this: "I want you to know that the things we talk about together are private and I will not discuss them with anyone else without your permission. There are a few exceptions you should know about. For example, if you talk about harming yourself or someone else, or if you talk about being in danger, I may have to involve someone else to help." It is necessary for trainees working under supervision to tell the client that a supervisor may also hear some of the sessions and that the supervisor will also respect the client's privacy (Welfel, 2002). This discussion assures that the client has given informed consent for the counseling and the supervision to proceed. Although counselors often take confidentiality for granted, a client who wishes to share highly personal information will be reassured by explicit statements that his or her story will not be treated casually.

Discussion of the time frame for counseling tells the client what to expect and provides a perspective for how he or she will choose to use counseling. A statement such as "We will have 45 minutes to talk together today" at the beginning of the first session lets the client know it is not going to be a hurried contact. If it is determined that additional counseling is needed, the client should be told that a specific time period (time and day) will be reserved for future contacts. This allows the client to look forward to future sessions and to anticipate how he or she will use them, while at the same time communicating the expectation that the client will be independent and not seek daily contact. Many counselors also set a target for completing counseling after assessment of the client's needs and establishment of counseling goals. This might be framed like this: "Let's plan to meet for about six sessions and then take stock of where you are. Often people are able to sort out concerns like yours in about that amount of time."

The most complex structuring skills are those that convey to the client what to expect of the counseling process itself. Wallace (1986) proposes that "clients should leave the initial interview with a clear understanding that therapy is a collaborative effort, that they are expected to be active participants in the therapeutic process, and that, although there is certainly reason to hope, there is no promise of success" (p. 71). The client's part of the collaborative effort includes sharing important and sometimes threatening material, making a sincere commitment to changing those things that can lead to problem resolution and growth, working with the counselor to develop alternatives, and taking action as plans develop. The counselor's role is to help the client tell his or her story; to facilitate the client's understanding of his or her feelings, motives, and behaviors; to help the client to reframe aspects of his or her perspective on reality; and to build action plans with the client. Although the client may learn these complementary roles through experience with counseling, it is useful if the counselor starts the process in the first session with statements like this: "I can see that you are troubled by what is happening in your relationship with your son, and I will try very hard to help you understand where the problem is coming from and what you might be able to change." The key element here is that the client must clearly understand that he or she will be left in charge of his or her own life. The counselor helps to enhance the client's coping skills but does not take over solving the problems presented.

A well-structured first counseling session begins the initial-disclosure process. It also helps the client understand what to expect from counseling (and what not to expect), how he or she should participate, and something of the time frame involved.

Some practical aspects of structuring can take place prior to the initial face-to-face meeting with the client though written materials, telephone conversations, or audiovisual or Internet-based resources. For example, a counselor may use this precounseling interaction to communicate to the client information about fees, length of sessions, and the logistics of counseling. Some counselors also provide clients with introductory information about confidentiality and its limits prior to the initial meeting. This approach can increase the productivity of the initial session and maintain the focus on the central issues that are bringing the client into counseling (Welfel, 2002). However, no materials can substitute entirely for a face-to-face discussion of the structure of counseling. Counselors must still clarify that the client understood this material and does not have unresolved questions about it.

Structuring Later in the Counseling Process

When structuring is used later in the counseling process, its purpose is to reassure the client about confidentiality, to reaffirm or renegotiate time parameters, to remind the client of the nature of the process, and to reinforce the appropriate roles of the participants or to move counseling forward to a new stage. A client who is about to reveal particularly sensitive material may want to hear his or her counselor reiterate the conditions of privacy that prevail. Some clients do not comply with stated time parameters, arriving late for sessions, appearing at unscheduled times when no emergency exists, or perhaps delaying the introduction of important material till near the end of a session in hopes of either extending their time or of escaping any authentic work on the new agenda. In any of these instances, it is necessary to reopen a discussion of the value and appropriate use of counseling time. Even in the absence of such problems, prudent counselors periodically discuss the client's progress related to the initially planned duration of counseling and revise the plan as needed.

Examples of structuring to reaffirm the process and to move to a new stage may be drawn from Carl Rogers' (1965) classic demonstration film with a client named Gloria. (These examples appeared late in a first session, not at the beginning of counseling.) Gloria was trying to decide whether or not to tell her young daughter about her own sexual behavior. Would it be more harmful to the relationship to tell her daughter about having sex or to lie to her about sex? She directly asked Dr. Rogers for his opinion. He responded, "I surely wish I could give you an answer, because an answer is what you want. . . . But that would be no damn good." Rogers went on to make clear that there are risks involved with both courses of action and that only Gloria could decide which risks she was more willing to take. He could help her clarify the consequences of each of the choices, but she must make the choice because she must live with the consequences. Later, the counseling session seemed to bog down. Gloria had carefully explored what appeared to be the only two courses of action available to her, but she seemed unprepared to take any action. Rogers gently moved her to the action stage by suggesting that he believed she knew what she wanted to do. He sensed that she placed a higher value on being honest than appearing "pure." Gloria affirmed his perception and began thinking about how to proceed. With this communication, Rogers provided a structure for his client's continued progress in the session.

LEADING

A counselor is typically confronted every few seconds during a counseling session with a choice about how to respond to the content and affect of what the client has just said. The potential range of choices is infinite, and there are usually several responses that have positive potential for advancing the counseling. Other responses may not contribute much to progress, and still others may actually delay progress or disrupt the counseling process altogether. Many potential counselor responses (e.g., paraphrases, statements of empathy, confrontations, interpretation, and ability potential responses) were discussed in Chapters 2 through 5. The purpose of this section is to assist counselors in the moment-to-moment selection of specific responses based on the anticipation of client readiness.

Robinson (1950) coined the term *leading* to describe the counselor's selection of a response that anticipates the client's readiness to benefit from a particular kind of response. As discussed in Chapter 4 (on in-depth exploration), responses that include elements of confrontation and interpretation may be valid but nevertheless destructive to the purposes of counseling if introduced before the client is ready to accept and integrate the information contained in them. The concept of leading includes the proposition that there is "a critical region, just ahead of but not too far ahead of the client, where therapy takes place most efficiently" (Martin, 2000, p. 25).

Robinson (1950) uses a football analogy to describe what he means by leading. When throwing the football, the passer anticipates where the receiver will be when the ball arrives and throws the ball out ahead of the receiver (leads the receiver) so that the ball and the receiver arrive at the same place at the same time. Analogously, Robinson advises the counselor to estimate where the client is going next and to formulate a response that will intersect with the client's path and further his or her progress. The analogy can be extended to include the concept of *length of lead*. If a counselor underestimates the pace of a client's progress, he or she forces the client to slow down and react to a statement that from the client's viewpoint needs no further work—much like a pass receiver must slow his pace or retrace his footsteps to catch a pass that is underthrown. If a counselor overestimates a client's pace, he or she may make a statement that is beyond the client's ability to comprehend and internalize, and the client may become confused and defensive. Progress is then impeded—much as in the case of a receiver who can't make it to the football because it has been overthrown. When trying to estimate a client's *leading edge*, a counselor includes everything that has occurred in his or her experience with the client that the client intended as signs. "This includes verbal and nonverbal cues, as well as all the material that the client has 'put on the table' and assumes you know from previous discussions" (Martin, 2000, p. 26).

In this chapter, we use the word *lead* to mean any response that is based on the counselor's estimate of the likelihood of making contact with the client's next awareness. We do not intend to suggest that the counselor leads the client as one might lead a small child by the hand through a crowded store. Nevertheless, the counselor does select responses (overtly or covertly) that he or she thinks will encourage the client to continue moving ahead in the process. "The term *lead* implies an active collaboration with the client, a partnership in which the counselor's remarks seem to clients to state the next point they are willing to accept" (Shertzer & Stone, 1980, p. 272).

Continuum of Lead

Some responses stay close to what the client has just said and introduce little of the counselor's thoughts and feelings; other responses take a large step from the client's most recent statement and introduce a considerable amount of the counselor's perspective (Hansen, Rossberg, & Cramer, 1994). Robinson (1950) suggests that it is useful to arrange all types of response on a continuum from least leading to most leading, thereby creating reference points that facilitate the choice of slightly more or less leading responses as they are needed in counseling sessions. Such a continuum provides a convenient system for comparing the impact of different counselor responses.

So many different terms have been used over the years to describe various kinds of counselor response that it is not possible to include all of them. Table 8.1 illustrates the usefulness of placing responses on a continuum; it is based on Robinson's early work but introduces the more contemporary terminology for several counselor responses as it appears in Chapters 2 through 5 of this text. Benjamin (2001) includes a similar continuum in his useful description of the helping process.

It is important to realize that all categories of response indicated on the continuum of lead are useful and appropriate at some time in the counseling process; none should be thought of as good or bad, right or wrong (Benjamin, 2001). The degree of lead—that is, the distance the counselor moves toward the most leading end of the continuum—depends on the client's readiness, the kind of concern being discussed, and the predisposition of the counselor. If a client seems particularly defensive, as in the case of a student referred to a school counselor after starting a fight in the cafeteria, the counselor is well advised to take it easy and try to learn the client's view of the incident. On the other hand, a student who is seeking information and guidance about selecting of a college may be well served by counselor-initiated ideas and information and frustrated by a lot of restatements of his or her need. It is the nature of some counselors to listen a lot and be cautious about reaching *any* quick conclusions about another person. These counselors maintain minimal lead in working with clients, using a lot of paraphrase and primary empathy responses and occasionally remaining silent. Other counselors believe they can size up clients fairly quickly, and they become impatient with listening to further iterations of a problem once they think they understand it. These counselors are likely to share their perceptions with clients earlier and thereby maintain a longer lead. They make rapid progress with clients whose defenses are moderate and who have good cognitive skills, but their leading may be threatening or simply confusing to clients who lack ego strength or cognitive skills. To some degree, a counselor's preference concerning the use of leads is influenced by his or her theoretical training. (See Chapter 10 for further development of the relationship between theoretical systems and preferences for leading.)

Table 8.1   Continuum of Lead

Least leading response	Silence	When the counselor makes no verbal response at all, the client ordinarily feels some pressure to continue and chooses how to continue with minimum counselor input.
	Acceptance	The counselor simply acknowledges the client's previous statement with a response such as "yes" or "uh-huh." The client is verbally encouraged to continue, but without content stimulus from the counselor.
	Restatement	The counselor restates the client's verbalization, including both content and affect, using nearly the same wording. The client is prompted to reexamine what has been said.
	Minimal encourager	The counselor directs the client to talk more about a specific subject with a statement such as "Tell me what you mean," or "Please say some more about that." The client is expected to follow the counselor's suggestion.
	Primary empathy	The counselor places himself or herself in the client's shoes and tries to capture what it would be like to have the client's experience. She or he then describes those themes that are readily apparent, using some new language and seeking to verify and clarify the client's meaning.
	Advanced empathy	The counselor states what the client has implied but perhaps not directly stated in his or her disclosures, thereby evoking some new meanings. Sometimes elements of several of the client's statements are brought into a single response. The counselor's ability to perceive accurately and communicate clearly is important, and the client must test the fit of the counselor's lead.
	Affirmation	The counselor affirms the correctness of information or encourages the client's efforts at self-determination by saying, "That's good new information" or "You seem to be gaining more control." The client may follow up with further exploration as he or she sees fit.
	Organizing lead	The counselor directs the client's attention to some aspect of experience that is important to developing a complete picture of the problem or issue at hand, but which the client has overlooked or avoided.
	Immediacy	The counselor calls the client's attention to what is happening in the relationship between the client and the counselor or changes in the client's behavior as certain topics are broached.

(Continued)

Table 8.1   Continued

		Consideration of these immediate behaviors often creates insight into the client's behaviors (and related meanings) outside of counseling.
	Interpretation	The counselor uses psychodiagnostic principles to suggest sources of the client's stress or explanations for the client's motivation and behavior. The counselor's statements are presented as hypotheses, and the client is presented with potentially new ways of seeing the self.
	Confrontation	The counselor directly challenges discrepancies, contradictions, or omissions in the client's disclosures while maintaining a nonjudgmental manner, thereby encouraging the client to resolve the discrepancies.
	Ability potential response	The counselor encourages the client to engage in a specified form of activity by stating an opinion that affirms the client's potential for success.
	Advice	The counselor supports or discourages a specific action based on his or her belief that it would not be in the client's best interest.
	Reassurance	The counselor states that, in his or her judgment, the client's concern is not unusual and that people with similar problems have succeeded in overcoming them. The client may feel that the reassurance is supportive but may also feel that his or her problem is being discounted by the counselor as unimportant.
Most leading response	Introducing new information or a new idea	The counselor moves away from the information in the client's last statement and prompts the client to consider new material.

The counselor's decision about length of lead is related to effectiveness and efficiency. On one hand, it is important to keep length of lead modest enough to stay in contact with the client; on the other hand, the longer the lead that can be achieved while still maintaining contact, the more rapid the progress. Minimum distance leads (e.g., paraphrases) are least threatening to the client because they do not pull him or her from a current level of understanding to some surprising hypothesis about self. On the other hand, there is efficiency in pulling a client toward a new perspective if his or her defenses will permit the assimilation of the new material; a longer lead (e.g., interpretation) may result in quicker development of insight if the client is ready. It is generally recommended that inexperienced counselors make conservative judgments (short length of lead) while gaining experience, because excessive numbers of longer leads can frighten clients and preclude effectiveness of counseling. Longer leads become safer once diagnostic abilities have been honed through experience.

Leading and the Stages of Counseling

Counselor responses usually become increasingly leading as counseling proceeds through the three stages. In the early phase of counseling, when relationship building is of prime importance, the counselor's responses tend toward the least leading end of the continuum. In-depth exploration is prompted by responses in midrange. Commitment to action often requires some counselor-initiated reinforcement as well as counselor-supplied information—both examples of responses toward the most leading end of the continuum.

A review of the material in Chapter 3 reveals that the counselor most often uses responses from the least leading end of the continuum during the initial-disclosure stage of counseling. The following example involved a worried 8-year-old girl.

> CLIENT: I don't know what I'm going to do. My mother doesn't live here any more, and my grandma says she is not going to be my mom.
> COUNSELOR: You're scared that there won't be anyone to take care of you, and you are too little to take care of yourself.

The counselor accurately perceived the emotion and the basis for that emotion. Such a statement is said to be *interchangeable* with the client's statement and communicates primary empathy.

By restating the material for the client, the counselor showed understanding and encouraged the client to continue with the disclosure process. The client went on to say that her mother had left town with a man after leaving her with her grandmother. Although the grandmother had been providing basic care, she had made it clear to the girl that she wasn't interested in getting back into the business of raising a child. Using primary empathy, acceptance, and silence, the counselor was able to acquire a fairly complete picture of the problem from the child's point of view.

Because the child could not be expected to arrive at her own solution to the problem of who was going to take care of her, counseling did not proceed to the second and third stages. Instead, the grandmother was invited for consultation, and the counselor helped her understand that the client took her statements about not wanting to have another child to care for as a threat that she too would abandon the child. Fortunately, the grandmother was committed to providing care for as long as the daughter was gone, and she was able to be more supportive with the child, saving her anger to express to the daughter when she could do so.

The second stage of counseling, as described in Chapter 4, promotes in-depth exploration by the client, and responses toward the middle of the continuum are likely to be most useful. For example, a counselor employs advanced empathy statements to encourage the exploration of ideas that may have been implied but not explicitly stated by clients. In the following example, the client is a 27-year-old woman.

> CLIENT: I got tired of just sitting around, so I went down to the bar to see if Frank was there. I almost hoped he wouldn't be there, but I had to get out.
>
> COUNSELOR: It sounds like you didn't want to stay home alone, and you didn't want to see Frank either. You were pretty desperate just to have some human contact.
>
> CLIENT: Yeah. When I sit around alone for a while, I begin to wonder if I'm okay. I don't seem to know what I want. I know Frank's a bum, but at least when he's around I don't feel so lost.
>
> COUNSELOR: When Frank is around, you don't feel quite so incomplete as when you are alone, and that is less frightening even though you know Frank isn't the kind of man you really want in your life.

In this dialogue, each counselor response added perspective and clarity to the client statement. In the first instance, the counselor magnified the affect of the client's statement by responding to the sense of desperation. In the second instance, the counselor labeled the sense of incompleteness that was at the root of the desperate feeling. This led to further in-depth exploration in which the client affirmed that the feeling she had when she was alone caused her to accept the company of virtually anyone who would spend time with her. This had led to a series of unsatisfying and abusive relationships with men whom she had met in bars. The responses in this example are referred to as *additive* because they add perspective from the counselor's assessment of the client's concern. Long-term counseling was required for this client to begin to feel a sense of personal integrity and worth that enabled her to begin to select more satisfying company and feel comfortable when alone.

Interpretation is also used heavily to promote in-depth exploration. Interpretation can be seen to appear on the continuum of lead toward the most leading end. In fact, interpretations are distinguished from advanced empathy statements because the frame of reference for interpretation is the counselor's diagnostic perspective, not the client's personal frame of reference. An example of an interpretive response follows. The client is a 15-year-old boy.

> CLIENT: I don't know why everyone keeps bugging me about getting good grades to get into college. I can always pull wire. (The client smiles as he makes the last statement and makes a hand-over-hand motion as though pulling wire into a structure.)
>
> COUNSELOR: Yeah, you could really get even with your dad by messing up in school.

As is characteristic of many interpretive responses, this counselor's statement seems harsh and irrelevant without information on the background of the client and the history of the relationship with the counselor. The client's father was a self-made entrepreneur who owned his own electrical contracting business. The father had placed a great deal of pressure on his son to "make something of himself"—that is, to become an educated man who would not have to do work that his father considered unfulfilling and often demeaning. The son resented this pressure and his wire-pulling pose was a passive-aggressive cliché he used to anger his father. The client saw nothing demeaning about pulling wire or running a contracting business. However, he had little awareness that his motivation to work in the family business came more from his rejection of his father's wishes than from an intrinsic interest in the business. What the counselor said was an attempt to stimulate the client to consider the motives underlying his behavior. By definition, interpretation goes beyond the client's present conceptualization of a problem and into the counselor's frame of reference, and it will therefore present the client with a new idea.

Techniques closer to the most leading end of the continuum are used more frequently in the third stage of counseling—commitment to action. By this stage, the counselor understands the nature of the client's concerns and has a good sense of the client's goals. With that background, the counselor may help specify action plans, provide active encouragement through ability potential responses, reassure the client about his or her progress, or provide new information or occasional advice. The focus is on helping the client to act on what he or she wants to do. As one problem or issue reaches resolution, the counselor may introduce other agendas that have come up during counseling to determine whether there is work to be done. (See Chapter 5 for a more specific discussion of counseling skills to promote client actions.)

The following principles relate the degree of lead to the stage of counseling:

- Minimum-lead responses are excellent for relationship building.
- Minimum-lead responses are low-risk responses, because they do not frighten the client with startling new perspectives.
- Responses toward the center of the continuum increase the client's in-depth exploration.
- Responses toward the center of the continuum can be somewhat threatening and may produce defensive reactions if used prematurely.
- Maximum-lead responses are directive, reinforcing specific behaviors that relate to the client's goals.
- Maximum-lead responses are likely to seem irrelevant or highly threatening to the client unless the counselor has taken time to know the client and his or her goals.

THE USE OF QUESTIONS IN COUNSELING

Counselors use questions frequently—according to several researchers they amount to between 9% and 13% of all counselor responses in session (Hill & O'Brien, 1999). Questions, depending on their formulation, can embody a minimum, middle, or maximum degree of leading. A minimum-lead question, such as "What happened next?" simply asks the client to continue with his or her own story. A medium-lead question incorporates information that the client has provided and implies that the information has significance, for example, "What meaning did you attach to your husband's repeated late nights at the office and occasional failures to come home at all?" A maximum-lead question often includes a counselor hypothesis, for example, "Do you see how your anger at your wife when she pressed you to do more was rooted in self-disgust at your own inability to deliver?" Each of these questions could be appropriate at a given moment in counseling, and each could be stated in a declarative way.

Questions are useful in opening new aspects of the client's situation for discussion (such as history, strengths, or prior attempts at alleviating the problem), in clarifying vague or conflicting comments from the client, or in focusing the client's attention on specific thoughts, feelings, or behaviors related to an issue or problem. They can also be used to acquire specific information needed to arrive at a diagnosis, as in seeking more information about the duration of a depressed mood and nature of the client's symptoms. Well-structured and well-timed questions move the counseling process ahead and promote insight and motivation to change, but poorly worded or mistimed questions interfere with that process. Well-planned questions follow from the client's prior statements without an abrupt change of topic or tone (like any other lead). For example, if a client has been discussing his ambivalence about seeking a more satisfying job and risking his current security, questions about his family might seem irrelevant. Any question about current stresses in his marriage, for example, should be related to his career concern (e.g., "To what extent do you think your worry over security has been tied up with your wife's attitudes about money?"). In addition, effective questions should deal with content that the client can comfortably handle (like any other lead), given the level of trust established and the depth of self-understanding achieved at the point at which the question is asked. Questions that address painful material must be stated with empathy for the client's feelings to minimize resistance.

An uninterrupted sequence of questions creates a distorted process where the counselor appears to be grilling the client and can actually prevent the client from disclosing what he or she needs to discuss by channeling attention onto issues that may seem pertinent to the counselor but not the client. Further, premature questions may rush the client to define the problems too quickly or hurry the process of identifying solutions. A counselor who hears himself or herself asking questions beginning with "Have you tried . . ." or "Do you think your problem is . . ." should examine whether he or she is hurrying the client. Another clue to hurrying the client is the feeling that the counselor is guessing at what the client is experiencing rather than encouraging the client to describe it in his or her own way.

As a general rule, questions should be open-ended—phrased so that they encourage the client to answer them in long phrases or full sentences. Closed-ended questions that have yes/no or one-word answers are less useful and may result in a pattern in which the counselor needs to respond again after the client's one-word answer. Consider the following interactions:

Interaction A

CLIENT: I feel so uncomfortable with my family lately. I'd rather be alone or at the office working.
COUNSELOR: What feelings are included in that discomfort?
CLIENT: Mostly I feel like such a failure, and I think that they can't really love or respect me.

Interaction B

CLIENT: I feel so uncomfortable with my family lately. I'd rather be alone or at the office working.
COUNSELOR: Do you feel distant with them?
CLIENT: Yes, often.

The second interaction generated little new information from the client and set up a pattern that required the counselor to ask something more to get the client to keep disclosing. Closed-ended questions tend to close off discussion of an issue. Asking the client in these interactions whether he felt distant or angry at his family would not lead to a much better result. The client can still respond with a one-word answer—"Distant," "Angry," or "Neither," placing the counselor in the position of needing to prompt further. Hill and O'Brien (1999) note that open-ended questions are particularly helpful when clients seem to be repeating themselves without moving to explore their concerns more deeply. Open-ended questions can also be used to assist clients in examining their problems from various perspectives. For instance, when a client seems to be going "round in circles" about what makes her roommate act so irritated with her, a counselor may ask, "What kind of reactions do you think a stranger observing the interactions between you and your roommate would have if that stranger had no knowledge of this history of your relationship?" Research supports the use of open-ended questions with adults and with children, indicating that they foster deep exploration moderately well and that they encourage children to talk longer and more deeply about their concerns (Hill & O'Brien, 1999). Either/or questions such as "Did you feel hurt or angry toward your roommate when he said that?" are really a type of closed-ended question as they often result in one-word responses and reduce the client's consideration of other alternatives.

Counselors sometimes fall into the habit of using questions that are not really questions. The following example with a fifth-grade girl who is resisting efforts to help her adjust to her parents' move to another state provides an illustration:

> CLIENT: It's just not fair that I have no say in this decision. I want to stay and live with my friend, Lucy, but my dad won't even consider it.
> COUNSELOR: Don't you think you'd miss your parents after a while?
> CLIENT: No. Besides, I could visit them at school vacations.

In this case, the counselor's question was really a statement of her opinion about the girl's reaction to such an arrangement, even though it was worded as a question. The counselor's hidden agenda may have been to get the girl to see another point of view, but it backfired when approached in this fashion. A question that begins "Don't you think . . ." or "Don't you feel . . ." probably should be rephrased. In this example, an open-ended question such as "How do you think it would work out if you lived with Lucy?" would show more respect for the client's viewpoint and help her explore the reality of such a situation.

In the final analysis, we suggest sparing use of questions because of the many pitfalls we have enumerated. Furthermore, beginning counselors usually think of questioning as a familiar process and fail to practice and learn other techniques if permitted to rely on questions. Nevertheless, an occasional question may be the most efficient way to seek a specific piece of information or to guide a client to deeper exploration. What is key is flexibility so that the counselor's response is determined by the client's needs at the moment. When a counselor is peppering a client with question after question, it is unlikely that the counselor is choosing a response based on the client's need or counseling goals.

SUMMARY

This chapter discussed techniques of counseling—specific statements to be used with a client at a specific moment. Structuring statements are designed to help the client learn to use counseling and learn the role and responsibilities of the client and the counselor. Leading responses are statements that prompt the client to develop his or her own picture of life events, issues, and problems. The counselor attempts to judge what degree of leading the client is ready for and to provide a response to the client's most recent statement that will move the process forward. Typically, in the early stages of counseling, leading is at the minimum end of the continuum.

In-depth exploration is best promoted by responses toward the center of the continuum, and commitment to action may involve responses at the most leading end, including the use of new information and reinforcement of selected behaviors. Questions can occur at any time in the counseling process. If they are open ended and well timed, they promote deeper client self-exploration. However, poorly formulated or badly timed questions interrupt client progress.

≈≈≈ *DISCUSSION QUESTIONS* ≈≈≈

1. Both structuring and questioning become problems when they are used too much. In what situations do you think counselors would be vulnerable to overusing these types of responses?
2. The authors suggest that some tasks defined as structuring the counseling relationship may be accomplished prior to the first session. They cite the explanation of fees and logistics as one example of information that may be appropriate to communicate through written, taped, or Internet-based media. What are the advantages and disadvantages of this approach? What content do you think would be better communicated in the face-to-face meeting?
3. Rogers advocated avoiding questioning as much as possible. He conducted some demonstration sessions in which he never asked a client a question. Do you see this as a strength or a weakness in counseling? What is your position on the advisability of questioning in counseling?
4. Responses toward the high end of the leading continuum can be threatening to the client because they delve into painful or uncomfortable material. Such high-lead responses also are at greater risk for misinterpreting the client's experience. What counselor reactions would be appropriate if a leading response generated either client defensiveness or the client's denial of their accuracy?
5. Research supports the contribution of open-ended questions to clients' exploration of issues. How common do you think open-ended questions are in ordinary conversations? How frequently do you use them, and what gets in the way of their use?

REFERENCES

Benjamin, A. (2001). *The helping interview: With case illustrations* (3rd ed.). Boston: Houghton Mifflin.

Brammer, L. M., Abrego, P., & Shostrum, E. L. (1993). *Therapeutic counseling and psychotherapy* (6th ed.). Englewood Cliffs, NJ: Prentice-Hall.

Corey, G. (2001). *Theory and practice of counseling and psychotherapy* (6th ed.). Pacific Grove, CA: Brooks/Cole.

Hansen, J. C., Rossberg, R., & Cramer, S. H. (1994). *Counseling theory and process* (5th ed.). Boston: Allyn & Bacon.

Hill, C. E., & O'Brien, K. M. (1999). *Helping skills: Facilitating exploration, insight and action.* Washington, DC: American Psychological Association.

Ivey, A. E., & Ivey, M. B. (2003). *Intentional interviewing and counseling: Facilitating client development in a multicultural society* (5th ed.). Pacific Grove, CA: Brooks/Cole.

Martin, D. G. (2000). *Counseling and therapy skills* (2nd ed.). Prospect Heights, IL: Waveland.

Patterson, C. H. (1974). *Relationship counseling and psychotherapy.* New York: Harper & Row.

Robinson, F. P. (1950). *Principles and procedures of student counseling.* New York: Harper.

Rogers, C. R. (1965). Client-centered therapy. In E. Shostrom (Producer), *Three approaches to psychotherapy* [Videotape]. Orange, CA: Psychological Films.

Shertzer, B., & Stone, S. C. (1980). *Fundamentals of counseling* (3rd ed.). Boston: Houghton Mifflin.

Wallace, W. A. (1986). *Theories of counseling and psychotherapy.* Boston: Allyn & Bacon.

Welfel, E. R. (2002). *Ethics in counseling and psychotherapy: Standards, research and emerging issues* (2nd ed.). Pacific Grove, CA: Brooks/Cole.

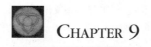 CHAPTER 9

WORKING WITH AMBIVALENT, INDIFFERENT, AND OPPOSITIONAL CLIENTS

The content of the preceding chapters applies most readily to voluntary, or self-referred clients who are willing to initiate discussion on an issue of concern. Starting the counseling process with these clients is relatively easy—the counselor simply begins with a statement that provides the client with an opportunity to share information. "How can I help?" is one example. Responses such as summaries or reflections of feelings and beliefs, leads such as "Tell me more about . . ." and "I" messages facilitate further exploration. However, many clients are neither motivated for counseling nor comfortable with the process when they arrive for counseling. This chapter discusses these harder-to-help clients, the nature of their reluctance and resistance, how counselors may react to them, why it is important to work with them, how to help them, and how to communicate with those referring them.

WHO ARE THESE HESITANT CLIENTS?

Ambivalent, indifferent, and oppositional clients are those who are mistrustful of counseling or who feel unready to change. If given a choice, many would choose not to be in the presence of a counselor and would prefer not to talk about themselves (Doyle,1998). To understand the hesitation of these clients, it is useful to consider their *reluctance*—conscious reservations about being in counseling—as well as their *resistance*—unconscious defensive reactions to the counseling situation. Their hesitation can vary from moderate difficulty in getting started at one end of the continuum, to perfunctory participation or to outright refusal to cooperate with counseling at the other extreme.

Many are not self-referred but are instead required or urged to engage in counseling by court action, school officials, spouses, or parents. Some self-referred clients also have a lot of ambivalence about seeking help from others and may be mistrustful of the counselor or their own capacity to achieve their goals even though they have tentatively decided to give counseling a try.

In certain settings, "these [hesitant] clients represent the major proportion of the counselor's caseload" (Ritchie, 1986, p. 516). Dyer and Vriend (1973) stated that a large proportion of students who visit school counselors are not there entirely voluntarily. These include students whom parents, the counselor, or other school staff have identified as academically or behaviorally deficient. Referrals from teachers and parents are often made with the implicit understanding that the counselor will straighten out the client's "silly" thinking and show the child a proper course of action. In clinical settings, many clients appear for counseling at the behest of significant others, including spouses, lovers, parents, or children. In relationship counseling, one party in a relationship often brings his or her partner to counseling. Parents frequently schedule their children for counseling, and, increasingly, adolescent and adult children are responsible for bringing their parents to counseling. Agendas such as substance abuse and family violence, among others, lead family members to insist that other family members attend counseling sessions. Physicians frequently refer their patients for counseling to help them with issues such as quitting smoking, managing stress, or reducing compulsive eating, and some patients reluctantly agree out of worry about alienating the physician or compromising access to medical care if they refuse. Finally, the criminal justice system may make counseling a requirement for juveniles or adults who have violated various laws. Some clients referred by the justice system are incarcerated, and others are required to seek counseling as a condition of remaining out of confinement while working toward rehabilitation. Typically, the literature refers to clients whose presence in counseling is demanded by the legal system as "mandated" or "involuntary" clients (Riordan & Martin, 1993; Rooney, 1992).

Another way to understand the variability in clients' openness to counseling is to use the model developed by Prochaska, DiClemente, and Norcross (1994) that defines six stages of client readiness for change. Although originally developed to understand clients' difficulties in changing addictive or other unhealthy behaviors, it has clear application to the counseling process and client attitudes toward therapeutic change. Their research on this model has shown that it can effectively predict clients' success with changing addictive behaviors, with managing chronic mental illness, and with making other mental health changes. They identify the lowest level of readiness for change as *precontemplation*. Because this stage means that people are not actively considering changing their behavior in the near future, few voluntary clients fall into this category, but it can be applied to clients who are pushed to enter counseling by a third party. People at this stage tend to avoid thinking about their problems and may be defensive when others initiate discussion of them. They appear unaware of the effects of their difficulties on other aspects of their lives and on their relationships. In some cases they may have attempted to change on their own and have failed, so they are hopeless about the success of future efforts. When entering counseling, people at this stage tend to underestimate the potential benefits of counseling and overestimate the difficulties involved. Unless they can progress to the next stage of readiness, counseling is not likely to be helpful. These clients clearly fit our definition of reluctant clients.

The second stage in this model is called the *contemplation* stage. Here clients are intending to make changes in their lives within the next 6 months. They are more conscious of the benefits from change than people in the precontemplation stage but are still very aware of the difficulties inherent in change and the work involved in succeeding with change. In other words, they experience real ambivalence about committing to the change process, hence they fit well into our definition of hesitant or ambivalent clients. People can remain at the contemplation stage for long periods as they wrestle with their ambivalence toward change. The emotions associated with this stage are tension and conflict within the self.

Clients at the third stage, *preparation,* want to take action for change soon, have often developed a personal plan for change, and are ready to engage in the work of self-discovery and behavior change. They are likely to have volunteered to start counseling. Because they are much less ambivalent about counseling, they fit the definition of voluntary clients.

At the next stage, the *action* stage, people have already implanted changes in their lives that move them toward their goal. When people at this stage enter counseling, they are likely to be seeking professional advice to speed up or maintain the changes they have already achieved. They may also wish to generalize the changes they have made in one problem area to another. At the *maintenance* stage of readiness, clients have achieved their goals and are now seeking to make them permanent. When clients enter counseling at this level of readiness, they are seeking deeper insight into the triggers for old patterns and a wider repertoire of coping skills. At the final stage, called the *termination* stage, people feel no risk at all of ever returning to the old behavior. Needless to say, few people reach this stage, and virtually no one who is entering counseling is at this point.

UNDERSTANDING CLIENT RELUCTANCE AND RESISTANCE

Reluctance, as previously noted, is simply a disinclination to participate in counseling. Reluctant clients are aware of their reasons for being reluctant, though they may not have focused on or articulated those reasons. Each of the following can contribute to reluctance:

- Embarrassment and the wish for privacy
- Unfamiliarity with counseling
- Lack of faith that talking can help
- Belief that one doesn't need help or ought to be able to "stand alone"

- Fear that one will lose autonomy over life issues and that the counselor will take control
- Belief that only crazy people need counselors
- Discomfort with the setting (the setting may seem too exposed, may be associated with a disliked entity such as the justice system, or may simply be physically uncomfortable)
- Discomfort with the personal characteristics or counseling style of the assigned counselor
- History of a negative experience with a helping professional
- Concern with fees and expenses of counseling

Chapters 2 and 3 examined several of these issues of relationship building. Reluctant clients may be thought of as having exaggerated trust issues, often reinforced by chaotic and unrewarding relationships with others outside of counseling.

Many clients, especially adult males, consider it a sign of weakness to need professional help in resolving life's problems (Addis & Mahalik, 2003; Mintz & O'Neil, 1990). Even if such persons initiate counseling, they may resent having to do so and behave as reluctant clients. Some culturally diverse clients may be socialized to be private about their concerns and have difficulty with disclosure (Atkinson, Morten, & Sue, 1998). Other diverse clients who feel they have been wronged by the majority culture may bring anger about racism to the counseling situation, especially if the assigned counselor is of another racial or ethnic background. (See Chapter 12 for a more complete discussion of working with the reluctance of culturally different clients.) Sometimes clients simply have a sense of futility because all their contacts with others seem to end in unproductive conflict. In some cases, clients have been unsuccessful so many times in their own attempts to change behavior that they have concluded that change is probably hopeless and that counselors are unlikely to do any better than they did on their own.

Reluctance can be exacerbated by ineffective and insensitive counselor behaviors. Counselors who push for behavior change prematurely, confront client inconsistencies too frequently or too harshly, or fail to appreciate the emotional and systemic components of clients' problems can actually create reluctance where none had existed before. Rather than conceiving of reluctance and resistance entirely as internal processes within the client's psyche or history, many scholars and researchers include an interactional perspective, asserting that client opposition can be situational and a product of inappropriate counselor behavior during counseling (see Beutler, Moleiro, & Talebi, 2002 for a summary of this literature). In other words, indifferent, judgmental, or unskilled counselors can actually trigger reluctance and resistance in a client. Others argue that reluctance is not necessarily limited to circumstances when a counselor acts in an unskilled or inappropriate way, but is a more universal consequence of the counseling process. They describe it as a "phenomenon that emerges between client and therapist in the unfolding interaction between differently organized subjective worlds" (Cowan & Presbury, 2000, p. 413).

Resistance is an unconscious process whose purpose is to protect the client from having to explore and claim feelings and motivations that have roots in his or her past. "Resistance includes everything in the words and behaviors of the client that prevents access to unconscious material" (Ivey, Ivey, & Simek-Morgan, 2002, p. 257), and thus resistance opposes the purposes of counseling (Brammer, Abrego, & Shostrum, 1993). It is an intrapsychic process that is experienced by all clients (not just reluctant ones). A client who has urges toward growth and completeness nevertheless still fears the pain of recalling traumatic material (Pipes & Davenport, 1999) and resists abandoning the certain present—with all its limitations—in favor of facing the past or anticipating an unknown future. A reluctant client such as we have discussed is quite aware that he or she does not have much trust in the counseling process and would prefer not to participate. In addition, these clients usually have strong unconscious defenses that create an unwillingness to participate in the process of counseling.

The most important manifestation of resistance underlying the behavior of ambivalent, indifferent, and especially oppositional clients is *transference*. Transference (Brammer, Abrego, & Shostrum, 1993, p. 200) is the "repetition of past relationships with significant others such that these earlier feelings, behaviors, and attitudes are 'transferred' or projected onto the therapist or others outside the therapeutic setting." According to transference theory, a person may build a pattern of negative and self-defeating response to authority over an extended period of time. The pattern usually begins with parent–child relationships in which the child perceives that the parents make arbitrary demands and make their love conditional on the child doing their bidding. The child experiences hurt, deprivation, frustration, and eventually anger because the parents perceive his or her behaviors as wanting and love from the parents is not dependable.

As children expand their world of social contact, teachers are the next authorities with direct influence over their lives. If the parent–child relationship does not improve and a child remains insecure about whether he or she is competent and loved, any demand a teacher may make is a further threat, and some of the resentment originally held for the parent is transferred to the teacher. Even reasonable expectations of teachers may prompt this transference if the situation with parents is strongly negative, and the situation may get worse if the teacher makes unreasonable demands or reacts hostilely to the resentment the child holds. Sometimes this kind of sequence is repeated as young people meet more new authority figures, and by adolescence they may perceive all adults as controlling and uncaring. A self-fulfilling prophecy develops. Anticipating negative responses from adults, the young person behaves in a way that tends to elicit such responses. If these authority problems are not resolved during adolescence, they are likely to manifest themselves through the adult years in situations involving family life, employment, and other socially defined roles. Even though a counselor may not perceive himself or herself as an authority figure, to clients with authority problems, the counselor is one more person trying to get them to change. However kindly the counselor may proceed, clients are likely to employ the strategies that they usually use with authorities.

Clients who have a history of conflict with parents, teachers, employers, and other persons in positions of authority tend to expect conflict as a new relationship begins with a counselor whom they perceive as another authority figure. Cowan and Presbury (2000) characterize this as an expectation of "retraumatization." Clients exhibit the attitudes and behaviors that they have learned and practiced in their earlier dysfunctional relationships with people who were in positions to exert influence over their lives. "It is as if the client is so certain that what he or she is experiencing is unacceptable that the therapist is presumed to be unaccepting and critical, all evidence to the contrary" (Pipes & Davenport, 1999, p. 173). These oppositional feelings toward the counselor have origins that the client does not fully understand, but the client's attitudes about counseling and the counselor are often expressed very directly.

When a counselor meets an oppositional client for the first time, what occurs often seems irrational to the counselor, as it would to an impartial observer looking in on the session. The counselor offers an accepting welcome, attends caringly to the client's communications, shows genuine interest in the client and the difficulties he or she is experiencing, and expresses empathy for his or her situation. In return, the client is often initially sullen, silent, belligerent, or overly compliant ("Just tell me what you want from me").

To understand why the counselor is treated like an enemy when he or she acts more like a friend, we look to the client's predisposition that the counselor will be uncaring and demanding. Two kinds of reactions are typical. The first and more common is a hostile stance testing each new authority figure and putting him or her at a distance. The other is excessive compliance, perhaps initially based on the misguided hope that doing exactly what is requested will win elusive acceptance. But compliant personalities lose control of their own lives, and when things do not work out, often respond, "I only did what you told me to do." Either reaction is detrimental to counseling because the former militates against the quick formation of a trusting relationship (therapeutic alliance) and the latter leads to dependency. Dependent clients look to the counselor for answers, are not able to form a true partnership with the counselor, and tend to do little productive work on their concerns.

THE COUNSELOR'S EMOTIONS TOWARD THE AMBIVALENT, INDIFFERENT, OR OPPOSITIONAL CLIENT

The ambivalent client may not present in ways strikingly different from the motivated client. Counselors may sense some holding back, passivity, or feel more powerfully the need to prove themselves trustworthy to the ambivalent client. Upon the initial encounter with an ambivalent or oppositional client, the counselor may feel a sense of rejection and even receive verbal abuse from the client, whom the counselor does not yet know and to whom he or she has done nothing offensive. The natural human response to such attack is to be angry, and indeed the counselor may experience a flash of anger toward such a client.

As Dyer and Vriend (1973) describe, counselors often experience relationship-blocking emotions when faced with an oppositional client. The counselor has a reality-based concern about whether counseling will succeed and the noxious experience of feeling rejected by another person. Even when a client is merely ambivalent, the counselor experiences real concern about whether he or she will really be able to help this client. On the other hand, the counselor may experience countertransference reactions to the client that call forth his or her tendency to respond in authoritarian (controlling parent) or dependency-building (solicitous parent) ways. Such countertransference reactions are based on the counselor's unresolved feelings about the nurturing process, and as with transference, the roots of the feelings may be largely beyond the counselor's awareness. The sources of the counselor's emotions when working with reluctant clients and some strategies for managing those emotions are developed in this section.

It is natural for a counselor to experience some anxiety when faced with a reluctant and resistant client. The client can be a threat to the counselor's sense of professional competence and is potentially capable of blocking the counselor's goal of being a successful helper. Opening communication, building trust, stimulating exploration, developing insights, and changing behavior are all made more difficult. If the counselor's anxiety about the possibility that counseling might fail is not managed successfully, his or her ability to respond sensitively and insightfully may be impaired. Counselor anxiety can lead to frustration and even anger at the client who is obstructing successful helping. Ironically, this amounts to blaming the client for his or her resistance rather than accepting it as a natural part of counseling that must be worked through.

As the encounter with a poorly motivated client takes shape, the counselor should monitor his or her self-talk about the client. One possible perspective is "This client has a lot of nerve. What right has this client to treat me so disrespectfully? I don't see how I can be of much help with his or her attitude as it is." The focus here is on the counselor's offended feelings and fear of failure. The counselor is blaming the client for these feelings, and counseling will be difficult. On the other hand, consider this counselor self-talk: "This client has barriers that are very strong. I will have to work hard to earn his or her trust and to remember that his or her behavior makes sense when viewed from his or her experience. I can't take his or her attacks personally if I want to be able to help." The focus here is on the client and demonstrates an emotionally neutral acceptance of the client's behavior. Additional efforts to comprehend how the client's disappointments and frustrations in past relationships have set the stage for his or her response to the counselor will also assist the counselor in avoiding hurt feelings that are translated into ineffective practice.

Counselor feelings that are countertransference reactions are hardest of all to manage, for they stem from the counselor's unconscious predispositions about authority relationships. Fundamentally, the problem begins when the counselor at some level decides that the client is incapable of handling or learning to handle his or her own life situation and so assumes an authority role with respect to the client. Having made this decision, the counselor responds as a controlling parent might, telling the client what he or she should do. With a dependent client, the counselor's response may be to try to do everything for the client rather than urging self-direction. Either way, the counselor loses sight of the fact that the client cannot grow in his or her ability to handle life situations unless he or she is an active participant in decisions that are made. Even very skilled counselors are sometimes overcome by their needs to be parental, especially in interactions with children and youths.

Perhaps the greatest problem with countertransference is that it exacerbates the client's transference behaviors. With a hostile client, a counselor who acts in an authoritarian way fulfills the client's expectation that the counselor is an authority figure who is trying to manipulate. The counselor can no longer offer the unique relationship (caring, genuine, and unconditional) that characterizes the helping process. When this set of events unfolds, we say that the counselor has fed the transference and reinforced the client's self-defeating views that all people who are "part of the system" are controlling and insensitive. If the conflict is not resolved, such a client will be even more reluctant to seek counseling again.

If a client tends to be dependent on authority figures, a counselor acting as a solicitous parent will increase the client's tendency to avoid responsibility. There are many examples of clients who hound their counselors for advice about the smallest move, "hang out" in the guidance office, or call counselors at home about inconsequential matters. This is the result of the counselor feeding the client's dependency needs, perhaps to satisfy his or her own countertransference needs to be a caretaker.

Countertransference has the potential of reinforcing dysfunctional client behavior and making the client less confident that the counseling process can be helpful. Consultation with or supervision by another counselor is usually the most effective way of coping with serious countertransference problems. As a general rule, any time a counselor thinks "If I could only control that crazy behavior" or "If I could only take that poor dear home," that is the time to talk with a colleague. By discussing his or her feelings with another counselor, a counselor in this situation can come to a better understanding of his or her own needs and restore his or her ability to place the client's needs first. Some counselors-in-training may find that their need to assume responsibilities that should be the client's is strong. In such cases, the counselor himself or herself may need counseling to resolve countertransference needs. Unmotivated and oppositional clients create stress for all counselors. The counselor's response to this stress is influenced by the persistence and degree of dysfunction in the client's behavior as well as countertransference based on the counselor's unresolved needs. In many instances, counselors can improve their work with difficult clients through skill development or through self-reinforcing talk. In other instances, consultation or counseling with a more objective third party (another counselor) is needed.

WHY WORK WITH UNMOTIVATED AND OPPOSITIONAL CLIENTS?

Whether or not counselors should be expected to work with unmotivated and oppositional clients is an important issue. Some say counselors should work only with those who appear to want a counselor's help. Others argue that, as professionals, counselors should be expected to work with anyone who stands to benefit from their services.

Counselors in schools or colleges are expected to work with students whose academic performance is unsatisfactory, whose behavior is disruptive, or who seem to have no sense of personal direction or commitment to the future, whether or not those students seek help. These behavior patterns are often important indicators of poor self-esteem. A counselor working within the framework of a developmental guidance program will extend counseling services to these students with the goals of encouraging them to identify and resolve underlying problems, to identify motivating forces, and to come closer to fulfilling their human potential.

Counselors who work in the criminal justice system know when they sign an employment contract that many of their clients will be reluctant about counseling. The decision to work with such clients is based on the belief that persons who commit crimes can learn to fulfill their needs in ways that don't violate the rights of others and that avoid future incarceration. To the degree that this occurs, both the individual and society benefit.

Many clients in substance abuse counseling have lost control of their lives to the substance (alcohol or other drugs) they are using. Their motivation is to maintain their habit even though they may recognize that they are losing their grip on work and family. It is often the family or the employer who insists that the client seek counseling—for the client's own welfare and that of the family.

Finally, some clients are referred or brought to counseling by family or friends who are concerned about the client's mood, behaviors, decision making, or performance. Many times these clients do not acknowledge that they need help even though their behaviors seem self-defeating and ineffective to others. These are clients whose actions may interfere with their own daily lives and potential development (e.g., persons who are disaffected and exert little effort in life), or they may fail in their responsibilities to others (e.g., parents who pay little attention to their children or fail to provide basic needs). Although they may experience unhappiness with their lot in life, they mistakenly assume that there is nothing they can do about their situations and they often see the referring person and the counselor as people who are pressuring them to be "better."

Some important assumptions underlie a counselor's decision to work with an unmotivated or oppositional client. One is a moral and ethical obligation to help others live more fully if one has the capacity to do so, whether or not those others seek help. This assumption is supported by the knowledge that an individual who has not experienced counseling cannot know its value.

A second assumption is that the counselor has the capacity to recognize ineffective behavior or unhappiness that may be amenable to alteration through counseling. The counselor's model of the mentally healthy individual forms a standard by which to evaluate client behaviors and emotions and to identify unhealthy or undesirable patterns. What may appear as unhealthy on the surface may turn out to be reasonable coping upon further understanding of the client and his or her situation. For example, a person currently being battered by a partner may refuse to leave that partner, a behavior that on the surface appears inconsistent with all notions of mental or physical health. However, many such victims intuitively recognize that the danger they face is likely to increase significantly if they attempt to leave the batterer. Reports of violence and murder after separating are legion in the news. Ultimately, staying with the batterer often has survival value if a clear safety plan for leaving is not in place.

Another assumption is that early intervention for dysfunctional behavior is likely to lead to more rapid and more complete resolution of the problem. This may serve as justification for a counselor to begin working with a client before the client recognizes the need for help. Examples include intervention with academic problems before skills deficits make it difficult to catch up and intervention with an alcoholic prior to the time the person hits rock bottom. Counseling is used to help prevent problems from becoming more serious or from extending their debilitating influence from one aspect of the client's life (e.g., work) to another (e.g., marriage).

When a counselor decides to work with an unmotivated or oppositional client, he or she concludes that it would be better to try to influence
the client than to allow things to go on as they are going. To this degree,
the counselor assumes some control over what happens. The counselor
determines that the client will benefit from counseling, even though there is
also a risk that the client will see the counselor to be like others who have
judged him or her to be insufficient. The counselor's effectiveness lies in his
or her ability to communicate caring and trust, to avoid a moralizing posture, and to avoid using coercive tactics to get the client to conform to
someone else's norms. The reluctant client, like any other, deserves the
opportunity to design his or her own solutions to life's difficulties.

WORKING WITH THE CLIENT'S RELUCTANCE

Earlier in this chapter we defined reluctance and the related concept of
resistance. These processes oppose the purposes of counseling when mani-
fested by the client, even though the client is usually aware of reluctance
and not aware of resistance. Fear of trusting and fear of changing underlie
these processes. Because all clients experience some resistance in counseling, it is reasonable to assume that a client who is actively reluctant is experiencing resistance as well. Authors who discuss reluctance and resistance as
separate issues often conclude that treatment is similar whichever process is
occurring (Egan, 2002; Pipes & Davenport, 1999). It is essential that the
counselor join the client in exploring what is making it difficult for the client
to trust the counselor and to begin work on his or her problem (Pipes &
Davenport, 1999). The counselor must avoid an adversarial relationship and
never fight with the client (Hackney & Cormier, 2001). The key principle is
to start where the client is. If the counselor remembers that the reluctant
client is fearful of what may happen in counseling and angry at having been
coerced into participation, it is easier for the counselor to avoid responding
to client affect as though it were intentionally directed at himself or herself.
If the counselor can truly join the client's struggle about being in counseling
and possibly needing to change, and can keep the focus on the client's
experience, little of the counselor's attention will be directed to feelings of
being manipulated by the client in hostile or dependent ways. Both the
counselor's conscious emotional responses and his or her countertransference will remain under control.

Accepting a reluctant client involves accepting the client's reluctance as
a part of the agenda of counseling. The counselor should recognize that
reluctance is "a normal by-product of the process of changing complex
behaviors" (Moyers & Rollnick, 2002, p. 187). One might begin with "Help
me understand what has been happening to you." The counselor accepts
the perspective that the client "does not want to talk with me right now, and
that is his or her right." At the same time, the counselor persists with leads

that show genuine caring and involvement. Eventually, the client may begin to observe that the counselor is not behaving like authority figures typically do when he or she is resistant. At that point, the client has to find other ways to interact that make sense in the new environment, and the beginnings of trust are established.

Bugental (as cited in Pipes and Davenport, 1999) recommends a three-step process of helping the client to become aware of his or her reluctant behavior. The first step is simply to observe the behavior, for example: "You seem to be very angry." The second step is to place the feeling into some kind of context: "You are angry because you were required to come here and you don't see how I can help." The third step is to openly invite the client to discuss his or her feelings: "Would you care to explore what it is that upsets you so much?" In actual experience, we have found that many clients respond so fully to the first lead that the subsequent leads become unnecessary.

For the client with an authority problem, "the client's feelings . . . are used to demonstrate how the client perceives, interprets, and responds to the present in the same ways he or she responded to significant persons in the past" (James & Gilliland, 2003, p. 24). It may take a number of sessions for the client to build an understanding of the nature and target of negative feelings and to understand how he or she projects those feelings onto others. It is usually helpful for the counselor to identify when the client is projecting feelings onto the counselor or other persons who have not earned them—though such responses are confrontive and thus are most effective once the client has begun to trust the counselor and the process. Through such discussion, the client can learn to discriminate between people who have perhaps committed wrongs against him or her and those who have simply been assigned "bad guy" status. Then the process of working through feelings toward the original objects of the anger (usually parents or siblings) may proceed. The counselor can help the client to develop an understanding that the past—no matter how deplorable—need not continue to affect the present. With a client whose resistance relates back to family relationships, change will be slow, and the client will require much support before trying new behaviors. The client will experience failures with his or her new behaviors and will have intense feelings about failure. The path to more positive feelings about self will be slow.

Counselors need to remember that all reluctant clients are a challenge to the counselor and that the chances of success are smaller than with self-referred clients. A counselor who undertakes working with reluctant clients must have the commitment to stick with the process and not become just another person who eventually gives up. Giving up will be seen as just one more rejection that further builds the client's view that authorities can't be trusted. On the other hand, many reluctant clients leave counseling of their own volition before the process reaches fruition. It is important that the counselor recognize this likelihood and acknowledge such failures as the incvitablc outcome of reaching out to those who are hard to help. It is important to take satisfaction from successes rather than castigating oneself for failures.

Along with the high level of empathy already mentioned, Moyers and Rollnick (2002, p. 186) emphasize the importance of using the following counselor responses to reduce client failure and maintain counselor commitment to this work:

- *Exploring the discrepancy between the client's deeply held values and his or her current behaviors that led to the referral for counseling.* Frequently the behaviors that others have labeled problematic are inconsistent with the client's own values, and self-definition, but the client has not recognized that discrepancy. To the degree that counselors can help clients explore their own values the clients may become more motivated to achieve the changes that others have sought for them. Outcome research supports that self-directive and nondirective approaches produce better counseling outcomes with reluctant clients (Beutler et al., 2002).
- *Rolling with the resistance rather than directly confronting it, just as a canoeist in whitewater rafting goes with the power of the water and uses the power of the water to go forward rather than directly opposing it.* Directly confronting resistance with a reluctant client backfires and produces higher levels of resistance.
- *Supporting the client's self-efficacy by building confidence that change is possible.* This is best accomplished by focusing on the client's strengths and the instances, however infrequent, when the client has already found some measure of control over the problem.

Brodsky and Lichtenstein (1999) advise counselors to avoid questioning as much as possible with involuntary and reluctant clients. Questions reinforce the reluctant client's tendency to be passive, and they often increase defensiveness and the sense of the counselor as invader of the client's personal space. Statements, observations, and reflections are preferable. Similarly, Moyers and Rollnick (2002) caution against using the word *but* in compound sentences. For example, rather than saying, "You really want to stop losing your temper at work and with your wife, *but* you can't seem to use the calming techniques the social worker recommended in court," a counselor can say, "You really want to stop losing your temper with your wife *and* you can't seem to use the calming techniques the social worker recommended in court." Although this may appear as merely a semantic change, it may reduce the defensiveness of a client who is already oversensitive to criticism for his behavior and increase his willingness to explore what gets into the way of making those changes.

WORKING WITH THE PERSON MAKING THE REFERRAL

Because a large number of poorly motivated clients are referred to counseling by a third party, we conclude this chapter with some important principles for managing contacts with these referring parties. Most often, the referring party has a relationship of some duration with the client and is in a position to provide information that will be useful in counseling. In some cases, the reason for referral is disruption in the relationship between the client and the referring party. At other times, the referring party has observed client behaviors that have caused concern for the client's welfare.

When a third party makes a referral, the counselor tries to learn as much as possible about why the referral is being made and should inform the referring party of the nature and scope of services that may be made available. A discussion of confidentiality and its limits may also avoid later misunderstandings.

Often referral sources are vague about their reasons for wanting a counselor to work with an individual. Just as it is necessary for counselors to help clients clarify their problems, it is also important to help people making referrals to state their observations in clear and specific terms and to distinguish between their observations and inferences. It is not sufficient for a teacher referring a student to say, "Lucinda has changed a lot during the last marking period. She used to be carefree, but now she seems to be very worried about something. I think you should see her." The counselor should help the teacher describe the behaviors and circumstances that led to the inference that Lucinda is worried. "Can you tell me about some of your observations of Lucinda's behavior that have given you the impression she is worried?" is an example of a counselor response that can facilitate clarification.

The counselor has many options in referral situations. In any setting, there are boundaries on the types of clients who may be accepted. Certain agencies will accept most clients who need mental health counseling but may not have the resources to manage severely disturbed clients who pose a danger to themselves or others. Other agencies specialize in career counseling, marriage counseling, or some other specialty and accept only clients who fit their identified niche. School counselors work with students with a wide variety of learning, decision-making, and personal problems but generally refer those whose emotional problems lie outside the range of normal functioning. Similarly, school counselors often provide consultation to parents but usually refer families that need extended family counseling. Instances of child abuse must be reported to child protective services but parents may be referred for counseling as well.

If the referring party describes a client whose concerns are obviously outside the scope of service of a counselor, that counselor may suggest another resource without ever meeting the client. More frequently, in general mental health facilities as well as school counseling offices, an initial meeting is scheduled with the client (often referred to as an intake interview), and a determination is made at that time as to whether the client could benefit from the services available at that location or should be encouraged to go else-where. The referring party should always be assured that the counselor will make every effort to ensure that the referred party will receive the needed help but that he or she may not be the service provider.

In many instances, the identity of the referring party is obvious to the client, such as when a judge makes counseling a condition of probation. Likewise, if a parent brings a young person into a counselor's office, there is little doubt in anyone's mind that it is the parent who thinks that the young person needs help. In other cases, though, the referring individual may not have discussed the referral with the client. This frequently happens in schools: a parent or teacher will approach the counselor without talking with the young person about it. A supervisor may contact a counselor in an employee assistance office to report that a worker seems to be experiencing a problem with alcohol or simply that his or her work habits have changed.

It is usually desirable for the counselor to tell the client who has been referred why the session has been arranged and who was responsible for initiating it. Disclosure places the cards on the table and contributes to a genuine interchange—which is especially important with a client who is initially indifferent or oppositional. The referring party should be told about the disclosure during the referral discussion and should participate in deciding how much the client should be told and how.

The referring party and the counselor must also agree in advance about what kind of feedback the counselor will offer after counseling has begun. This can be a difficult dilemma for the counselor. Referring parties, especially parents and spouses, generally want some feedback, yet the counselor wants to offer the client an opportunity for private communication. Some counselors handle this dilemma by simply explaining it to the referring person: "I understand your desire for feedback. You care for Lucinda and want to know that something is being done to help her. But it is also important for me to help Lucinda develop a sense of trust. This means I must let her know that I will keep private whatever she shares with me unless she makes reference to hurting herself or others. Of course, she may agree to share certain information with you (or release information to others in a position to be helpful), but I hope you understand that I won't be able to share with you everything that Lucinda and I discuss." Sometimes referring parties are especially concerned about what the prospective client may say about them. The counselor can indicate that he or she will try to find ways of working on the relationship between the referring person and the client if that proves to be an important issue. Nevertheless, it is still necessary that the referring person understand that the client will have choices about what information is shared once the counseling begins. Unless the potentially conflicting roles of counselor to the individual, and resource person to the referring party, are clarified, either the client or the referring person may feel betrayed by the counselor.

Case: Eddie

Eddie, a 12-year-old seventh grader, was referred to the counselor by his teacher. Eddie attends an eight-grade elementary school with self-contained classrooms. He was doing passing work, but his behavior suggested that something was wrong. He rarely spoke to other children in his class and spent his free time brooding by himself. He occasionally showed bottled-up anger by responding violently with little provocation and striking out physically at nearby people and objects. The referring teacher regarded these "tantrums" as somewhat dangerous. Furthermore, when they occurred, they seemed to increase Eddie's isolation even more. Eddie would respond to verbal questions from the teacher in class if he knew the answers to the questions, but the teacher had been unsuccessful in establishing any conversation with Eddie on an informal level outside of class.

The counselor in this case was in his mid-20s and exuded caring as he worked with young people. He dressed informally and behaved in a fashion that allowed most seventh-grade boys to see him as a "cool" role model rather than an authority figure.

Initial Counseling Session

COUNSELOR: Hello, Eddie. How's it going?

EDDIE: Okay.

COUNSELOR: I imagine you're wondering why I wanted to see you. Your teacher asked me to talk to you. She seems to think you have some things on your mind that you'd like to talk to someone about.

EDDIE: Well, I don't.

COUNSELOR: Everything's fine with you then.

EDDIE: Yeah. (The counselor allows a fairly long silence to occur before continuing.)

COUNSELOR: Your teacher says that you hardly ever talk to anyone and that you seem sad or worried or something. Do you think that describes how you are in her room?

EDDIE: Ain't got nothing to say.

COUNSELOR: So it is true that you don't buddy around much with the kids in your class?

EDDIE: They are stupid.

COUNSELOR: It must seem kind of lonely not to have anyone to talk to or do things with.

EDDIE: (Silence, but visible emotion in the form of tears welling in his eyes.)

COUNSELOR: Well, maybe you'd like to think about whether, at a later time, you can tell me how it is for you. Would you like to shoot a few baskets with me for the rest of our time today?

The counselor and Eddie adjourned to the playground, where they spent some time playing basketball. By mutual consent, the conversation was restricted to short comments about the game.

Subsequent Events

Two days after the counselor's initial meeting with Eddie, the boy became involved in another classroom incident that resulted in a conference with the teacher, the school principal, the counselor, and Eddie's mother. The mother described how difficult it was for her to "manage" Eddie by herself. She expressed the opinion that a boy needs a father to keep him under control and that she did not know what to do with him.

Because the problem seemed to indicate personal adjustment and development issues, the principal and the teacher left the counselor and Eddie's mother alone to consider what might be done. There was a history of family violence, and both the mother and Eddie (an only child) had suffered physical abuse. The mother revealed that Eddie's father was in prison, having been convicted of second-degree murder. After the publicity of the arrest and conviction, the mother had moved with Eddie to a new town, where they and their history were not known. The incidents of Eddie's violent behavior at school occurred when other students tried to get close, tried to learn more about him or his family, or made any comments that he construed to reflect on his parents.

Eddie's mother told Eddie that the counselor knew about his father, and the counselor continued to meet with Eddie. At first, the sessions were still difficult, with Eddie sharing little of his thoughts or feelings. He did eventually show signs that he liked the attention from the counselor and enjoyed some of the activities they did together. The first indication that counseling was having an effect occurred after about a month, when Eddie's mother called to say how cooperative Eddie had become at home and that the evening before he had kissed her for the first time since his father had been arrested. Through his relationship with the counselor, Eddie slowly recovered his ability to trust and love other people, his interaction with other students improved, and he progressed toward a more satisfying lifestyle. (He never did discuss his feelings about his father with the counselor, and this could be unfinished business that may create further difficulties later.) Eddie gained from counseling in spite of some reluctance that persisted throughout the 6-month period during which he worked with the counselor.

Discussion

Eddie's reluctance to work with the counselor was an extension of his reluctance to interact with other people. He had a history that was too painful to discuss even after the counselor was informed about it by the boy's mother. Eddie chose to keep his feelings about his father private, even through extended contact with the counselor. Therapeutic movement nevertheless occurred, presumably as a result of a caring and respectful relationship with the male counselor, who served as a person to be emulated. The fact that the counselor could accept and care for him, even knowing the dark secret of his father's crime, was in itself supportive. Counseling conversations eventually included content about day-to-day relationships as they began to build. Future-oriented discussions about education and career planning also took place.

Eddie's reluctance to share his world with others is easy to understand. Clearly, it would have been inappropriate and counterproductive for the counselor to respond in anger or frustration to Eddie's initial rejecting behavior. Through patience, persistence, and understanding, the counselor was eventually able to experience a measure of success in helping Eddie to lead a fuller, more satisfying life.

Questions for Further Thought

1. To what extent do you believe that transference may have been a factor in Eddie's reluctance to become involved with the counselor?

2. How important do you believe it was that Eddie and the counselor never openly discussed Eddie's feelings about his father?
3. Can you account for Eddie's reaction when the counselor observed that he seemed lonely? How lonely was he? What do you think about the counselor's decision to disengage from the counseling session at that point?
4. In the case study, the counselor had a personal charisma that made him popular with young people. How important do you think that was? Your own personal characteristics are different in some ways from the counselor's. If you were Eddie's counselor, how might you vary the approach to take advantage of your own personality in building the relationship?

SUMMARY

A certain proportion of the clients any counselor sees will be ambivalent, indifferent, or oppositional people who would not seek counseling if the choice were left to them. They are requested or required to see a counselor by a spouse, parents, teachers, or the legal system, or the counselor may see them as part of a routine session in a school setting. They express reluctance by failing to participate fully in the counseling process and sometimes are hostile, discourteous, unpleasant, or dependent in their relationship with the counselor. In addition to the conscious interpersonal element that we have referred to as reluctance, these individuals experience resistance, or intrapsychic fears of change, that oppose the work of counseling.

A client may be reluctant to participate in counseling because he or she feels there is little to be gained by sharing private thoughts with another person. Perhaps he or she has been hurt in the past when trying to discuss personal thoughts and feelings, or perhaps failure has resulted from repeated independent efforts to change, resulting in hopelessness about the possibility of success. Most of the time a client's defensiveness centers on previous and current relationships with authority figures. Anger, frustration, alienation, or dependence that have been experienced in relationships with authority figures, usually parents, are transferred to the counselor. The counselor, who has offered help and kindness, is likely to experience feelings of frustration and/or rejection when faced with a reluctant client. Furthermore, the counselor may feel anxious about the possibility that counseling may fail. Nevertheless, the commitment to work with reluctant clients is important because it constitutes a reaching out to individuals who have built barriers when it comes to relating with others and who need help in establishing better interpersonal contacts. Using a model of readiness for change, such as the one developed by Prochaska and his colleagues, can help a counselor assess client readiness and develop an appropriate pace for the counseling process.

The counselor can manage his or her own feelings of rejection by focusing on the client. Instead of personalizing the rejection, the counselor must see it as the client's present need and begin to work where the client is with his or her reluctance to become involved. Having established such an initial approach, the counselor takes special care in using the relationship-building skills of the first stage of counseling. Consultation or supervision to help the counselor manage countertransference is often helpful. Many initially reluctant clients will eventually respond to the counselor's caring and genuineness and begin to trust him or her. To the degree that this change occurs, the road to other kinds of change opens. However, the success rate with reluctant clients is lower than with self-referred clients.

Working with the referring party is another delicate aspect of working with reluctant clients. The counselor should help the referring person to understand the nature of counseling and the importance of confidentiality. The degree to which the referring person is involved after counseling begins depends on where he or she fits in the life of the client and the client's need and readiness for that person to be a part of the change process.

≈≈≈ *DISCUSSION QUESTIONS* ≈≈≈

1. The authors present a long list of possible reasons that clients may be reluctant to enter counseling. Which of these do you think occur most frequently? What others might you add to the list? Which of these do you think are most challenging for a counselor to respond to?

2. The model of readiness for change presented by Prochaska and his colleagues has sparked much interest among counselors and psychologists to help explain why so many clients drop out of counseling prematurely and why other clients seem to make so little progress. What do you see as the potential strengths and weaknesses of using this model with clients? Can it be applied to students sent to the school counselor's office for behavioral or academic problems as well as to mental health clients?

3. When one of the authors was in graduate school, a clinical supervisor regularly stated, "Resistance is a form of integrity." What does that statement mean to you? Does it seem to fit with the way resistance is discussed in this chapter?

4. The brief therapy approach of the managed care system of mental health appears to operate with the assumption that clients are ready and willing to implement change. Based on what you have read in this chapter, what do you see as the problems with that assumption?

5. Do you think that the recommendations of scholars to avoid questioning reluctant clients and to "roll with the resistance" may also be useful ways

to cope with the counselor's negative countertransference reactions? If yes, why? If no, why not?

6. Can a person become a competent counselor if he or she cannot learn to work effectively with reluctant or oppositional clients?

REFERENCES

Addis, M. E., & Mahalik, J. R. (2003). Men, masculinity and the concept of help seeking. *American Psychologist, 58,* 5–14.

Atkinson, D. R., Morten, G., & Sue, D. W. (Eds.). (1998). *Counseling American minorities: A cross-cultural perspective* (5th ed.). Madison, WI: Brown & Benchmark.

Beutler, L. F., Moleiro, C., & Talebi, H. (2002). Resistance in psychotherapy: What conclusions are supported by research. *Journal of Clinical Psychology, 58,* 207–217.

Brammer, L. M., Abrego, P. J., & Shostrum, E. L. (1993). *Therapeutic counseling and psychotherapy* (6th ed.). Englewood Cliffs, NJ: Prentice-Hall.

Brodsky, S. L., & Lichenstein, B. (1999). Don't ask questions: A psychotherapeutic strategy for treatment of involuntary clients. *American Journal of Psychotherapy, 53,* 215–221.

Cowan, E. W., & Presbury, J. H. (2000). Meeting client resistance and reactance with reverence. *Journal of Counseling and Development, 78,* 411–419.

Doyle, R. E. (1998). *Skills and strategies in the helping process* (2nd ed.). Pacific Grove, CA: Brooks/Cole.

Dyer, W. W., & Vriend, J. (1973). Counseling the reluctant client. *Journal of Counseling Psychology, 20,* 240–246.

Egan, G. (2002). *The skilled helper: A problem management approach to helping* (7th ed.). Pacific Grove, CA: Brooks/Cole.

Hackney, H., & Cormier, L. S. (2001). *The professional counselor: A process guide to helping* (4th ed.). Boston: Allyn & Bacon.

Ivey, A. E., Ivey, M. B., & Simek-Morgan, L. (2002). *Counseling and psychotherapy: A multicultural perspective* (5th ed.). Boston: Allyn & Bacon.

James, R. K., & Gilliland, B. E. (2003). *Theories and strategies of psychotherapy* (5th ed.). Pacific Grove, CA: Brooks/Cole.

Mintz, L. B., & O'Neil, J. M. (1990). Gender roles, sex, and the process of psychotherapy: Many questions and few answers. *Journal of Counseling and Development, 68,* 381–387.

Moyers, T. B., & Rollnick, S. (2002). A motivational interviewing perspective on resistance in psychotherapy. *Journal of Clinical Psychology, 58,* 185–193.

Pipes, R. B., & Davenport, D. S. (1999). *Introduction to psychotherapy: Common clinical wisdom* (2nd ed.). Englewood Cliffs, NJ: Prentice-Hall.

Prochaska, J. O., DiClemente, C. C., & Norcross, J. C. (1994). *Changing for good.* New York: Morrow.

Riordan, R. J., & Martin, M. H. (1993). Mental health counseling and the mandated client. *Journal of Mental Health Counseling, 15,* 373–383.

Ritchie, M. H. (1986). Counseling the involuntary client. *Journal of Counseling and Development, 64,* 516–518.

Rooney, R. H. (1992). *Strategies for working with involuntary clients.* New York: Columbia University Press.

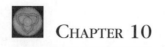 CHAPTER 10

MAJOR THEORIES OF COUNSELING

The early chapters of this book presented a generic model of counseling. That model traced the flow of the counseling process as it typically occurs, from relationship building and initial disclosure through deeper exploration to action planning. We emphasized elements of counseling that are accepted by most professional counselors. Because we have blended compatible elements from several theories, we call our model multitheoretical and integrative.

This chapter examines some of the differences in the counseling process that arise from the various theoretical positions on counseling. Each theory includes certain assumptions about the nature of human beings, and these assumptions influence the counseling interventions that adherents of a particular theory select to promote client progress. Because of their varying emphases, each theory elaborates more on certain aspects of the generic multitheoretical-integrative counseling model. The special contributions of each theory are discussed in the material that follows.

If you are using this book as the sole source in a first counseling course, the brief summaries of the several theories will also elaborate on the theoretical foundations of the book presented in Chapter 1 and suggest a path for further reading. If you are using the book in combination with a counseling theories text, this chapter will help you to link your more extensive study of the theories to the generic model.

The chapter begins by presenting a structure that shows a relationship among the theories on a continuum according to, among other criteria, the emphasis on affect or cognition in the counseling process. The first section also provides some historical perspective on the development of counseling during the 20th century. Introductions to six of the more important counseling theories and a synopsis about brief therapy follow. We acknowledge that the task of condensing the significant elements of six theories of counseling into a single chapter is challenging, and thus the presentations are necessarily skeletal. A serious student of counseling will want to study a comparative theories text (Corey, 2001; James & Gilliland, 2003; Patterson & Watkins, 1997; Prochaska & Norcross, 2003; Sharf, 2000), as well as original works by the key authors of each of the theoretical approaches.

STRUCTURE FOR RELATING COUNSELING THEORIES

The counseling profession traces its origin to the work of Frank Parsons (1909), who was concerned about helping young people make effective career choices in a work environment diversified by the Industrial Revolution. He regarded career decision making as primarily a rational process of guided self-appraisal, analysis of work opportunities, and matching self with opportunities. From 1909 until the 1940s, much of the progress made by the counseling profession involved the development of better means of assessing people's aptitudes and interests through testing, and the collection and publication of occupational information. In many respects, counseling became more "rational" and more scientific during that period. E. G. Williamson (1939) and others described the decision making process as an application of the scientific method. The counselor, as an expert in measuring skills and abilities as well as in sharing career information, directed clients toward the careers for which they were best suited. This rational approach to counseling came to be known as *directive counseling* because of the counselor's role in advising clients about career choices. It was also referred to as *trait-factor counseling* because personal traits were matched with factors needed for success in various jobs. Though not totally ignored, clients' feelings were treated as second in importance to their thoughts, and "irrational" feelings were to be controlled rather than worked through.

In 1942 Carl Rogers published *Counseling and Psychotherapy*, a book that was destined to change the counseling profession profoundly. Rogers described an approach to counseling that assumed that the clients had capabilities within themselves for knowing best how to manage their affairs. The role of the counselor was to facilitate the client's process of self-exploration and personal growth by providing a nurturing relationship within which the client could express self freely and develop new insights. This approach came to be called *nondirective counseling*, because the counselor was not an adviser. The client was seen as self-directing, and the counselor had no advice to give. The client's feelings about self were the central concern of counseling, because these feelings were the elements of self-concept. According to Rogers, a person's concept of self shapes how he or she responds to the challenges of life.

For 20 years after the publication of Rogers' initial work, a battle raged within the counseling profession over which of the viewpoints, directive or nondirective, was "right." Slowly many counselors came to the view that there were elements of truth in each viewpoint, that some clients might be helped most by the one approach and others by the alternative, and that many aspiring counselors were more adept at one approach or the other. Furthermore, since Rogers' approach had opened the door to the inclusion of the full range of human experience as appropriate material for counseling, counselors began looking toward theories that had previously been regarded as the territory of psychotherapists. Counseling and psychotherapy launched their journey toward merging into a single discipline. Ironically, even though Rogers was as vocal in his objections to Freudian therapy as to trait-factor counseling, the work of Sigmund Freud and his psychoanalytically oriented descendants became incorporated into the counseling literature largely as a result of Rogers' expansion of the horizons of the problems with which a counselor could help. Freudian counseling (also referred to as psychoanalytic or dynamic counseling) took up a position between the rational and affective viewpoints; its practitioners regarded both thoughts and feelings as important. Other theories that have subsequently been developed lie on a continuum whose extremes are defined by the initial arguments over directive and nondirective counseling.

Patterson and Watkins (1997), after reviewing a number of classifications systems for counseling theories, concluded that contemporary approaches could be arranged on a continuum with primary emphasis on cognitive process at one extreme and primary emphasis on affective concerns at the other. Figure 10.1 shows a continuum similar to that proposed by Patterson and Watkins, with the theories to be discussed in the remainder of this chapter placed in appropriate locations. Generally, those counselors who focus heavily on affect are also nondirective and see the client as controlling the content of the sessions. Counselors who are more cognitive in orientation are more inclined toward directive approaches, in which the counselor is more in control of content of the session. We have chosen to present summaries of six theoretical positions that are frequently cited as the germinal thinking on which counseling practice is based and from which other theoretical variations arise. Although their placement on the continuum cannot be regarded as precise, it was purposeful.

Person-centered counseling (originally called client-centered) places great emphasis on affect and client autonomy and thus appears at the extreme left. *Gestalt counseling* was positioned to the right of person-centered counseling because the counselor is more inclined to manipulate conditions in order to elicit exploration by the client. *Psychoanalytic counseling* is found

Figure 10.1   Continuum of Counseling Theories

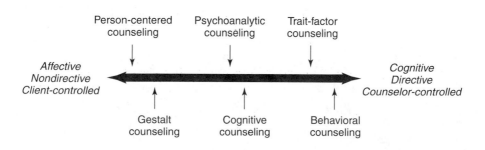

near the center of the continuum because it emphasizes both affect and thought processes. The right side of the continuum shows those theories that emphasize cognitive process, with each system being progressively more directive and counselor centered as one moves toward the far right of the continuum. *Behavioral counseling* appears at the extreme right because it pays little attention to affect and is heavily counselor controlled.

PERSON-CENTERED COUNSELING

Carl Rogers (1942, 1951, 1961, 1980, 1986) is known as the founder of the person-centered approach to counseling. Two other names, nondirective counseling and client-centered counseling, were attached to this approach in Rogers' earlier writings, and a majority of the references to his work are found under the headings "client-centered counseling" or "client-centered therapy." The change to a person-centered approach reflects Rogers' (1980) later recognition that his system worked in any setting in which a helper sets out to promote human psychological growth and that many of those who are helped (e.g., students in a classroom) do not think of themselves as clients.

Rogers' approach to the counseling process was presented initially as an alternative to psychoanalytic psychotherapy, in which he was first trained. Because his views of human nature (1942) appealed to educators and his method of counseling did not require extensive psychological training, many practicing counselors adopted the person-centered approach, and it had a great influence on the preparation of new counselors. Rogers' work is regarded as one of the principal forces in shaping current counseling and psychotherapy.

The Nature of People

In person-centered counseling, human beings are seen as possessing positive goodness and the desire to become "fully functioning"—that is, to live as effectively as possible. This view of human nature contrasts with the Freudian view that people possess impulses that, if not adequately socialized, will lead to behavior that is destructive to self and others. According to Rogers, if people are permitted to develop freely, they will flourish and become positive, achieving individuals. Because of the faith in human nature expressed in Rogers' theory, it is considered a humanistic approach to counseling.

Person-centered counseling is based on a theory of personality referred to as *self-theory*. An individual's view of self within the context of environment influences his or her actions and personal satisfactions. If provided with a nurturing environment, people will grow with confidence toward self-actualization—becoming all they can be. If they do not receive love and support from significant others, they will likely come to see themselves as lacking in worth and to see others as untrustworthy. Behavior will become defensive (self-protective), and growth toward self-actualization will be hampered.

An important principle of self-theory is the belief that a person's perceptions of self and environment (including significant others) *are* reality for that person. Thus, if an individual sees himself or herself as incompetent or parents as mean, he or she will act on that belief, even if others view him or her as brilliant or the parents as kind. Telling an underachieving student that he or she is capable seldom makes much difference, because the assessment probably conflicts with the student's personal reality. Personal reality may be changed through counseling, but usually not by such a direct intervention as substituting the judgment of the counselor for that of the client.

The Counseling Process

Because Rogers viewed humans as positive and self-actualizing by nature, he conceived the counselor's role as providing conditions that would permit self-discovery and encourage the client's natural tendency toward personal growth. The nurturing conditions described by Rogers are essentially those presented in Chapter 3 as vital to the initial-disclosure stage of counseling. If the counselor is totally accepting of each client as a person, relates empathically to the client's reality, and behaves in a genuine way (behavior is congruent with feelings), the client will be free to discover and express the positive core of his or her being. As clients come to perceive themselves more positively in the nurturing environment, they will function more effectively. Counselors not only provide the nurturing environment missing elsewhere in clients' lives, but also serve as role models of how fully functioning persons relate with others.

The underlying philosophy of human nature in person-centered counseling is far more important to its practice than any particular set of techniques or any body of knowledge. It has been said that in person-centered counseling, helpers learn how to *be* counselors rather than how to *do* counseling. Counselors must be comfortable enough within themselves to become fully involved with the worlds of their clients without fear of losing their own sense of wholeness, and counselors must care enough about their clients to be willing to experience their pain. Through all this, counselors must be able to retain their own sense of separateness and emotional perspective on the client's difficulties. Because clients are seen as having the potential to solve their own problems, counselors are not perceived as having expert knowledge to share with clients.

The person-centered counselor functions with the techniques that are toward the least leading end of the continuum of lead (see Table 8.1, p. 175). Silence, acceptance, restatement, empathy, and immediacy responses occur most frequently, with the client taking the lead on what is discussed and being responsible for outcomes. If a counselor perceives a need for information in the course of a discussion, he or she may encourage the client to seek information outside the counseling session. A purely person-centered counselor would not be likely to use tests, although a counselor who uses some person-centered procedures might include some testing at the client's request. Person-centered counselors encourage careful self-exploration, but they tend to avoid confrontation and interpretation as tools for hastening insight. There is little focus on specific action planning except as initiated by the client. It is assumed that as the client becomes free to actualize his or her potential through the exploration process, behavior change will occur naturally and without prompting from the counselor.

Contribution to the Multitheoretical Integrative Model of Counseling

The work of Carl Rogers has made a great contribution to the generic model of counseling that is presented in this book. The obvious contribution is his clear description of the counseling relationship that forms the substance of the first stage of the counseling process and sustains trust through the second and third stages as well. Because of Rogers' work, counselors have learned to become better listeners. Even counselors who prefer more active and counselor-initiated methods have come to appreciate the importance of employing relationship-building conditions to encourage clients to reveal significant elements of their personal reality. It has been said that counseling must begin where the client is—and to learn where the client is, most counselors employ methods that Rogers defined.

A second important contribution, which owes its origin to Rogers' statements about the nature of people, is the view that clients are ultimately responsible for their own lives. Even though some counselors may not be as optimistic as Rogers in believing that all persons are fundamentally good, most counselors recognize that the counselor cannot and should not attempt to control a client's actions (except in instances where physical safety is a real concern). Counselors of essentially all theoretical persuasions now agree that they are working to help clients achieve their own goals.

Person-centered counseling, then, is based on a positive view of human nature consonant with Western views of freedom and self-determination. Rogers has described a methodology that people who are themselves "fully functioning" can learn relatively easily. Because Rogers and his colleagues have demonstrated through a strong research program that person-centered counseling can be effective with a wide variety of clients, many of his ideas have been incorporated into other counseling models. For example, they are an important element of the generic model of counseling presented in this book.

GESTALT COUNSELING

Gestalt counseling was developed by Frederick (Fritz) Perls, who, like Carl Rogers, was educated as a Freudian psychotherapist. Though a dynamic and effective counselor, Perls was not as diligent as Rogers in writing about his work, and there are probably more conceptual loose ends in his system. When considered together, several publications by Perls and others (Fagan & Shepherd, 1970; Perls, 1969; Perls, Hefferline, & Goodman, 1951; Polster & Polster, 1973; Van de Riet & Korb, 1980; Wheeler, 1990; Yontef & Simkin, 1989) provide an adequate basis for understanding his contributions.

Nature of People

The name of this approach to counseling comes from the German word *Gestalt,* which can be translated as "form or figure." A central concept of this view of human nature is that the whole form is greater than the sum of the parts and that the organism functions as a whole. In addition, humans are seen as constantly striving for balance in their lives, this balance being threatened by events outside of self as well as by internal conflict. Regardless of the source or nature of threats to the individual's balance, the whole organism is disrupted when imbalance occurs. Thus, difficulty in one's marriage will influence one's job performance; failure in school is likely to affect interpersonal relationships; and success in sports will have an impact on friendships. The concept of the whole also applies to interaction between the physiological and psychological aspects of a person; thus, emotion often is expressed through physical means. Understanding nonverbal behavior is important to understanding the whole person.

Perls believed that instinct plays a part in motivating behavior, but he emphasized a "hunger" instinct rather than sexual instinct as in the Freudian theory. This hunger instinct motivates persons to "take in" elements of the environment. Although this instinct drives the organism, it is not seen as bad or good. In fact, Gestalt theorists tend to see behavior not as "bad" or "good" but as "effective" or "ineffective."

As persons live and experience, they often develop elements of personality that differ and that "want" different things. For example, one's "fighting self" might want to battle with perceived enemies, but one's "loving self" wants to make peace. An abused child might seek revenge against the abuser at one time and seek only to be loved at another time. According to Perls, an important part of understanding any individual is appreciating the polarities that exist simultaneously within the personality. Part of the counseling process is encouraging the client to address these polarities and to work toward a more unified set of motives.

Gestalt counseling is placed toward the affective and client-centered end of the continuum of counseling theories because client feelings are emphasized and because the client is viewed as responsible for his or her own coping behavior. As in person-centered counseling, the counselor is defined primarily as a facilitator of the client's growth toward self-responsibility; the private reality of the individual is regarded as the basis for his or her inter-actions with the world at large; and the growth of awareness, which alters that private reality, results in more effective functioning. Gestalt counseling, like person-centered counseling, is classified as a humanistic approach, but differ-ent emphases among its adherents result in distinct counseling procedures, as will become clear in the next subsection.

The Counseling Process

In the Gestalt system, the purpose of counseling is to encourage per-sonal growth. Neurosis is seen as an interruption of the growth process, and defensiveness as a process that pulls energy away from living effectively. Growth is defined as a sequence of occurrences that proceeds from experi-ence (with a life situation) to sensing (taking in the qualities of the situation through the senses) to excitement (becoming involved with the event) to Gestalt formation (integrating the experience into one's stored perspectives of the world). Stagnation occurs when a person uses defenses to isolate self from new experiences.

At the beginning, Fritz Perls advocated that counselors frustrate the client's efforts to hide from new experience by deliberately pointing out when the client retreats into defensive behavior. Over time, other Gestalt counselors became less directly confrontive, but nevertheless they still encourage their clients to consider discrepancies that occur in their thoughts and feelings about life and that block experience and growth. In current practice, confrontation is an important counseling technique, though most contemporary Gestalt counselors are decidedly more gentle in their approach than Perls was.

Frequently, confrontation is based on discrepancies between the client's verbal statements and his or her nonverbal behavior. For example, it is common for people to laugh when embarrassed in an attempt to dis-miss the embarrassment. A Gestalt counselor would observe, "You say you were embarrassed but you are laughing." Confrontation is also used in response to discrepant components of verbal statements the client makes and to omissions—what the client is not saying (e.g., about the significant others in his or her life). Through this kind of intervention, the client is moved closer and closer to an authentic awareness and acceptance of his or her own experiences.

A number of techniques used by Gestalt counselors focus on bringing "then and there" experience into the "here and now." If a client is con-cerned about a disagreement with his or her spouse, the client may be asked to reenact some aspect of the dispute, alternately taking the roles of self and spouse. Instead of *talking about* what has occurred, the client reexperiences the occurrence, and the affect is recreated. New understandings often lead to new behaviors or new acceptance of self or others. When such reenactments of life events reach back to earlier phases of the client's life, the process is referred to as *finishing unfinished business*. For example, a young adult may bring the residue of conflict he or she had with parents during the growing years into relationships with legitimate authorities of adult life, such as employers. By reprocessing and "digesting" the old conflict, the client is freed to interact more objectively with persons currently present in his or her life.

Gestalt counselors use many techniques, or *experiments,* to bring the client into clearer touch with himself or herself. Only a few of these will be described here. Role-playing is perhaps the most important. This can be done with the counselor playing the part of a significant other and the client playing himself or herself, with the counselor playing the client and the client playing the significant other, or with the client playing both roles. Sometimes the client is asked to change chairs as he or she shifts roles. Another variation of the empty-chair technique occurs when the client is asked to play separate parts of self, perhaps the "assertive" self and the "weak" self. With all role-playing techniques, the counselor permits only enough talking about the situation to be able to structure roles and then moves to bring the action into the here and now.

Still other experiments are the exaggeration game and the "I take responsibility" game. In the first of these, the client is asked to exaggerate a view that has been expressed and that the counselor sees as defensive. As the affect and content become exaggerated, the client comes to see the inaccuracy and may retract part of the original defensive statement. The "I take responsibility" game works in much the same way. The client is instructed to repeat a questionable statement and follow it with the words "and I take responsibility for what I have said." If in retrospect the client has doubts about the original statement, he or she must alter it in order to be able to take responsibility for it.

Though Gestalt counseling is not interpretive—that is, the counselor does not interpret behavior—the Gestalt counselor needs diagnostic skills that will allow him or her to recognize clients' defensive strategies. To make observations that cause a client to look into self, the counselor must be able to recognize the client's defensive attempts to hide. As the counselor works with a given client, themes emerge that outline the client's characteristic ways of coping with life and with other people. The counselor calls the client's attention to attempts to hide within counseling sessions and may refer to such defensiveness as "phoniness." The counselor continually encourages the client to move toward authentic behavior that reflects his or her internal state accurately, while recognizing that such authenticity can be difficult.

As counseling proceeds and the client finishes unfinished business and approaches an understanding of his or her authentic self, he or she is able to establish effective contact with other people and participate more fully in daily life experiences. The growth process is contagious, in the sense that success in life situations builds the client's belief that he or she can safely reach out rather than hide. At some point, the client's tendency to reach out exceeds his or her tendency to hide, and the growth process reaches a momentum that makes further counseling unnecessary.

Contribution to the Multitheoretical Integrative Model of Counseling

Gestalt counseling is a client-oriented approach that suits the temperament of counselors who wish to intervene more actively than is typical in the person-centered approach. Much of the leading is characteristic of the second stage of counseling, as described in Chapter 4, but the Gestalt counselor stops short of interpretation (which is more characteristic of systems further toward the active end of the continuum of theories). One of the important contributions of Gestalt counseling to the generic model presented in this book is its elaboration of many techniques that can help the client see himself or herself more clearly. The client is still in charge of the outcome, but the counselor can use active techniques in promoting self-insight.

Because of its attention to the client as a total being, the Gestalt approach also extends the counselor's focus to the client's physiological response to experience. Gestalt counselors frequently ask clients to be aware of the tension or relaxation in their muscles, the responses of the circulatory or digestive systems, or their overt and observable physical behavior as they discuss stressful (or happy) life events. Training in Gestalt work enhances any counselor's ability to integrate cues from the client's nonverbal behavior into the counseling process, whether or not the counselor chooses to confront such behavior directly.

Finally, we reiterate that Gestalt counseling is a growth-oriented approach that, like the Rogerian approach, emphasizes human potential. The counselor attempts to remove barriers to permit the client the freedom to become more fully functioning. Unlike person-centered counseling, Gestalt counseling includes more statements about the nature of barriers and thus has a more diagnostic orientation.

PSYCHOANALYTIC COUNSELING

Psychoanalysis was originated by Sigmund Freud, who developed his theory from his experience as a therapist and wrote about his work for a period of nearly 50 years prior to his death in 1939. An edited multivolume collection of Freud's complete works (Freud, 1953–1974), compiled by Starchey and published over a period of years, facilitates reference to this important germinal material. Psychoanalytic theory is also sometimes referred to as psychodynamic theory because of its emphasis on the interactions (dynamics) of unconscious processes "where conflicts arise between the need for tension reduction and the inhibition of basic instinctual drives" (Baker, 1985, p. 25).

As indicated earlier in this chapter, Freud's works were not initially considered important to the practice of counseling. His work focused on the alleviation of serious emotional problems; counseling in its early years centered on decision making and career choice. The introduction of person-centered counseling opened the door for counselors to deal with a broader range of human concerns and emotions, and the counseling profession has subsequently moved steadily toward increased involvement with clients with emotional disturbances so that today counselors are licensed to diagnose and treat emotional disorders in many states. Counselors have embraced psychoanalytic theory as an important stream of thought, and many psychoanalytic concepts (e.g., the unconscious, defenses, ego) have, in fact, entered the common language.

Freud's form of psychoanalysis was a thorough, long-term helping process that placed heavy emphasis on the client's historical psychosexual development; the goal was for the client to gain insight on all aspects of his or her personality. Today, few practitioners offer that kind of treatment. Modern psychotherapists generally question whether such total analysis of the personality is necessary for a majority of clients, and the time and financial investment in such a process exceeds most people's resources. Consequently, shorter-term counseling based on psychoanalytic theory is now a more common form of treatment (Messer & Warren, 1998), and many counselors who practice with other theories as a base also use some psychoanalytic principles.

It would be difficult to overestimate Freud's contributions to the understanding of the human psyche and to the process of helping people resolve emotional problems through talking about them. Burke (1989) points out that much of the theoretical basis for current psychotherapy is either a further development of Freud's work (Adler, 1927; Alexander, 1963; Erikson, 1963; Fromm, 1941, 1976; Jung, 1954; Sullivan, 1953) or a reaction against it in the form of the person-centered, Gestalt, cognitive, and behavioral systems. Psychoanalytic counseling and psychotherapy account for a large proportion of helping services.

The Nature of People

Freud saw humans as biological beings driven by an instinctual desire for personal pleasure (gratification). The life force, or *libido,* was postulated as the energy source that propels people toward behavior that satisfies the pleasure motive. Only through the process of socialization are humans redirected toward behavior that allows for the satisfaction of personal needs in ways that are not destructive or unacceptable to others. If allowed to grow and develop without controls, people would serve their own selfish pleasures without regard for the rights of others or the accomplishment of useful work. Freudian theory contains no reference related to any tendency on the part of humans toward self-actualization: rather, humans are seen as operating by the pleasure principle and in need of shaping toward positive endeavors.

Psychosexual Development. In Freud's theory, pleasure is linked with sexuality, and libido is a driving force toward gratification. Freud proposed that the desire for sexual pleasure is a lifelong drive that begins in infancy and is first satisfied by sucking the mother's breasts. This first stage is called the oral stage; if the baby's oral needs are not met, later greediness or acquisitiveness may result (Corey, 2001). Anal, phallic, latency, and genital stages each follow in turn, bringing needs that, if satisfied, allow growth toward psychological maturity. If the child's needs are not accepted by the parents and are not satisfied in acceptable ways, the probable consequence will be "fixation" on meeting these needs at a later period in ways that are not effective.

Freud's views on sexuality have resulted in a great deal of controversy over the years. Many people object to the idea that all pleasure has a sexual component, and to many, the idea that humans are sexually motivated beings who begin seeking satisfaction at birth is offensive. Some have seen Freud as not only incorrect but perverted. Others see truth in the theory of infantile sexuality but place less emphasis on sexual pleasure as the primary motivator of all human behavior. Many women have seen his views of female sexuality, heavily influenced by the social strictures of the 19th century, to be offensive and inaccurate.

Whether or not one chooses to accept Freud's ideas about psychosexual development, there is much to be learned from his work on the unconscious, the structure of personality, and the defense mechanisms (summarized next). Unfortunately, many counselors have discounted this important work because his views on sexuality seem extreme or because his views on women and mental health, developed in Victorian times, do not pass muster today. We suggest that instead of rejecting Freud's contributions, it is wise to use his work selectively in those areas where it can be applied in a contemporary context.

The Unconscious. One of the most important ideas introduced by Freud was the concept that people are unaware of much of their mental processes—that mental activity can be unconscious. A person's unconscious motivation is based on instinct as modified and socialized by interaction with significant others, mainly parents, during the formative years. If satisfaction of instinctual needs is blocked through ineffective parenting so that acceptable means of expression cannot be found, then unconscious motivators will propel the individual to satisfy those needs by whatever means available. The key concept is that people frequently do not understand why they behave as they do, because motivation can be unconscious. This may be true even when a person seems to have a plausible explanation for particular behaviors. The plausible explanation may simply be a socially acceptable defense covering a motive of which the person is not aware. All behavior is understood to be purposeful (as a means of satisfying drives), though the individual may not be aware of the purposes. Discovering motives and developing effective means of meeting needs is one of the tasks of counseling.

The Structure of Personality. Freud postulated that the personality is made up of three interacting components: the id, the ego, and the superego. The *id* is the source of psychic energy and the locus of instinct. It propels the individual toward the search for pleasure, without regard for consequences. The *ego,* often referred to as the "executive" of the personality, is in touch with external reality and through experience gains strength to help the individual satisfy needs in acceptable ways. The ego is the seat of rational thought. The *superego* consists of learned principles of right and wrong and serves also to control instinctual gratification. When born, the individual is motivated by an unfettered id, instinctively seeking immediate gratification of needs. As time passes, the ego builds a repertoire of strategies for coping with life so as to satisfy needs in positive ways, and the superego develops a store of attitudes about right and wrong that regulates behavior. Both the ego and the superego establish control over the direct expression of id impulses.

Contemporary practitioners of psychoanalytic counseling tend to emphasize the development of the ego as the key to effective functioning. This leads to a sociocultural perspective on development, which emphasizes the role of interpersonal relationships and cultural institutions in the development of normal and pathological behavior (Burke, 1989). One major branch of psychoanalytic thought today addresses the effects of object relations (bonding with others during infancy and childhood) on the development of personality (Patterson & Watkins, 1997).

Defense Mechanisms. When an individual is confronted with demands for which the ego has no solutions, anxiety results. The person becomes afraid because, without ego-mediated solutions, he or she may directly express unacceptable impulses. The resulting behavior may be both ineffective and embarrassing. In such circumstances, defenses come into play to soften the blow on the ego and reduce stress. For example, a student who is failing in school may use the defense of denial to dismiss the problem or the defense of rationalization to explain why he or she can't do better. A defense mechanism works in the sense that it takes the pressure off the individual. Unfortunately, if defense mechanisms are used repeatedly, the result is that the person dismisses many demands to perform and thus misses many opportunities to succeed at life tasks. According to psychoanalytic thinking, a neurosis occurs when an individual uses defense mechanisms in interaction to such an extent that he or she experiences few or no rewarding interpersonal relationships. Psychosis results if the ego becomes so overwhelmed that its contact with external reality is severed and distorted thought patterns result.

Defense mechanisms are employed as a part of the unconscious process of a person's mental functioning. Therefore, it would rarely be useful to tell a client, "You are just being defensive." Counselors need to be able to recognize defenses and to help clients explore troublesome circumstances to find coping responses that can replace or reduce the defensive ones. It is also important to realize that there are times when everyone needs the temporary respite that a defense provides and that moderate defensiveness in the face of tough circumstances is healthy and necessary.

Common defense mechanisms include denial, rationalization, intellectualization, projection, and regression. It is beyond the scope of this chapter to define and describe these and other defense mechanisms; you are urged to refer to virtually any general psychology text for further information.

Freud described humans as instinctually motivated beings, seeking pleasures that have sexual roots. Development through the psychosexual stages in a nurturing environment allows the individual to develop a healthy personality in which the ego is strong. When the ego is not strong enough to face life's challenges, defenses are developed to protect the ego. Defenses serve a useful purpose, provided they are not overused as substitutes for coping with challenges. The dynamic process of personality includes unconscious thought; thus, people are not fully aware of all the motives behind their behavior.

The Counseling Process

Fundamental to the psychoanalytic counseling process is the belief that people relegate material they cannot tolerate to the unconscious, using defense mechanisms (e.g., repression). Because crucial issues have been pushed out of awareness without being resolved, unmet needs keep intruding into the fabric of life. The process of counseling, then, encourages the client to dislodge unconscious material and resolve the conflicts contained therein. The client is encouraged to talk as freely as possible about troublesome situations. Talking about these issues often leads the client to recall related thoughts that were repressed. In some cases, *free association* is used. In free association, the client suspends control over what he or she says and just lets speech flow—regardless of how disconnected or bizarre the material seems. Sometimes dreams are also analyzed for clues to the unconscious.

Regardless of the method of disclosure—problem discussion, free association, or dream analysis—the counselor seeks to understand the client's motives and to interpret to the client his or her thoughts, feelings, and behaviors. The counselor relies on his or her knowledge of psychodynamics to lead the client toward new insights. The counselor also uses events from the therapeutic interaction as samples of the client's behavior that can be interpreted (see the description of transference in Chapter 9). The client often discharges substantial emotion (referred to as catharsis) as painful circumstances are explored and new insights are achieved. With interpretation serving as an important counselor lead, psychoanalytic counseling depends heavily on the counselor's knowledge of personality dynamics. Psychoanalytic counseling places the most emphasis on the second stage of counseling, in-depth exploration.

Contribution to the Multitheoretical Integrative Model of Counseling

The greatest contribution of the psychoanalytic approach to the practice of contemporary counseling is its theory of personality and its application to the diagnostic process. The structure of personality as posited by Freud provides a convenient framework for analyzing human functioning and unconscious motivation. It helps the counselor consider the comparative contribution of impulse, reason, and conscience to a client's behavior. Along with the tripartite structure of personality comes the concept that the ego develops strength through positive experience with the external world (environment). At times, the strength of the ego is not equal to the demands placed on it, and the client becomes defensive. The nature of defense mechanisms, the purposes they serve, and the problems they cause are all important to the diagnostic process. Transference, countertransference, and resistance are manifestations of the process of ego defense (see Chapter 9).

Elements of Freud's original methods of conducting therapy certainly survive today. Many counselors use interpretation as a predominant lead, attempting to help clients see their experiences using a psychodynamic structure of personality. These counselors work primarily with clients' reports of their experiences in everyday life, and they also use observations of the client's interaction with the counselor as material for interpretation. Dream analysis and free association are used less as material for the interpretive process than they once were, but they remain a window on the client's unconscious experience. Much of psychoanalytic counseling is in-depth exploration, with comparatively less emphasis on relationship building or action plans. However, all three stages of the counseling process will receive some attention from most psychoanalytic counselors.

We have placed psychoanalytic counseling near the middle of the continuum of counseling theories because it focuses on both cognitive and affective material and both the counselor and the client are active in the process of counseling. A psychoanalytic counselor will not be content to have a client talk about feeling without meaning, or meaning without feeling. The client's task is to reveal self as freely as possible. The counselor's responsibility is to interpret the client's experiences so that the client gains greater insight and the ego can increase its coping capacity, directing effective rather than defensive responses to environmental demands.

COGNITIVE COUNSELING

Cognitive counselors regard erroneous thinking as the source of emotional upset and ineffective behavior. Events occur in each person's life that involve loss, disappointment, and failure to accomplish valued goals. Cognitive therapists believe that people who are able to think effectively about their experiences are able to put negative events in perspective and get on with life, and those who do not think effectively tend to perseverate on negative happenings and allow them to disrupt their happiness and effectiveness.

Albert Ellis (Ellis, 1962, 1973, 2001; Ellis & Bernard, 1986; Ellis & Dryden, 1997), founder of rational-emotive behavior therapy, is probably the best known of the cognitive therapists. Like Rogers and Perls, he was trained as a psychoanalytic therapist, but he came to believe that the traditional approach was inefficient and that the process sidetracked clients from learning how to live more effectively. Influenced by learning theory, Ellis began to develop a new approach to counseling in which clients are taught to think rationally about blocks to accomplishing love and work goals. Psychiatrist Aaron Beck (Beck, 1972, 1976; Beck, Rush, Shaw, & Emery, 1979) and psychologist Donald Meichenbaum (1977, 1985) have both gained recognition for their development of related theories of cognitive counseling and psychotherapy.

The Nature of People

For cognitive theorists, humans are thinking beings with the capacity to be rational or irrational, erroneous or realistic, in their thinking. According to Patterson and Watkins (1997), "Cognitive therapy is based on the commonsensical idea that what people think and say about themselves—their attitudes, ideas, and ideals—are relevant and important" (p. 223). Cognitive therapists subscribe to the view that what people *think* about their experiences determines how they *feel* about those experiences and what they will *do*. Ellis, Beck, and Meichenbaum all posit internal dialogue that mediates a person's reactions to stressful events.

Ellis explains that negative emotion and ineffective behavior are the results of irrational thinking. It is not the events in people's lives that create bad feelings, but how they think about those events. For example, suppose a person is snubbed at a party by someone he or she thinks is attractive.

Such an event might be unpleasant for almost anyone, but it becomes a problem, according to *rational-emotive behavior therapy (REBT),* when the snubbed individual "catastrophizes" about the event. The individual may have such "irrational" thoughts as "I can't stand being snubbed" or "If this person can't like me, no one else ever will." If the person simply thinks, "It's too bad that person snubbed me; I'd like to spend time with him or her," then negative emotion will not get out of hand and the person can plan to work toward another opportunity for contact. However, if the person catastrophizes about the incident, negative emotion and ineffective behavior result. Energy is wasted in self-pity and in either avoiding contact with or planning retaliation against the other person. Clearly, such behavior does not achieve the desired result of having further opportunity to spend time with the person.

The REBT view of personality is often referred to as an ABC theory, in which A is an activating event, B is the person's thought about the event, and C is the emotional and behavioral reaction. If the thinking at B is irrational, the emotional reaction will be negative and the behavior is likely to be inappropriate and ineffective for accomplishing the desired outcome.

There are many similarities between Beck's and Ellis's views of how humans come to behave ineffectively. Ellis has listed eleven specific irrational thoughts any one or more of which may lie at the source of an individual's difficulties. Examples include "[I] must be unfailingly competent and perfect in all [I] undertake," and "It is horrible, terrible, or catastrophic when things do not go the way [I] want them to go" (Ellis, 1977, p. 10). Ellis has identified all the statements as applying to love and/or work motives, and in that sense he repeats Freud's view of human priorities. It is easy to see how extreme ideas like those just quoted would result in feelings that one could not be successful and behaviors that are not well designed to bring about success. Beck (1972) has focused more on the nature of erroneous thought processes than on specific life events. He identified several patterns of erroneous thinking (Patterson & Watkins, 1997) including the following:

- Selective abstraction—focusing only on certain details while ignoring others
- Dichotomous thinking—believing that everything is either good or bad, black or white, with nothing in between
- Overgeneralization—arriving at far-reaching conclusions on the basis of little data
- Magnification—overestimating the importance of an event (essentially the same as the REBT concept of catastrophizing)
- Arbitrary inference—drawing conclusions that things are bad with no evidence
- Personalization—viewing events as related to oneself when they are not

Ellis speaks of "rational and irrational thoughts," Beck of "automatic thoughts," and Meichenbaum of "self-instructions"—all of which are spontaneous thought processes that occur when an individual is confronted with experience. These thought processes derive from adults' instructions that children internalize while growing up and later apply to new situations. Thus, from this perspective, parenting practices influence one's subsequent ability to think effectively, to feel confident and competent, and to behave using the maximum amount of one's resources. For clients to change their behavior, they must learn new ways of thinking, which is the means by which cognitive counseling achieves its purpose.

The Counseling Process

The counseling process has similar elements in each of the cognitive systems, and cognitive restructuring is the principal mechanism of change. The first step is to have the client describe the stressful situations in his or her life and to identify the faulty thinking that underlies the feelings. The counselor identifies the irrational thoughts, automatic negative thoughts, and silent assumptions that the client uses to interpret (erroneously) his or her experience. The cognitive errors and distortions may be explained to the client, as frequently occurs in REBT, or discussion is structured so that the client comes to see his or her errors of reasoning, as is common with Beck and Meichenbaum's approach. Then more adaptive alternative patterns of thinking can be developed.

In REBT, the alternatives are relatively easy to construct once the irrational thinking is identified because they are direct modifications of Ellis's list of irrational thoughts—which reduce the compelling nature of the client's thinking to a more reasoned version. For example, the thought "I must be loved and accepted by almost everyone" might be modified to "It would be nice to be widely cared for, but there are some significant people who like me and I can get along okay even if I don't get the attention I want from everyone else." It was stated above that REBT is an ABC theory of personality, where A is the precipitating event, B is the client's thought about the event, and C is the emotional and behavioral response. The counseling process adds a DE component (Ellis & Dryden, 1997), where D is the disputing intervention. The scientific method is used to identify new rational thoughts (E) about the client's situation. When this occurs, the client will change in cognition, affect, and behavior. Ellis has referred to this process as "depropagandizing" because it results in the client's giving up irrational beliefs that he or she was taught (as propaganda) during the formative years. Techniques such as persuasion, suggestion, instruction, and discovery of new ways of thinking through the Socratic method are common in the cognitive therapies. Planning of specific actions to take place outside of counseling, rehearsing the client's role in these new actions, and reviewing success are also parts of the cognitive counseling process. Thus, clients are given homework assignments in order to experiment with their environment between sessions and acquire new learning.

Beck's cognitive approach leads to examination of the client's story for examples of selective abstraction, dichotomous thinking, overgeneralization, magnification, arbitrary inference, and personalization in the client's response to troublesome circumstances. Seeing that a client looks at behavior in an all-or-nothing manner, makes *mountains of molehills,* or jumps to conclusions, the counselor helps the client understand the erroneous nature of his or her thinking. Meichenbaum also suggests that it is important to look for self-talk that, if present, would lead to better conclusions. Thus, it is important to consider what the client has overlooked as well as the cognitive errors that he or she has made.

The cognitive approach to counseling is placed near the rational and counselor-controlled end of the continuum of counseling theories. The counselor enters the client's world of experience through his or her thinking (cognitive) processes, and the counselor takes charge of the counseling. Nevertheless, it is the client's goal of coping more effectively with troublesome experience that shapes the content for counseling. Although Ellis places little importance on first-stage counseling skills, the other cognitive therapists see the conditions of the first stage as important to establishing a therapeutic alliance with the client, creating a climate of trust so that the client will respond to the interventions the counselor suggests. None of the cognitive therapists would see the first-stage conditions alone as sufficient for effective and efficient treatment.

In cognitive counseling, the in-depth exploration process of the second stage allows the client to identify issues with which he or she is experiencing difficulty and to examine the thought patterns that underlie the unpleasant feelings and ineffective behaviors. The counselor helps the client identify fallacies in perceptions, inaccuracies in information, and self-defeating behaviors. Although the affect attached to certain circumstances signals where the client is experiencing difficulty and the severity of that difficulty, discussion focuses more on thoughts and actions than on feelings. The client's goal of becoming more effective in managing troublesome aspects of his or her life becomes clearer. Some cognitive counselors (e.g., Ellis) tend to move fairly quickly through this stage; others engage in more discussion, and their exploration process may not seem very different from that of a person-centered or psychoanalytic counselor, except for the emphasis on thoughts.

The third stage is more elaborate in the cognitive approach than in others. The client is instructed to go out and behave differently, either by implementing newly discovered rational thinking or possibly by experimenting with finding new information about his or her beliefs about others. Scientific problem solving, led by the counselor but with the client as an active participant, leads to plans of action. As with any new learning experience, new patterns may not be implemented perfectly at first, and reinforcement and refinement are necessary. Cognitive counseling aims to bring about changes in actions in a comparatively short time.

Contribution to the Multitheoretical Integrative Model of Counseling

Cognitive counseling provides a model for understanding and intervening in human behavior in which the point of entry is through the thinking process. The fundamental assumption is that more effective thinking will result in more satisfactory (to the client) behavior and feelings. For certain clients, indentifying faulty thinking and learning more effective ways of viewing life experiences can result in rapid improvement. The REBT approach in particular bypasses a complicated historical diagnostic process and moves directly to supporting change in the client. Cognitive restructuring gives the client direct help in changing self-defeating thoughts and feelings. Just as person-centered counseling provides the clearest view of the first stage of counseling, cognitive counseling—with its emphasis on action planning—provides the strongest descriptions of the third stage. In addition, it adds a diagnostic process based more on learning theory than on personality theory.

TRAIT-FACTOR COUNSELING

As described in the introduction to this chapter, trait-factor counseling was considered to be *the* counseling method for many years during the early part of the 20th century. Although originated by Frank Parsons (1909), the trait-factor approach was more clearly articulated by E. G. Williamson (1939, 1950, 1965). Because Williamson was a professor at the University of Minnesota, the method is sometimes referred to as the Minnesota school of counseling. Although a number of newer humanistic, psychodynamic, cognitive, and behavioral approaches to counseling have emerged to help people with emotional and behavioral problems, the trait-factor approach remains the most common method for assisting people with educational and vocational choices. It is the mainstay of career counseling in educational, business, and government settings.

The Nature of People

Proponents of the trait-factor approach to counseling do not take a position that human beings are either innately good or innately bad. They share the view of their cognitive colleagues that what people learn serves as the basis for their behavior. People are treated as rational decision makers, and children are seen as naive and inexperienced—in need of adult guidance toward effective decision making. Each individual is endowed with a unique set of abilities and develops particular skills, interests, and attitudes that have implications for decision making. The better an individual knows his or her particular characteristics and the demands of the world, the more effective he or she will be in planning and having a good and useful life.

The Counseling Process

Trait-factor counseling is sometimes referred to as counselor-centered counseling because so much of the process depends on the counselor's activity. The counselor uses his or her expertise to help the client *objectively* assess various traits that have implications for problem solving and decision making. This objective assessment includes the use of test scores that reflect the client's skills, abilities, interests and personality. The counselor shows the client how he or she compares with other persons on specific scores so that he or she can choose a course of action that will lead to success and satisfaction. The counselor actively introduces information about the world of work and about educational opportunities so that the client can become more aware of alternatives. Guidance about such things as how to study and how to get along with others may also be offered.

Williamson described the counseling process as a six-step sequence including analysis, synthesis, diagnosis, prognosis, counseling, and follow-up. Each of these steps refers to the counselor's role. Analysis is collecting all relevant data about the client, including test scores and information from school records if available. Synthesis is the process of bringing the data together into a comprehensive picture of the client. Diagnosis, based on the synthesis of the information collected, indicates where any impediment to progress or decision making may lie—dependency, lack of information, inaccurate self-concept, choice anxiety, or no problem at all. Prognosis consists of predicting further developments relating to the client's progress. Counseling is helping the client take steps that will bring about adjustment or readjustment. These steps include conforming with societal expectations, changing environments, selecting new environments, learning new skills, and changing attitudes. Finally, follow-up is the process whereby the counselor watches the client's progress and repeats the other steps if the client is not developing positively. From this description, it is clear that the system is directed toward helping individuals find their spot in the larger scheme of things and that the counselor often sees the best course of action more clearly than the client.

Problem solving in the trait-factor approach also follows the scientific method: a problem is clearly defined, data (information) are collected, courses of action are defined, one course of action is selected and implemented, and evaluation takes place that may lead to the repeat of the cycle. The appeal of this approach lies in its optimistic belief that people can figure out how to handle their lives better. Generally, if emotional disturbance is not a significant factor in the client's problem, the process of carefully reviewing a problem or decision with the help of a counselor results in clarification of the choice to be made and improvement in decision-making skills. Trait-factor counseling was devised for work with developmental and decision-making problems, and Williamson advised that more disturbed clients should be referred to other mental health professionals. In contemporary counseling settings, most counselors have training in trait-factor methods as well as other approaches described in this chapter, and they select specific techniques depending on the nature of the client's presenting concern.

Contribution to the Multitheoretical Integrative Model of Counseling

Trait-factor counseling is the method of choice for clients who seek help with educational and vocational choices when the problem can be resolved by rational decision making and when the level of emotional complication is low. The trait-factor approach provides the counselor with tools for collecting objective data about the client and about opportunities that may be available to the client. This information, often stored in and sorted by computer, is fed into the client's decision-making process.

Trait-factor counseling offers little emphasis on the first or second stages of the generic model of counseling presented in this book. Relationship building is seen as rapport building and makes the client more receptive to the counselor's information and advice. In-depth exploration is concentrated on a systematic exploration of client traits in order to inform the problem-solving and decision-making process. Goals that are directly related to the problem or problems the client presents are discussed and clarified. The counseling interventions are primarily those of the third stage, which emphasizes action steps. The counselor is active in formulating some of the action steps and may offer advice if he or she believes the client lacks the perspective to make good choices on his or her own.

We note that a basic philosophical position stated by Williamson conflicts with the generic model presented in this book. He believed that counselors are responsible for perpetuating societal values. This viewpoint supposes that all counselors know what society values and that what society values is good for everyone. Because humankind is in a constant state of finding new truths to replace old ones, different cultures hold different values, and there are many different ways of living a happy and productive life, we find it inappropriate for counselors to espouse the majority culture's value system in their counseling. The role of helping clients find values to mediate conflicts between personal freedoms and the rights of others is a much more complex activity than Williamson construed it to be.

However, the importance of information (knowledge) in making good decisions is widely accepted and is the major contribution of trait-factor theory to contemporary counseling. Modern computer and psychometric technology has greatly increased the availability and accuracy of information available for decision making. In counseling settings that focus on career decisions and job-search strategies, trait-factor counseling enjoys a renewed emphasis, and there is the capacity for greater thoroughness of analysis than was possible before. In most settings where counselors work, trait-factor counseling will be useful for some problems of some clients.

BEHAVIORAL COUNSELING

Behavioral counseling is based on learning theory. Its fundamental assumption is that all behavior is learned and therefore can be changed by implementing strategies to produce new learning. The personality is regarded as the product of accumulated learning.

The purpose of behavioral counseling is to change ineffective and self-defeating behavior, and only measurable behavior change is regarded as evidence of successful counseling. Generally, behavioral counselors do not regard hypothetical concepts about mental functioning, such as the unconscious, as important to the counseling process. Self-understanding is not an outcome goal.

No single author is credited with the development of behavioral counseling. Joseph Wolpe's (1958) work on reciprocal inhibition applied the principles of classical conditioning to changing neurotic behavior. B. F. Skinner (1971) is widely recognized for his work in developing operant conditioning techniques used in behavioral counseling, although he was not a therapist himself. Together with modeling, operant conditioning and classical conditioning are the principal methods employed in behavioral counseling. Lazarus (1989), Wolpe (1990), and Kazdin (2001) offer contemporary applications of behavioral methods. Interest in behavioral methods increased during the late 1960s, when many people became disenchanted with Rogerian methods as a predominant approach to counseling. More recently, narrowly conceived behavioral approaches have declined in popularity, and some behavioral counselors (e.g., Meichenbaum, 1977) have turned their attention to the thought processes that mediate behavior, blending their work into that of cognitive counselors. Lazarus (1989) has described a broad array of behavioral techniques, each of which provides clients with new opportunities for learning strategies of self-management.

The Nature of People

Behaviorists see human behavior as a function of heredity and environment. This view is often called deterministic, because both elements that shape behavior are largely beyond the control of the individual. One is born with certain inherited equipment that cannot be changed, and so the only variable left to alter after birth is the environment. What one learns from the environment determines behavior; changing the environment changes behavior.

Behaviorists hold no general view that humankind tends toward good or evil. Given adequate hereditary characteristics, any individual can become good or evil depending on what he or she learns from the environment.

Constructs such as the self-concept, the ego, and the unconscious have no meaning in describing human nature in a strict behavioral system. Behaviorists do not necessarily deny that such mechanisms exist, but they say that if the mechanisms exist, it is impossible for the counselor to observe or manipulate them. The description of humans as capable of learning is sufficient for behavioral counseling. A lot of knowledge about how people learn exists, and it makes sense to use it to influence them toward effective behavior.

The Counseling Process

Goal Setting. Behavioral counseling places great emphasis on a clear definition of goals. Goals are stated in terms of behavior change so that observation will provide evidence that can be measured. A goal such as "I'd like to get along better with my parents" would not be acceptable. A more specific goal, such as "I will be home for dinner at least four nights a week to share some part of my life in pleasant conversation," would be seen as a step toward a better relationship with parents. Because the goal is a specific behavior, the counselor and the client are able to assess the extent of accomplishment. Krumboltz (1966) stated that many nonbehavioral counseling efforts fail because of a lack of specific enough goals.

Frequently, clients are referred for counseling by significant others who are dissatisfied with the clients' behavior. Behavioral counselors are perhaps more amenable than other counselors to the suggestions of significant others about the need for clients to change. For example, a child may be referred to counseling because she fails to meet her parents' curfew standards. A behavioral counselor might center his or her work on changing the unwanted behavior without devoting a lot of time to understanding the client's affective experiences in historical relationships with parents or peers.

The client is provided with the opportunity to participate in the goal-setting process, even when problem behaviors are obvious to the counselor from the outset. In some instances, the client may come with his or her own goals in mind, as in the case of a person seeking to gain control over eating habits or to be free of a fear (e.g., of heights).

Because goals are specific, the counselor and client have direct means for documenting change. It is possible to identify and count specific *target behaviors* that are to be eliminated or increased as a result of counseling. The frequency of the target behavior at the outset of counseling is considered to be the *baseline* against which progress is measured.

Strategies for Change. Counseling strategies are based on the principles of learning. The client is taught to think differently about his or her behavior (in cognitive-behavioral approaches) or simply conditioned to behave differently. Operant conditioning is one of the most common procedures used in behavioral counseling. The procedure, which can be used to eliminate undesirable behaviors or to develop positive behaviors, uses reinforcement techniques. If the counselor is helping a client eliminate an undesirable behavior, he or she first determines what environmental conditions are supporting the behavior and then arranges for the reinforcers to be eliminated. A child who acts out at home or in school is frequently seeking the attention of parents or teachers. Often parents and teachers pay attention to the child only when he or she is misbehaving. In an operant conditioning plan, the counselor would teach parents or teachers to withhold attention to misbehavior and to provide attention instead when the child does something positive, such as doing his or her chores or homework. If significant others consistently reward positive behavior with attention and fail to respond to negative behavior that is attention seeking, the child will learn new behaviors that succeed in attracting the attention he or she wants. In operant conditioning, the client's behavior is selectively reinforced to increase desired behaviors in a variety of ways—for example, through positive attention, free time after the completion of tasks, or candies. Undesirable behaviors may be discouraged through negative consequences, such as isolation or withholding of privileges.

Desensitization training (Wolpe, 1958, 1990), used to help clients reduce or eliminate irrational fears or phobias, was developed using the principles of classical conditioning, though research has shown that classical conditioning does not really explain its effectiveness (Sharf, 2003). In this procedure, the client is first asked to be as specific as possible about the anxiety-producing condition, such as being in high places. A list is developed that arranges frightening conditions on a hierarchy from least frightening (e.g., standing on a chair) to most frightening (e.g., standing at the edge of a cliff though safely behind a railing). The client is then taught to relax his or her body through breath control and muscle control. When completely relaxed, the client is asked to think about the frightening circumstances, starting with the least frightening, while the counselor continues to encourage relaxation. Eventually, the client can tolerate the more frightening thoughts while still remaining relaxed. The feared circumstance becomes paired with relaxation and the positive feelings that accompany relaxation. Finally, the client is encouraged to experiment with real feared circumstances while practicing self-relaxation techniques.

Modeling is yet another process whereby the client is taught new behaviors. A model (the counselor, a peer in group counseling, an assistant) demonstrates effective behavior in a situation with which the client has difficulty, and the client observes the model's behavior. The models may also report their thinking aloud as they are performing, giving the client access to the thought processes that lead to behavioral consequences. This procedure may be applied more informally by placing the client with effective models in real-life situations, such as work or school. Public television's Fred Rogers effectively used modeling in his program for children.

As mentioned previously, cognitive restructuring is closely related to behavioral methods in that it attempts to change behavior by changing how one thinks. However, it is more appropriately considered with cognitive counseling.

The sampling of behavioral procedures presented here is far from exhaustive. The common thread in these and other behavioral strategies is the establishment of conditions for new learning to take place. This often requires the manipulation of circumstances in the client's life external to counseling, and significant others may become involved in consultation on how to support the client's behavior change.

Contribution to the Multitheoretical Integrative Model of Counseling

Behavioral counseling places little emphasis on how a problem developed, except for an assessment of the learning conditions in the environment that have sustained an unwanted behavior or failed to support a desired one. This approach depends on learning theory, rather than personality theory, as a basis for understanding a client's behavior. In that respect, it differs substantially from the other approaches discussed in this chapter, with the exception of its close relative, cognitive counseling. Self-understanding and insight into developmental issues are not a focus of behavioral counseling.

The process of behavioral counseling moves quickly from the first stage (initial disclosure) to the third stage (action planning). The first stage is accomplished without special emphasis on empathy, acceptance, or genuineness. These conditions are simply helpful in learning what the client's problems are. Once the problems are identified, goals are set quickly and as specifically as possible. Goals all address specific target behaviors, and behavioral counselors emphasize the development of specific goals more than any other system of counseling. The major emphasis of behavioral counseling lies in third-stage strategies that develop commitment to action, often through environmental manipulation. The procedures of behavioral counseling are effective in relieving irrational fears (phobias), in modifying the behavior of children who have difficulty adapting to and making use of classroom environments, and in helping clients overcome various addictions. Counselors whose primary allegiance is to approaches that are more insight oriented often use behavioral methods for these specific problems, and it is with these issues that a counselor using our model might employ behavioral techniques.

We have presented behavioral counseling in its most conservative conception in this chapter to show how much it can contrast with some of the other theoretical orientations presented earlier. However, it is important to understand that behavioral counselors are as concerned and committed to helping their clients as are other counselors and that they are aware of the affective states of their clients. A common perception that they are cold and mechanistic toward their clients is unfounded. In fact, research has demonstrated that behavior therapists are viewed as equally warm and empathic as other counselors (Sloane, Staples, Cristol, Yorkston, & Whipple, 1975). Their procedures are dictated by their belief that the most effective means of helping is through setting conditions for new learning rather than through an extensive discussion of feelings rooted in developmental experiences.

BRIEF THERAPY

Most readers, as they consider the various theoretical approaches to counseling, will have heard of brief therapy and may wonder where brief therapy fits in the spectrum of theoretical approaches. Brief therapy works best when the client trusts easily, is capable of introspection, and is ready to change. Warnick (1995) notes that individuals who can achieve their goals in a short time have one or more of these characteristics:

- They are basically stable individuals with a specific problem.
- They have an acute problem rather than a long-term condition.
- They may need confirmation that their problem is not solvable and must be lived with.
- They may be stuck in a process and want to resume a more normal lifestyle.

Unlike the other theories presented in this chapter, brief therapy is not a general-purpose theory that is applicable to "people who have had a lifetime of problems, of living on the edge" (Warnick, 1995, p. 170). In fact, there is no one approach to brief therapy which, according to Sharf (2003), may vary widely from 3 to 40 sessions in length. Hoyt (1995) notes that brief therapy is defined "by the intention of helping patients make changes in thoughts, feelings, and actions in order to move toward or reach a particular goal *as time-efficiently as possible*" (emphasis added) (p. 1) more than by any specific number of sessions. Limits on the length of psychotherapy are often attributed to the cost containment efforts of insurers in a managed care environment (Hoyt, 1995), but many clients also prefer brief treatment and most will not choose longer treatment even if it is available to them (Cooper, 1995; Warnick, 1995). Warnick points out that clients who stop attending therapy after a few sessions often do so because their goals have been met.

Brief therapy focuses on identifying a specific issue or problem, maintaining limited goals, and working toward clearly defined outcomes (Cooper, 1995; Quick, 1996). Quick (1996) uses a technique of focusing on one problem at a time and avoiding rambling by repeatedly asking the client to talk about the problem "that you are here for." Restructuring of personality is not the goal of brief therapy, though clients who learn to cope better with one segment of their lives may generalize their coping skills to other sectors.

Because of the focus on specific problem resolution, the theoretical base of most brief therapies is cognitive behavioral and thus related to the work of Ellis, Beck, and Meichenbaum as presented earlier in this chapter. Sharf (2003) indicates that there are some psychoanalytic short-term therapies, but that existential, client-centered, and Gestalt therapy do not have specific short-term guidelines.

Quick (1996) has combined two of the more popular forms of short-term therapy to form what she calls *strategic solution focused therapy*. She defines the approach as a three-part theory as follows:

1. "What's the trouble?
2. If it works, do it more.
3. If it doesn't work, stop doing it. Do something different." (p. 2)

One begins by defining as specifically as possible what is troubling the client. Then an effort is made to identify times when there are exceptions (Molnar & deShazer, 1987) to the negative experience—when things work more as the client would wish. The client is reinforced to extend these good times by repeating whatever he or she does to create the good experience. By the same token, the client is asked to look at what doesn't work—what precipitates unwanted outcomes—and to avoid that behavior. Quick (1996) notes that brief therapy is similar to the intermittent care model often associated with physical medicine, where the client returns for treatment as needed when new problems arise. Systems of brief therapy focus on specific counseling procedures and are currently offered in continuing education formats for practicing counselors and in some counselor education programs.

SUMMARY

A variety of theoretical emphases in counseling relate to the multitheoretical integrative model of counseling presented in Chapters 2 through 6 of this book. Each emphasizes the conditions or techniques appropriate to one or more of the stages of the generic model, while deemphasizing conditions or techniques of the other stages. Person-centered counseling emphasizes first-stage conditions almost to the exclusion of third-stage techniques, and behavioral counseling emphasizes third-stage techniques almost to the exclusion of first-stage conditions.

Counseling theories can be arranged on a continuum from client controlled and affective in orientation to counselor controlled and cognitive in orientation. In presenting our generic model of counseling, we acknowledge that each of the more doctrinaire systems makes an important contribution in detailing procedures that are important to one or more of the stages. We believe that a student of counseling will benefit by understanding the generic model first and then adding techniques and procedures that can be learned by studying the various contributing theories. Through this process, the counselor-in-training first gains a broad view of available theory and technique and then chooses and practices what fits best with his or her personal style. Many counselors will retain an eclecticism based on the multitheoretical integrative model; others will gravitate to one system as the predominant source of diagnostic and helping tools. Most counselors recognize that certain client concerns respond better to one of the different counseling approaches. Brief therapy utilizes principles of one of the major theories (often cognitive) to resolve narrowly defined problems as quickly as possible.

≈≈≈ *DISCUSSION QUESTIONS* ≈≈≈

1. The authors have placed these six theories on a continuum of emphasis on affect or cognition and degree of directiveness of the counselor. How would the continuum differ if the theories were positioned according to the seriousness of the problems they seem best suited to help or according to the time needed to complete counseling?
2. Some have argued that the counselor's faith that a theory can be helpful to clients is more important than the actual truth value of that theory. What do you see as the strengths and limitations of this argument?
3. When many of these theories were developed, their originators were not explicitly thinking about applications for culturally and ethnically diverse populations. How much modification (if any) do you think each theory would require to be applicable across different cultural groups?
4. Ultimately, counselors must select counseling approaches based on the needs of the client and the evidence that a particular approach is likely to be helpful. To some degree, however, a counseling approach must "fit with" the personality and style of the counselor using it. Based on what you have learned about these six theories, where would each fit with your own personality? Explain your rationale for each theory.
5. Research has generally shown that the techniques the counselor uses have a relatively small influence on the effectiveness of counseling and that the counseling relationship and the characteristics the client brings to counseling are more important. Given that evidence, how much emphasis should be placed on learning theories and techniques during

graduate school? Should personal characteristics be weighed more heavily in admissions than intellectual ability?

REFERENCES

Adler, A. (1927). *The practice and theory of individual psychotherapy.* New York: Harcourt.

Alexander, E. M. (1963). *Fundamentals of psychoanalysis.* New York: Norton.

Baker, E. L. (1985). Psychoanalysis and psychoanalytic psychotherapy. In J. L. Lynn & J. R Garske (Eds.), *Contemporary psychotherapies* (pp. 19–67). Columbus, OH: Charles E. Merrill.

Beck, A. (1972). *Depression: Causes and treatment.* Philadelphia: University of Pennsylvania Press.

Beck, A. (1976). *Cognitive therapy and the emotional disorders.* New York: International Universities Press.

Beck, A., Rush, A., Shaw, B., & Emery, G. (1979). *Cognitive therapy of depression.* New York: Guilford.

Burke, J. E. (1989). *Contemporary approaches to psychotherapy and counseling: The self-regulation and maturity model.* Pacific Grove, CA: Brooks/Cole.

Cooper, J. F. (1995). *A primer of brief psychotherapy.* New York: W. W. Norton.

Corey, G. R. (2001). *Theory and practice of counseling and psychotherapy* (6th ed.). Pacific Grove, CA: Brooks/Cole.

Ellis, A. (1962). *Reason and emotion in psychotherapy.* New York: Lyle Stuart.

Ellis, A. (1973). *Humanistic psychotherapy.* New York: Julian Press.

Ellis, A. (1977). The basic clinical theory of rational-emotive therapy. In A. Ellis & R. Grieger (Eds.), *Handbook of rational-emotive therapy: Vol. 2* (pp. 3–30). New York: Springer.

Ellis, A. (2001). *Overcoming destructive beliefs, feelings and behaviors: New directions for rational emotive behavior therapy.* New York: Prometheus Books.

Ellis, A., & Bernard, M. E. (1986). What is rational-emotive therapy (RET)? In A. Ellis & R. Grieger (Eds.), *Handbook of rational-emotive therapy: Vol. 2* (pp. 3–30). New York: Springer.

Ellis, A., & Dryden, W. (1997). *The practice of rational emotive behavior therapy* (2nd ed.). New York: Springer.

Erikson, E. (1963). *Childhood and society* (2nd ed.). New York: Norton.

Fagan, J., & Shepherd, I. (1970). *Gestalt therapy now.* New York: Harper Colophon.

Freud, S. (1953–1974). *The standard edition of the complete psychological works of Sigmund Freud.* London: Hogarth.

Fromm, E. (1941). *Escape from freedom.* New York: Holt, Rinehart and Winston.

Fromm, E. (1976). *To have or to be.* New York: Harper & Row.

Hoyt, M. F. (1995). Characteristics of psychotherapy under managed health care. In M. Hoyt (Ed.), *Brief therapy and managed care: Readings for contemporary practice* (pp. 1–8). San Francisco: Jossey-Bass.

James, R. K., & Gilliland, B. E. (2003). *Theories and strategies of counseling and psychotherapy* (5th ed.). Boston: Allyn & Bacon.

Jung, C. G. (1954). *Collected works: The practice of psychotherapy.* New York: Pantheon.

Kazdin, A. E. (2001). *Behavior modification in applied settings* (6th ed.). Pacific Grove, CA: Brooks/Cole.

Krumboltz, J. D. (Ed.). (1966). *Revolution in counseling.* Boston: Houghton Mifflin.

Lazarus, A. A. (1989). *The practice of multimodal therapy.* Baltimore: Johns Hopkins University Press.

Meichenbaum, D. (1977). *Cognitive behavior modification: An integrative approach.* New York: Plenum.

Meichenbaum, D. (1985). *Stress inoculation training.* New York: Pergamon.

Messer, S., & Warren, C. S. (1998). *Models of brief psychodynamic therapy: A comparative approach.* New York: Guilford.

Molnar, A., & deShazer, S. (1987). Solution focused therapy: Toward the identification of therapeutic tasks. *Journal of Marital and Family Therapy, 13,* 349–358.

Parsons, F. (1909). *Choosing a vocation.* Boston: Houghton Mifflin.

Patterson, C. H., & Watkins, C. E. (1997). *Theories of psychotherapy* (5th ed.). New York: Harper Collins.

Perls, F. (1969). *Gestalt therapy verbatim.* Moab, UT: Real People Press.

Perls, F., Hefferline, R., & Goodman, P. (1951). *Gestalt therapy: Excitement and growth in human personality.* New York: Dell.

Polster, E., & Polster, M. (1973). *Gestalt therapy integrated.* New York: Brunner/Mazel.

Prochaska, J. O., & Norcross, J. C. (2003). *Systems of psychotherapy: A transtheoretical analysis* (5th ed.). Pacific Grove, CA: Brooks/Cole.

Quick, E. K. (1996). *Doing what works in brief therapy: A strategic solution focused approach.* San Diego, CA: Academic Press.

Rogers, C. R. (1942). *Counseling and psychotherapy.* Boston: Houghton Mifflin.

Rogers, C. R. (1951). *Client-centered therapy.* Boston: Houghton Mifflin.

Rogers, C. R. (1961). *On becoming a person.* Boston: Houghton Mifflin.

Rogers, C. R. (1980). *A way of being.* Boston: Houghton Mifflin.

Rogers, C. R. (1986). Carl Rogers on the development of the person-centered approach. *Person-Centered Review, 1,* 257–259.

Sharf, R. S. (2003). *Theories of psychotherapy and counseling: Concepts and cases* (3rd ed.). Pacific Grove, CA: Brooks/Cole.

Skinner, B. F. (1971). *Beyond freedom and dignity.* New York: Knopf.

Sloane, R. B., Staples, E. R., Cristol, A. H., Yorkston, N. J., & Whipple, K. (1975). *Psychotherapy versus behavior therapy.* Cambridge, MA: Harvard University Press.

Sullivan, H. S. (1953). *The interpersonal theory of psychiatry.* New York: Norton.

Van de Riet, V., & Korb, M. (1980). *Gestalt therapy: An introduction.* New York: Pergamon.

Warnick, J. (1995). *Listening with different ears: Counseling people over sixty.* Fort Bragg, CA: QED Press.

Williamson, E. G. (1939). *How to counsel students.* New York: McGraw-Hill.

Williamson, E. G. (1950). *Counseling adolescents.* New York: McGraw-Hill.

Williamson, E. G. (1965). *Vocational counseling.* New York: McGraw-Hill.

Wheeler, G. (1990). *Gestalt reconsidered: A new approach to contact and resistance.* New York: Gardner.

Wolpe, J. (1958). *Psychotherapy by reciprocal inhibition.* Stanford, CA: Stanford University Press.

Wolpe, J. (1990). *The practice of behavior therapy.* Elmsford, NY: Pergamon

Yontef, G. M., & Simkin, J. S. (1989). Gestalt therapy. In R. J. Corsini & D. Wedding (Eds.), *Current psychotherapies* (4th ed., pp. 323–361). Itasca, IL: Peacock.

PART THREE

ADAPTING THE COUNSELING PROCESS
TO SPECIFIC POPULATIONS

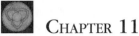 CHAPTER 11

WORKING WITH CLIENTS IN CRISIS

The counseling process, as described in the first 10 chapters of this book, provides opportunities for clients to ventilate emotions, to examine the factors that have led to unwanted emotions and unsatisfying behaviors, to explore alternative plans of action, and to implement and test selected plans. The goals include the resolution of troublesome emotional experiences, the discovery of previously unexplored aspects of self, the planning of new courses of action, the development of new skills, and the integration of new understandings about self in relation to others. Through a deliberate process that may require many sessions over an extended period of time, the client experiences growth in a range of interpersonal and instrumental functions of life.

When a client telephones or appears at the counselor's office in a state of crisis, priorities must be shifted to helping with the immediate crisis so that the client can regain the ability to manage the tasks of daily living as quickly as possible. Resolution of the crisis is sometimes all the help a client needs; in other instances, the client may have longstanding concerns that may become the content of further counseling once the crisis is handled. Sometimes an ongoing client experiences a crisis. For example, a client who has been seeing a counselor for help with depression may suddenly experience the loss of his family in a fire. This trauma needs to be dealt with differently than the ongoing counseling sessions for depression. Aguilera (1998) describes crisis intervention as offering "the immediate help that a person in crisis needs to reestablish equilibrium" (p. 1).

DEFINITION OF CRISIS

We say that people are in a state of crisis when they perceive "an event or situation as an intolerable difficulty that exceeds [their] resources and coping mechanisms" (James & Gilliland, 2001, p. 3). Solutions that have worked before are no longer sufficient. The difficulty involves one or more life goals that the person fears are being blocked. As tension and anxiety over the inability to resolve the problem increase, the person becomes less and less able to find a solution. He or she feels helpless, upset, shamed, guilty, and unable to act on his or her own to reach a resolution. Crises occur rather commonly. According to Hillman (2002), nearly 40% of men and 70% of women in the United States will experience at least one traumatic event in their lifetime.

Aguilera (1998) has developed a paradigm (Figure 11.1) that shows what happens when a person in a state of equilibrium is confronted by a stressful event. The person feels disequilibrium and the need to return to stability. If the person perceives the event accurately and has adequate support and coping skills, the problem is resolved and crisis is avoided. In the absence of accurate perception, situational support, or coping skills, the problem remains unresolved and crisis results.

It is important to recognize that a given event—for example, losing one's job—may precipitate crisis in some people but not in others. Whether losing a job will trigger a crisis depends on a variety of factors, including the individual's skills for seeking a new job, employability, financial reserves, the reactions of significant others to the job loss, the other stressors at the time, and the person's perceptions about each of these conditions (which may differ from reality). The centrality of career and the particular job to the person's sense of identity is yet another determinant of the potential for crisis, because centrality is related to the importance to the individual of the life goal being blocked. For a highly employable individual with good job-seeking skills, some financial reserves, and a supportive spouse, loss of a job may simply be an annoyance, not a crisis. In contrast, less serious negative events are more likely to precipitate crises for individuals with fewer coping skills, many stressors besides the precipitating event, and weak or absent support systems. Counselors cannot determine what constitutes a crisis for their clients by assessing whether the event would cause crisis in their own lives. Certain events, such as the loss of a person's entire family in a fire or being critically injured in a serious car accident, are highly likely to precipitate a crisis, regardless of the person's coping skills or support systems, because they are so traumatic. The attacks on the World Trade Center and the Pentagon on September 11, 2001, were experienced as traumatic by most

Figure 11.1   The Effect of Balancing Factors in a Stressful Event

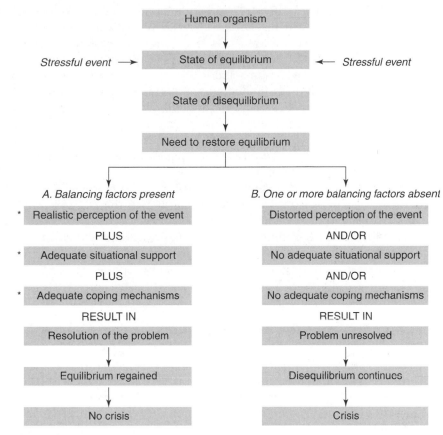

* Balancing factors

Reprinted from D. C. Aguilera, *Crisis intervention: Theory and methodology*, 8th ed. (p. 34). Copyright 1998 with permission of Elsevier.

Americans, though the intensity of the trauma varied not only with a person's location and connection to the victims but also with one's prior history of trauma and the time spent watching the reenactment of those events in the media (Galea et al., 2002; Silver et al., 2002). Generally though, as James and Gilliland (2001) emphasize, the term *crisis* refers primarily to "a person's feelings of fear, shock, and distress about the disruption, not to the disruption itself" (p. 3).

THE PURPOSE OF CRISIS INTERVENTION

According to Aguilera (1998), "The minimum therapeutic goal of crisis intervention is psychological resolution of the individual's immediate crisis and restoration to at least the level of functioning that existed before the crisis period" (p. 18). The goal is a limited one: "The individual must either solve the problem or adapt to non-solution" (p. 5). If the crisis was precipitated by the loss of a job, then finding another job is a solution. If the crisis was precipitated by a spouse's decision to move out of the house, there is potential for either mending the relationship or coming to accept that the spouse is gone. In the case of the death of a significant other, the only alternative available for resolving the crisis is acceptance of the loss and adaptation to life without that person.

The focus of crisis intervention work is the immediate problem, not the totality of the client's personality or life issues. In fact, the counselor must guard against allowing the sessions to ramble onto other issues that might distract attention from resolving the event that has resulted in the client's disequilibrium. Crisis intervention is oriented in the present; it involves the client's developmental history only to illuminate an understanding of the specific crisis and to gain knowledge of coping abilities that have served the client in previous situations.

STRESSFUL EVENTS THAT MAY PRECIPITATE CRISES

The pioneering work in crisis intervention (Lindemann, 1944) was generated in response to the needs of survivors and family members of the 493 victims of a fire at the Coconut Grove nightclub in Boston. Lindemann's interventions anticipated the needs of these individuals, encouraged them to allow themselves to experience their losses, and provided support. Currently, the literature on crisis intervention includes both group and individual approaches for working with situational crises (e.g., loss of life or health) and developmental crises (e.g., the midlife crisis). Some kinds of crisis (e.g., suicide) are common enough that they have been studied extensively and group programs have been designed that anticipate the crisis and focus on prevention. Our review of the literature identified at least 30 different kinds of occurrences that commonly overload human coping capacities and thus lead to crises.

Perhaps the best way of identifying the triggering events for crisis is to remember that crisis occurs when the client believes important life goals are blocked, and it is commonly stated that essentially all life goals relate to the love and work motives of human experience. Therefore, any event that jeopardizes success in either or both of these arenas has the potential to initiate crisis responses. Money and mortality, though not entirely independent of the love and work motives, are sometimes added as causes of crisis.

Table 11.1 lists many events that commonly precipitate crises in people's lives. It is important to realize that crisis is sometimes caused by an event that affects an important person in the client's environment. Any of the events listed in the table can seriously disrupt the quality and stability of life by depriving an individual of opportunities to love and be loved,

Table 11.1   Events That Trigger Crises

Type of Event	Examples	Those Affected
Death	Suicide Homicide Accidental death Natural death	Family Friends Associates Anticipated for self
Health and well-being	Physical illness Mental illness Injury Disability Abuse (physical, sexual, psychological) Substance abuse	Self, family, friends
Reproductive issues	Unwanted pregnancy Stillbirth Miscarriage	Self or significant others
Disruptions of intimate relationships	Arguments Infidelity Separation Divorce	Spouse, family, friends
Violence	Domestic Criminal (including rape) Civil (including war and terrorism)	Self, family, friends
Disruptions of work or school	Layoffs Firings Strikes Academic failure	Self or significant others
Natural and environmental disasters	Storms/Hurricanes Earthquakes Fires	Self or significant others
Financial emergencies and homelessness	Unexpected expense Bankruptcy Gambling losses Investment losses Theft or fraud	Self or significant others

to perform optimally in school or work settings, or to possess the necessities and amenities of a comfortable life. Though it could be established empirically that some of these events are regarded by people in general as much more serious than others, it is important to understand that one individual may be able to cope with the most egregious happening (e.g., the death of a child) with only temporary disruption of life activity. Even though the individual may experience a deep sense of loss, he or she is able to cope with the routines of life. Another person may be immobilized and propelled into crisis by an occurrence that might seem much less important to most people (e.g., failure on a school examination). Whether or not a crisis occurs depends not only on the severity of the loss, but also on the individual's coping resources.

Besides situational crises, crises may be precipitated by a range of developmental transitions, and these developmental crises are managed the same way. A developmental crisis occurs when an individual's coping skills fail under the stress of role transformations that are considered to be a usual part of maturing and aging. Examples include starting school, moving to a new school, changing one's college major, entering the world of work, marriage, having children, retiring, and many more. Often these events are challenges that people seek and that can bring joy. However, if a client perceives himself or herself as unready for an event that he or she sees as timely or culturally expected, emotions of fear and guilt may immobilize him or her. The crisis that is experienced will closely resemble those created by the situations of loss presented in Table 11.1.

STEPS IN CRISIS INTERVENTION

1. Establish a Helping Relationship

As James and Gilliland (2001) remind us, "Basic listening and responding skills are the prerequisites for opening gateways into all other therapeutic modalities" (p. xvii). In crisis intervention, it is crucial that the counselor develop a clear understanding of the event that precipitated the crisis and the meaning of that event to the client. At the same time, the client needs to feel the support that grows from being understood. Therefore, the basic relationship-building skills that were discussed in Chapter 3, including active listening and the core conditions of empathy, positive regard, genuineness, and concreteness, form the bedrock on which crisis intervention is built. The fact that there is some urgency about restabilizing the client as quickly as possible does not reduce the necessity for employing these skills.

Counselors who maintain a calm confidence and hopeful expectation will also facilitate a crisis interview (Hersh, 1985). A calm and confident manner is reassuring to the client, who observes that the counselor is not overwhelmed by his or her problem. If the client is very emotional and out of control, the counselor may need to encourage the client to settle down and try to talk calmly so that together they can figure out what to do. A direct statement such as "We will work something out that will help you face this situation better" bolsters hope. Hersh also recommends special attention to a comfortable environment, privacy, and the absence of time pressures. Catching the panic the client is experiencing is one of the most problematic behaviors counselors can exhibit in crisis intervention. What the client needs is a role model who is not also overwhelmed by circumstances.

2. Assure Safety

One of the first concerns about a client in crisis is how dangerous he or she may be to self or others (Aguilera, 1998; Hillman, 2002; James & Gilliland, 2001). The client may also be in danger from someone else. The conditions that may bring a client to a counseling office or motivate a telephone call for help include suicidal ideation or attempts, homicidal ideation, threatened or actual attacks upon self, and fear of attacking or hurting someone else. Fear that a loved one is in danger from a third party or from oneself may also motivate contact.

It is important for the counselor to ask direct, specific questions about any of these circumstances. If the individual is planning to kill himself or herself, the counselor should ask when and how. Is the client merely thinking about it, or is there a plan? How lethal is the plan? Does the plan include a time and place where the act is not likely to be discovered? Has the person been spending time alone brooding over problems? What is his or her support system like? There is no evidence that talking directly about suicide or homicide increases the likelihood that it will occur; in fact, talking about it may release some tension and reduce the likelihood. The decision to share the concern often represents an alternative to actually carrying out the act. Bongar (2002) and Shea (2002) are valuable resources in helping counselors to properly assess suicide risk and intervene responsibly when that risk is high.

Of course, the counselor must judge the risk based on the answers to the questions and, if the situation is dangerous, take steps to involve family and other sources of support, to help to obtain hospitalization for the client, and to protect any intended victims. In situations where the safety of the client or another person is a concern, the counselor should consult with a supervisor or colleague. Seeking a second opinion helps assure the best possible plan of action and alerts others in the agency or school that a crisis has occurred and that backup assistance may be needed. Failing to seek the support of colleagues and supervisors not only reduces the likelihood of a good resolution to the crisis for the client, it also places unnecessary stress on the counselor. Dealing with a client in crisis is one of the most emotionally and intellectually demanding situations a counselor can confront. Counselors who attempt to go it alone put themselves at risk for burnout and *secondary post-traumatic stress* (Figley, 1995). In other words, they can begin to experience some of the same symptoms of crisis as their clients. When counselors who work regularly with clients in crisis experience these symptoms, the term *compassion fatigue* has been applied (Figley, 1995). To avoid this experience, crisis counselors need to arrange a consultation and support network for themselves and to scale back their crisis work, at least temporarily, when they begin to feel overwhelmed by the pain and trauma of their clients.

In instances of telephone contacts about family violence, Roberts (1991) also recommends that the counselor ask specific questions about whether the client is personally in danger, whether children are in danger, whether the attacker is present, whether police or medical personnel are needed, and whether the client wants to leave and can safely do so. A client will sometimes come to a counselor's office anticipating family violence or after an incident has occurred, and similar questions aimed at assessing the safety of all persons involved are necessary.

Children and adolescents are increasingly at risk from violent acts by peers in school and in other settings, particularly attacks involving firearms (MacNeil & Stewart, 2000). If an individual approaches a counselor with concerns about his or her own safety, the counselor should explore the situation carefully to assess the risk. In addition to working with the young person to defuse whatever conflict exists, it may be necessary to involve family members and to notify appropriate authorities, especially if firearms have been seen in the hands of a potential attacker or other credible means of violence are identified. (See Sandoval, 2002, for an excellent resource on crises in the schools.)

Regardless of the nature of the destabilizing event, the client may be experiencing symptoms of stress that are sufficiently severe to disrupt normal patterns of eating, sleeping, and working. In such circumstances, consideration should be given to psychiatric evaluation for the purpose of prescribing appropriate medication for anxiety, depression, or psychotic symptoms.

3. Conduct an Assessment

In the assessment process, the crisis intervention worker secures information about the event that precipitated the crisis, what the event means to the client, the client's support system, and his or her functioning prior to the crisis (Aguilera, 1998; Hersh, 1985; Roberts, 2000). This information helps the counselor decide whether the consequences of the event might be moderated or reversed, whether the client's own coping skills can be mobilized to meet the challenge, who else might help and how, and what the counselor may need to do. Based on Caplan's (1964) germinal work on crisis intervention, Aguilera has developed a paradigm (Figure 11.1) show-ing how people react to stressful events that introduce disequilibrium.

The counselor should inquire first about what caused the crisis. Aguilera (1998) recommends opening with this simple direct question: "Why did you come for help today?" (p. 30). If the client skirts the issue by saying that he or she has been feeling upset for some time, it is important to persist in asking "Why today?" and "What happened that is different?" The purpose is to identify the "last straw" that overwhelmed the client's coping abilities; it might range in severity from a violent assault to rejection or humiliation (Roberts, 2000). The precipitating event usually would have occurred within the previous two weeks and often within the past 24 hours (Aguilera, 1998), but it may also "extend back as far as a few months or to an anniversary reaction of a major loss" (Hersh, 1985, p. 287).

The counselor working at crisis intervention employs concreteness (Chapter 3) and structuring, leading, and questioning techniques (Chapter 8) to narrow the focus of the initial discussion to the precipitating event. Many clients have a myriad of chronic problems that preceded the crisis and may lead to follow-up counseling; for other clients, life may have been stable prior to the crisis. In either case, the purpose of crisis intervention is to restore the level of functioning that existed prior to the precipitating event. Involvement with other preexisting problems will only complicate and delay the planning of an intervention that will reduce the state of crisis.

While focusing on one problem, it is nevertheless important to encour-age the client to expand on its personal impact. What feelings is the client experiencing (sadness, rage, panic, dread, embarrassment, guilt, etc.)? Has there been an impact on daily routines, sleep pattern, physical functioning, or relationships with others? How has the precipitating event threatened the client's life goals? By discussing these issues, the counselor seeks to under-stand the meaning of the destabilizing event to the client. "Unless the worker perceives the crisis situation as the client perceives it, all intervention strate-gies and procedures the worker might use may miss the mark and be of no value to the client" (James & Gilliland, 2001, p. 33). Taking into account the potential impact of culture, age, gender, ethnicity, sexual orientation, and related variables will help the counselor get a fuller sense of the impact of the event on a given client (Hillman, 2002). Although questioning is a neces-sary part of the assessment process in crisis intervention, the core listening skills of empathy, genuineness, and acceptance are also essential if the coun-selor is to gain access to the client's world of inner meaning. Remember also that feeling understood and accepted contributes directly to calming the client, instilling hope, and mobilizing his or her coping behaviors.

As the counselor comes to understand the meaning of an event to the client, it is necessary to "listen for and note cognitive distortions (overgener-alizations, catastrophizing), misconceptions, and irrational belief statements" (Roberts, 2000, p. 12). Premature direct confrontation of such distortions leads to resistance and impedes progress, but the counselor may try gentle attempts at cognitive restructuring. For example, a young man who has been dropped by his girlfriend may hold the views that he can't go on without her, is not a desirable person, and is doomed to spend his unhappy life alone unless he gets her back. The counselor might respond, "Right now you are consumed with thinking about her and can do nothing else." The phrase "right now" gently implies that this may not be a permanent condition. A more direct attempt at restructuring might be a question about whether he can name anyone other than the girlfriend who thinks he is nice. Although it would certainly be premature to attack or discount his girlfriend's action, the purpose of this question is to reduce any distortion that her decision reflects an accurate representation of his worth. Avoiding direct confrontation of distortions is especially difficult for the counselor who finds it uncomfortable to hear intense expressions of emotion or who wishes to rescue a client from pain. Counselors who become aware of such feelings need to remind themselves of the importance of calm support to a person in crisis. If such feelings become persistent, they should seek consultation and supervision to deal with the underlying issues that are provoking these feelings.

During the assessment process, the counselor observes the client's physical appearance, behavior, mood, speech pattern, attention span, and any outward signs of distress. The extent of the client's preoccupation with the crisis can be estimated from these cues.

Finally, it is important to develop an understanding of the client's functioning prior to the crisis. The purpose of this assessment is to determine how the client usually manages difficult situations and what skills have typically been available to him or her. Such a specific assessment of strengths provides direction as to what kinds of actions the client may be able to mobilize with the support and encouragement of the counselor. Brammer and MacDonald (1999, p. 24) list the following as skills that the client may possess:

1. Perceptual skills (seeing problematic situations clearly, as challenging or dangerous, and as solvable)
2. Cognitive change skills (restructuring thoughts and altering self-defeating thinking)
3. Support networking skills (assessing, strengthening, and diversifying external sources of support)
4. Stress-management and wellness skills (reducing tensions through environmental and self-management)
5. Problem-solving skills (increasing problem-solving competence through applying [decision-making] models to diverse problems)
6. Description and expression of feelings (accurate apprehension and articulation of anger, fear, guilt, love, depression, and joy)

The assessment process includes evaluating strengths in each of these six dimensions of coping skills. Plans for action should be designed to maximize the client's precrisis strengths and, where possible, to minimize dependence on skills that have not been a part of his or her repertoire. For example, one client may have a wide range of family and friends with whom to network for support, and another may be so isolated that emergency contact with a professional may constitute the bare beginning of a network. A given client may have perceived events and other persons accurately up to the point of the crisis and will usually be able to work out distortions related to the crisis with the counselor's help. A different client may routinely misinterpret the intent of others and perceive events in distorted ways; this client's habitual defensiveness will make it much more difficult to establish an accurate perspective on the event that precipitated the crisis.

4. Give Support

Assessing the client's support system involves finding out who in the client's environment cares what happens to him or her and has a favorable opinion of his or her worth. When self-esteem is low, calling on such individuals to be attentive and provide comfort is important. An unmarried woman with an unwanted pregnancy will usually find her strength to cope with the crisis strengthened if the father and/or her own parents are able to assure her that she is still loved and that the crisis event has not deprived her of important relationships. Sometimes the contributions of persons in the support system may be more tangible, for example, providing financial support for needed medical attention. James and Gilliland (2001) are emphatic in their recommendation that the crisis worker directly express his or her caring for the client. Even if other support persons are scarce, the counselor can make it clear to the client that there is one person right here who really cares. When support persons are not evident in the client's daily life, plans should be arranged so that emergency contacts can be made with the counselor personally or with an emergency worker in off hours. This is, of course, especially important if there is suicidal ideation but insufficient evidence to consider hospitalization.

5. Assist with Action Plans

It is in the action-planning step that crisis intervention is probably most different from other forms of therapy. The client is in such a state of distress that some action step that will return him or her to a precrisis level of equilibrium must be identified in the first session. By definition, the client's own coping mechanisms have failed; therefore, the counselor must be willing to take an active role and will often be more directive than in other forms of counseling (Aguilera, 1998). Because the client's ego function has been inadequate to the task of defusing the problem, the counselor may be seen as temporarily "lending" his or her ego function, which is unimpaired by the experience of the crisis, to the client. By the time the action-planning stage of crisis intervention begins, the client is likely to have experienced some calming as a result of catharsis and of sharing the problem. The folk wisdom that "a problem shared is a problem halved" describes the impact of the preceding work. Because of the calming effect, the client's own coping abilities are likely to be more available to him or her than was the case at the beginning of the session.

Although the precipitating event and circumstances surrounding it are discussed as a part of the assessment process, it is necessary to help the client gain an accurate cognitive understanding of the crisis before seeking a solution (Aguilera, 1998; Hersh, 1985; James & Gilliland, 2001; Roberts, 2000). The client's specific problem with the precipitating event—what consequence is so intolerable that the client cannot function—sets the parameters for determining what actions might provide relief. Because crisis intervention is not the time to try to resolve a myriad of concerns, the counselor must tenaciously hold the client's attention on one problem whose moderation will begin to restore equilibrium. It is often difficult to get the client to focus on one problem and to let go of the problems of some third party (e.g., a spouse) who is not present (James & Gilliland, 2001).

The search for possible actions begins with alternative ideas or solutions the client can think of. Even though many clients under stress may initially have a limited view of options, there are usually additional possibilities. Through the use of open-ended questions, the counselor tries to elicit, identify, and modify coping behaviors that have worked for the client before in similar situations. Some material that is initially at a minimal level of awareness for the client should become more available as the discussion of alternatives proceeds. When the client's ideas have surfaced, the counselor may add other possible actions to the list. Initially, it is useful to use brainstorming, where all possible actions that the two parties can think of are listed without evaluation. This process should expand the range of options and create the impression that there are many actions that have a possibility of making a difference.

Once alternatives have been listed, the counselor encourages the client to select one or more actions that he or she feels capable of accomplishing. The counselor "endeavors to develop a short-term plan that will help the client get through the immediate crisis, as well as making the transition to long-term coping" (James & Gilliland, 2001, p. 65). The counselor helps identify concrete positive actions that will help the client regain control of his or her life. The best plans are those that the client truly owns (James & Gilliland, 2001), but the counselor may have to give "specific directions . . . as to what should be tried as tentative solutions" (Aguilera, 1998, p. 31). Ideally, "the final part of the action plan involves cognitive mastery: restructuring, rebuilding, or replacing irrational beliefs and erroneous cognitions with rational beliefs and new cognitions" (Roberts, 2000, p. 12).

Among actions that may be appropriate are referrals to other sources of material assistance and support, such as housing, food, clothing, financial assistance, legal advice, or emergency contact. The counselor serves as a resource person to help the client in crisis find resources such as the Red Cross, public assistance, legal aid, hotlines, and other community agencies. Clients with a history of medical problems or in a crisis likely to affect their health (such as a physical attack) should also be referred to their physicians for an evaluation. Counselors rarely manage these resources but should be networked with agencies that do so.

Before concluding a crisis session, it is important to judge whether the client's anxiety has decreased, whether the client can describe a plan of action on his or her own, and whether there is a glimmering of hope in the client's demeanor. It is also a good idea to readdress the questions of who else knows how the client has been feeling and whether the client is willing for the counselor to make direct contact with that person (e.g., spouse, parent, friend, or roommate). The help of another individual in expressing caring and providing support and a sense of hope can reduce tension for the client and encourage him or her to take the actions that have been planned. Sometimes, it is quite useful to invite a friend or loved one to join the counseling session at the end to ensure that appropriate support will be available, assuming, of course, that the client agrees to such participation.

6. Arrange for Follow-up

A follow-up meeting or telephone call should be arranged at a designated place and time to check on the client's progress toward resolving the crisis (Roberts, 2000). Even though clients in crisis are usually well motivated to escape from the discomfort they are feeling, some plans are hard to execute and no plan comes with a guarantee of success. Roberts (2000) recommends that follow-up take place within one month of the crisis session. If the client has not begun to manage his or her problem by the time of the follow-up conversation, then recycling through any or all of the preceding steps may be in order.

Case: Carolyn

Carolyn, a 26-year-old single female of European-American background, sought counseling at a community mental health center. She was driven to the center by a friend who stayed in the waiting room while the initial session took place.

In an initial flood of information, Carolyn revealed that she "feels like she's in a box and can't get out" that she has never liked herself, that she feels like a "fat slob" even though her weight appeared near normal, and that she feels stupid even though she got good grades in high school and college. For the past 6 months, she had been forcing herself to vomit to try to gain control of her weight and has lost 30 pounds. Carolyn also said that she is tired all the time but even so has trouble sleeping.

When asked to explain what she meant by "feeling like she is in a box," Carolyn explained that she has rigid views of what is right and wrong and that she constantly finds herself doing things that are against her beliefs. She was especially disapproving of her active sex life with a variety of partners.

She has maintained employment as a medical records clerk and reported that her employer is satisfied with her performance, though she feels that she always has loose ends hanging around and should be more efficient. The client's language and behavior in describing her circumstances had a dramatic quality, punctuated by both nervous laughter and tears. She reported feeling very depressed and that recently she has been feeling like taking her life sometimes.

Initially, the counselor responded using mainly reflective responses that captured the meaning and feeling of the client's statements and open-ended questions to elicit more information. After much of the presenting situation had been disclosed, the counselor asked the client what brought her to counseling at this time. The client reported that she had been feeling like she was "increasingly out of control" and that she became frightened as she began dwelling on a suicide plan.

The counselor inquired about the plan and learned that the client had been stockpiling tranquilizers and had read that when these are taken with alcohol they can lead to sleep from which one does not awake. Furthermore, she lives alone, has no contact with her family, and has only the one friend who has brought her to the center. The likelihood that she would be discovered before death was not high. The counselor asked about the men with whom she had intimate relationships and learned that these were better described as sexual encounters than relationships and that it would be pure chance if she heard from one of these men during a suicide attempt. When asked whether she would consider relinquishing her supply of tranquilizers to her friend for safekeeping the client declined. The counselor concluded that the client was at considerable risk of suicide.

The counselor also reasoned that the client's vomiting, combined with the control issues that are typical of eating disorders, constituted a second source of risk. The counselor decided that the risk of allowing the client to return home was one that should not be taken. Indeed, the client's own statement that she was frightened about what she might do indicated that some tangible action was needed.

Clearly, two medical problems existed. First, an evaluation was needed to determine what medication would help with the client's depression and whether the client could be trusted to take an appropriate dosage of any antidepressant that would be prescribed. Second, the potential of an eating disorder must be evaluated. The counselor carefully explained that each of these problems was medical and that evaluation at the psychiatric unit of a local hospital would be the safest course of action. Though Carolyn felt anxious about going to the hospital, she agreed to go if her friend would accompany her. The counselor and client discussed what the friend should be told about the referral, and it was agreed that she should be told that the client was in danger and needed an immediate evaluation. The friend agreed to take the client directly to the hospital, and the counselor made a telephone referral to the hospital. With Carolyn's permission, the counselor spoke directly with the emergency intake worker on duty.

The hospital psychiatrist recommended inpatient treatment to more fully evaluate the client's mood, to fully explore her eating pattern, and to establish the client on antidepressant medication. The client declined to be hospitalized on a Friday afternoon, but by Sunday she became more frightened for her own safety and admitted herself to the hospital, where she was retained for treatment for 2 weeks. She was subsequently referred to an eating disorder specialist and continued to see the hospital psychiatrist on an outpatient basis to deal with her depression.

Questions for Further Thought

1. Identify ways in which this crisis intervention counseling is similar to and different from the generic model of counseling.
2. Do you agree with the decision that the counselor made to seek an immediate referral? Why or why not?

3. If the client had not chosen to cooperate with the referral, what actions would be open to the counselor?
4. If the indications of suicidal intention had been lower, what changes would you recommend as to the actions to be taken?

SUMMARY

This chapter addressed how a counselor should help a client who presents with a problem so distressing that it has destabilized the client's equilibrium and rendered him or her incapable of acting to resolve the problem. Many of the skills that are evident in all counseling are evident in crisis intervention work: the core conditions of effective listening and responding are employed, the client's environmental support system is reviewed, the client's strengths are identified, and problem analysis and action planning take place. However, little effort is devoted to developing a history of the client, and the resolution of precrisis emotional concerns is not among the crisis intervention goals. The process begins with careful listening that allows for problem identification and catharsis as well as sharing of the burden. It is useful to identify early in the session exactly what event caused the client to lose control of his or her coping abilities. Care must be taken to ensure the physical safety of the client and any others who may be in danger from the client. Together, the client and the counselor search for alternative plans of action, based on the client's coping skills in previous situations similar to the one that precipitated the crisis. The counselor is often more active in suggesting alternatives and structuring the discussion than he or she would be in other counseling circumstances. Some plan of action must be agreed upon within the session. Finally, it is necessary to follow up with the client to make sure that action has been taken and that it is beginning to moderate the crisis and to restore the client's precrisis abilities to deal with the challenges of living.

≈≈≈ DISCUSSION QUESTIONS ≈≈≈

1. Adequate support systems, a history of reasonable coping skills, and a realistic perception of the stress all act to influence the degree of disequilibrium a person experiences in the face of a crisis. Do you see all these factors as equally important? If you judge them to have varying impact on the experience of crisis, describe which you see as most important and why?
2. How do you account for the increased stress felt by many people who spent long hours watching the reenactment of the attacks on the World Trade Center even though they lived far from New York and personally knew no one victimized by that attack?

3. Compassion fatigue is an occupational hazard among professionals who spend a great deal of time doing crisis intervention. The chapter emphasizes the importance of support, consultation, and good self-care as ways to minimize compassion fatigue. What exactly should professionals do to take care of themselves while engaged in crisis intervention? What do you think motivates professionals to continue in this stressful form of counseling?

4. Crisis intervention requires a modified approach to the counseling process, with a more active counselor using a briefer model of intervention. What styles of counseling and what personality characteristics lend themselves most to this work?

5. The authors emphasize that the counseling approach for clients in crisis must build on the fundamental counseling skills discussed in earlier chapters and that the counselor in this situation must be active and guide the client back toward equilibrium without taking control away from the client or giving lots of advice. Do you agree with their view? If so, what training do you see as necessary to ensure that professionals have the skills needed to help in these situations?

6. Because crises are so common in people's lives, should extensive training in crisis intervention be a required component in counselor education programs?

7. Effective crisis counselors must be knowledgeable about other community resources if they are to help their clients. Which community resources do you see as particularly helpful with the following kinds of crises: sexual assault, school violence, natural disasters, and victimization from street crime.

REFERENCES

Aguilera, D. C. (1998). *Crisis intervention* (8th ed.). St. Louis, MO: C. V. Mosby.

Bongar, B. (2002). *The suicidal patient: Clinical and legal standards of care* (2nd ed.). Washington, DC: American Psychological Association.

Brammer, L. M., & MacDonald, G. (1999). *The helping relationship: Process and skills.* (7th ed.). Boston: Allyn & Bacon.

Caplan, G. (1964). *Principles of preventive psychiatry.* New York: Basic Books.

Figley, C. R. (1995). *Compassion fatigue: Coping with secondary traumatic stress disorder in those who treat the traumatized.* New York: Bruner/Mazel.

Galea, S., Ahern, J., Resnick, H., Kilpatrick, D., Bucuvalas, M., Gold, J., & Vlahov, D. (2002). Psychological sequelae of the September 11th terrorist attacks on New York City. *New England Journal of Medicine, 346,* 982–987.

Hersh, J. B. (1985). Interviewing college students in crisis. *Journal of Counseling and Development, 63,* 286–289.

Hillman, J. (2002). *Crisis intervention and trauma: New approaches to evidence-based practice.* New York: Kluwer Academic/Plenum.

James, R. K., & Gilliland, B. E. (2001). *Crisis intervention strategies* (4th ed.). Pacific Grove, CA: Brooks/Cole.

Lindemann, E. (1944). Symptomatology and management of acute grief. *American Journal of Psychiatry, 101,* 141–148.

MacNeil, G., & Stewart, C. (2000). Crisis intervention with school violence problems and volatile students. In A. R. Roberts (Ed.), *Crisis intervention handbook* (pp. 229–249). New York: Oxford.

Roberts, A. R. (1991). *Contemporary perspectives on crisis intervention and prevention.* Englewood Cliffs, NJ: Prentice-Hall.

Roberts, A. R. (2000). How to work with clients' strengths in crisis intervention: A solution-focused approach. In A. R. Roberts (Ed.), *Crisis intervention handbook* (pp. 31–55). New York: Oxford.

Sandoval, J. (Ed.). (2002). *Handbook of crisis counseling, intervention, and prevention in the schools* (2nd ed.). Mahwah, NJ: Lawrence Erlbaum.

Shea, S. C. (2002). *The practical art of suicide assessment: A guide for mental health professionals and substance abuse counselors.* New York: Wiley.

Silver, R. C., Holman, E. A., McIntosh, D. N., Poulin, M., & Gil-Rivas, V. (2002). Nationwide longitudinal study of psychological responses to September 11th. *Journal of the American Medical Association, 288,* 1235–1244.

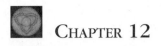 # CHAPTER 12

ISSUES OF HUMAN DIVERSITY IN COUNSELING

The human family is very diverse. The genetics of our creation determines certain physical characteristics, including race, size and stature, gender, and capacities. Our life experiences from the moment of conception continue the differentiation process, so that in the final analysis no two humans are exactly the same. Even twins with identical genetic material become different through their unique experiences. But we are all more like some of our fellow humans than others; we are most like those with whom we share a genetic similarity and an experience repertoire.

As humans, we also tend to be egocentric and ethnocentric with a predisposition to value most our own experience and our own kind. Each of us is limited in our experience and thus cannot know all of what is known and valued by others.

When, as counselors, we try to become the facilitators of others' development, problem solving, and mental health, we work to get inside our clients' frames of reference and to share their experiencing of the world. The more different the client is from us, the more challenging it becomes for us to "get inside the client's skin," to feel his or her joys and sorrows and know what she or he values and aspires to be. By the same token, the greater the difference between counselor and client, the harder it is for the client to trust that an understanding is possible or that the counselor has a genuine desire to create it.

The more a counselor can know about the ways in which people different from himself or herself live their lives, experience their worlds, and place value on their relationships and accomplishments, the more able that counselor will be to reach out to a variety of clients. While coming to recognize elements of our own enculturation with its related values and preferences, we can come to appreciate how a different way of living may be more valued by someone else.

We believe that a counselor who is experienced with a variety of ways of being human will

- succeed in establishing intimate and facilitative communication with more clients and

- come to value ways of living differently from oneself as valid and productive for others.

In this chapter, we ask the student of counseling to reflect in depth about his or her experience of living as male or female, and in his or her particular culture or station in life, in comparison with the spectrum of possible client experiences.

The chapter discusses the impact of many forms of diversity on the counseling process. Within diversity we include cultural, ethnic, gender, and sexual orientation variables. First, we examine why diversity has such a critical influence on the counseling process. Second, we focus on the specific attitudes and knowledge base that counselors need for effective diversity-sensitive counseling. Third, we identify several skills counselors should integrate into their counseling approach when working with diverse clients. We begin the chapter with issues especially relevant to culturally diverse clients, then proceed to topics related to issues of gender and sexual orientation.

It is important to note that the following recommendations represent adaptations of the three-stage model of counseling we advocate. Counselors need to build a trusting relationship, encourage the deep exploration of problems, assess client needs, devise appropriate intervention strategies, and end counseling on a positive note with all clients. However, the attitudes, skills, and techniques counselors use to progress along this process may differ somewhat, depending on the cultural, social, and individual characteristics of the particular client. For example, counselors need to take into account the possible impact of the experience of discrimination on the client's willingness to trust a counselor from a different cultural group and to intensify their efforts to build trust when dissimilarity may make trust harder to build. Nevertheless, as Fischer, Jome, and Atkinson (1998) assert, there are universal healing conditions present in all forms of counseling.

THE MULTICULTURAL FACE OF AMERICA

Because the United States is a nation of immigrants, its population has never been homogeneous in culture, race, or ethnicity. However, recent decades have seen a significant increase in the cultural, ethnic, and racial diversity of the nation. This increase has been attributed to higher rates of immigration by Hispanics and Asians and to lower birthrates among European Americans (Atkinson, Morten, & Sue, 1998). The specific percentages of change are dramatic. In the 1980s, for example, the Asian-American population rose by nearly 80%, the Hispanic-American population by 39%, the American Indian population by 22%, and the African-American population by 14%. During the same period, the European-American population increased by only 7%. Furthermore, demographic trends indicate that this diversity will be an enduring characteristic of the American people.

U.S. Census Bureau figures suggest that by the year 2050, European Americans will constitute only 53% of the population, a projection some believe underestimates the growth in diverse populations in the next 50 years. In some states, the rate of diversification is even greater. In California, for example, European Americans probably already are a numerical minority (Atkinson, Morten, & Sue, 1998).

This demographic shift is affecting many American institutions. Currently, women and culturally diverse populations represent 75% of the entering workforce (Sue, Arrendondo, & McDavis, 1992). Many students entering the school system come from homes in which English is not spoken. In California, 25% of entering students currently come from non-English-speaking homes, and European-American students represent less than 50% of the school population (Atkinson, Morten, & Sue, 1998). American colleges and universities are experiencing a significant increase in the number of international students along with increasing proportions of culturally diverse Americans.

For many years, American society was viewed as a *melting pot* in which diverse races, cultures, and ethnic groups were merged into one American culture relatively soon after their arrival on United States soil. Current scholars challenge that view of the society and believe that the terms *multicultural* or *pluralistic society* better describe this nation (Atkinson, Morten, & Sue, 1998). They argue that the melting pot image may have held some value to describe the experience of European Americans arriving on the shores of the United States but that it does not reflect the experience of others, partly because African Americans, Hispanic Americans, and Asian Americans have suffered from oppression and discrimination. For these reasons, a number of scholars prefer the term *cultural stew*, if any analogy is fitting. The notion that a single culture necessarily emerges from such diverse cultures is not only unrealistic, it also denies the potential value of diverse cultural traditions to the society.

Thus, it is clear that counselors in virtually every setting in the United States will serve a diverse clientele and must adapt their models of the counseling process to the needs of a multicultural society. Moreover, they must examine their own assumptions about race and culture to ensure that they do not inadvertently contribute to racist and stereotypic patterns of treatment of persons from non-European backgrounds.

People of color are not the only diverse groups in American society, nor are they the only groups who have experienced oppression and discrimination. People with physical challenges, sexual minorities, and women have long been treated in prejudicial ways. Partly in response to their common characteristics and partly as a reaction to oppression, each group has developed its own cultural identity. In each of these cases as well, the counseling process must be adapted to take into account these experiences.

CONSIDERATIONS IN COUNSELING
CULTURALLY DIVERSE CLIENTS

Why Is Culture Important in Counseling?

It is not uncommon to hear counselors say that they are "color-blind" or that "underneath, all people are the same." This attitude implies that culture is a relatively minor influence on human behavior and that the universality of human experience is the major influence. This emphasis on core human experience is termed an *etic* perspective. What usually follows from an etic perspective is a view that cultural heritage (either the counselor's or the client's) is much less important than the common human experience of the individuals who are interacting. The second consequence of an etic perspective is the belief that counseling theories and methods can be effective regardless of cultural differences. Both new evidence from scholars and the experiences of culturally diverse groups in counseling reveal the flaws of this perspective (Sue, Ivey, & Pedersen, 1996). Culturally diverse clients are less likely to seek out counseling services, are more likely to be given more serious diagnoses than their majority counterparts, tend to drop out of counseling earlier, and are less likely to have "positive outcomes" from the counseling they do engage in (Sue & Sue, 2003). In short, there is little evidence that the common human experience of people from different cultures is much more important than their cultural differences in producing good counseling outcomes. Scholars of cross-cultural counseling argue that the relative ineffectiveness of counseling can be explained by the fact that an *emic* perspective on culture is often left out of the mix. Ideally multicultural counseling allows for both emic and etic perspectives, examining issues from both the clients own cultural viewpoint and from the more universal viewpoint as well (Pedersen, 2000). The emic perspective acknowledges that culture does indeed influence a whole array of human experiences, including the following:

- The values one holds
- The language one uses and the nuances of meaning one attributes to words
- The use and interpretation of nonverbal behavior
- The definitions of what is normal and dysfunctional behavior
- The ways one seeks to get help for dysfunction
- The patterns of family and interpersonal relationships
- One's world view, or frame of reference for making sense of one's experience and set of deep assumptions about one's relationship with the outside world

One way that culture affects the counseling process is by influencing verbal communication and the understanding of the language used. When counselors and clients are of different cultures, they may not be equally comfortable using English or they may speak different dialects of the language. Even if English is the first language of each participant, subtle differences in usage exist, and there is no guarantee that nuances of meaning will be the same for the counselor and the client. Because verbal communication is the currency of counseling, language barriers can be an enormous roadblock to effectiveness. As discussed in Chapter 3, verbal communication is the primary means by which the counselor demonstrates empathy. Without a commonality of language, empathy is harder to attain and communicate to the client. In addition, verbal communication is the dominant means by which problems are assessed and the means by which intervention strategies are communicated and evaluated. Without shared language, then counseling is hampered at every turn. After all, as Sue and Sue (2003) remark, "The presupposition is that participants in a counseling dialogue are capable of understanding each other" (p. 47).

Second, culture influences many nonverbal behaviors. Some nonverbals, such as smiles or frowns, seem to have universal meanings, but others are culturally relative. For example, in European-American culture establishing eye contact with another person during a conversation is viewed positively as a sign of self-respect, respect for the other, and attention to the conversation. Conversely, failure to establish eye contact during a conversation is seen as a sign of shyness, low self-esteem, or lack of interest in the partner or the conversation. In some cultures, however, whether one establishes eye contact depends entirely on the status of the other person and not on self-esteem or interest in the topic. In this case, when the other person has a higher social status, to make eye contact is seen as aggressive or disrespectful to that person. For example, for a young person from some Native American cultures to make eye contact with an adult in authority would be seen as rude and presumptuous. In these cultures, eye contact is only appropriate between equals. Counselors from different cultural backgrounds who do not understand this influence of culture on nonverbal behavior are vulnerable to misinterpreting a Native American client's nonverbal behaviors. This simple misinterpretation of eye contact can lead to misdiagnosis of problems with self-esteem or assertiveness and misuse of counseling strategies such as assertiveness training. The research of Ivey, Ivey, and Simek-Morgan (1997) offers a good resource for additional examples of divergent meanings of nonverbal behaviors.

Third, culture affects the behaviors a person perceives as normal or dysfunctional and the kinds of self-help strategies a person will use to solve his or her problems. For example, Sue and Sue (2003) suggest that for Asian-American clients, it is typical and normal for parents' desires for their offspring's career to take priority over the child's wishes. Counselors who do not understand the impact of this cultural tradition on Asian-American youth may misinterpret the young person's deference to the parents' wishes as career immaturity. The likelihood of misunderstanding the client's reaction is greater when the counselor's culture emphasizes the "rugged individualism" that is a dominant philosophy in the European-American culture. As another example, in Asian-American cultures, a common self-help strategy for emotional distress is to distract oneself from the emotion or to ignore it; the assumption is that attending to it will make things worse. (Note that Sue and Sue, (2003), suggest that this is a common approach in Asian-American cultures, not an approach that characterizes *all* Asian Americans.) Again, counselors ignorant of this cultural message may misinterpret a client's avoidance of emotional content as repression or lack of insight and may overuse affectively oriented interventions. The tendency to misunderstand the avoidance of negative emotions is stronger if the counselor's culture or training emphasizes affective awareness and exploration as the only path to mental health. Clearly, in some circumstances, avoidance or repression of negative emotions can be a serious impediment to healthy functioning. In these circumstances, attention to such emotions is a legitimate counseling goal even with Asian-American clients who share the view that Sue and Sue describe. The counselor's central concern becomes sensitivity and skill in respecting the client's cultural tradition and possible difficulty with such an undertaking. The client needs to understand the rationale for this focus and to freely choose it in spite of the attendant discomfort.

Fourth, culture affects family dynamics and interpersonal relationships. In European-American culture, the autonomy of the individual takes precedence over the family or the group, and many counseling interventions rest on this principle of individual freedom and responsibility. In some other cultures, however, the needs of the family or group take priority over the rights of the individual. Using the example of an Asian-American student's career dilemma, not only does the cultural tradition define deference to the parents' wishes as normal, it also suggests that open expression of disagreement with those wishes is improper and disrespectful. Moreover, discussion of family tensions outside the family is typically seen as dishonorable and disloyal. Obviously, this view of family dynamics will color the client's responses to the counselor's exploration of family conflict and the counselor's selection of strategies that include assertive behavior by the child toward the parents. Counselors who fail to take this cultural difference into account in assessing client needs or designing intervention strategies are likely to misunderstand family and group dynamics and risk an unsatisfactory or premature end to the counseling process. Clients with culturally insensitive counselors will see the counselor's suggestions as impossible demands that risk the dissolution of family bonds.

Finally, culture influences the worldview of a person. Sue (1978) defined *worldview* as one's "psychological orientation in life" (p. 458) and identifies it as having two major components: locus of control and locus of responsibility. *Locus of control* refers to an individual's assumptions about his or her personal power to influence the events that happen. In European-American culture, a strong internal locus of control is assumed to be appropriate. An *internal* locus of control means that individuals see themselves as able to influence what happens to them, and an *external* locus of control places greater emphasis on the role of fate, luck, or historical accident in affecting human behavior. The latter orientation results in a more passive and accepting response to external events and is more frequently represented in non-European cultural traditions. Similarly, *locus of responsibility* refers to the placement of responsibility or blame for a person's plight on the person or on the system or institution. European-American culture places the locus of responsibility squarely on the individual. Other cultures view the environment or social system as more responsible for individual outcomes. Furthermore, European-American culture has come to define mental health almost exclusively in terms of an internal locus of control and an individual locus of responsibility. The risk of such a perspective is an underestimation of the real role that external events can play in a client's life circumstances and a minimization of the struggle involved in change and self-empowerment. A counselor with a narrow European-American worldview would have a difficult time understanding or helping clients whose perspective on control and responsibility was at the other end of the continuum. Similarly, clients with an externally focused worldview would be likely to see such a counselor's narrow focus on internal factors as blaming and blind to social and accidental influences. (For a more detailed discussion of the effects of culture on human behavior and the debate about an etic or an emic perspective, see the September 1991 issue of the *Journal of Counseling and Development* edited by Paul Pedersen.)

Counselors who understand how the client's worldview affects his or her situation and how it relates to the client's goals for counseling are more likely to establish an effective counseling relationship. In contrast, counselors who judge a different worldview as inherently inferior or problematic are unlikely to foster rapport. While working as a counselor in the Midwest, one of the authors sometimes saw European-American counselors make this mistake with Native American clients whose worldview tended to emphasize external locus of control and responsibility. Instead of understanding behavior in light of the clients' worldview, some counselors labeled their clients' behavior as passive, resistant, or unambitious. Needless to say, counseling was hampered under these circumstances. Clearly, where clients present problems of adjustment to the mainstream society because of a different worldview, the task of counseling may be to help them gain insight into the issue of differing worldviews. With this information, they can then decide how much they wish to change their behavior to function in the mainstream society. During this process, counselors need to help clients see how the different worldviews are operating and need to convey to them that the issue is the difference in perspective, without any suggestion that their worldview is flawed or inadequate. Counselors should acknowledge that human experience can be viewed through different lenses and no single lens provides an absolutely accurate view.

Self-Awareness: The First Step Toward Cultural Sensitivity

To avoid what Wrenn (1962) called "cultural encapsulation"—that is, the tendency to acknowledge only one cultural perspective or to define different cultures as deficient—counselors must first become fully aware of the influences of their own culture on their personal and professional behaviors. Understanding their own culture will give counselors both a clearer sense of their cultural identity and the capacity to identify values, beliefs, and behaviors that are culture specific. This exploration of cultural history can help the counselor move beyond cultural encapsulation, a critical need in this multicultural and often racist society.

If counselors have acquired negative views of other cultures, they need to identify what stereotypes underlie their attitudes. Confronting one's own racist and stereotyping attitudes is a painful endeavor, and the impulse may be to avoid it. After all, counselors naturally want to see themselves as helping people, truly devoted to the well-being of others. In our view, this impulse must be resisted because racist attitudes are insidious and often held unconsciously. Only one's commitment to their exploration will ferret them out and open them to change. Cultural elitism, the view that other cultures' values and practices are inferior to one's own perspective, is a related danger because clients from oppressed groups are alert to subtle racist messages, a sensitivity developed as a coping mechanism in a prejudiced society. Only counselors who have truly understood their own cultural heritage and dealt with their own biases will be trusted by those who have had many other experiences of racist attitudes in those of the majority group.

━━━━━━━━━━   *Exercise in Cultural Awareness*   ━━━━━━━━━━

With a partner, discuss the following questions:

1. What is your own cultural background? Include not only ethnicity and nationality but other relevant aspects of culture such as religion, gender, or urban or rural upbringing.
2. What strengths and weaknesses does this particular background provide in your capacity to interact in an open and nonstereotyping way with people from other cultural backgrounds?
3. Are there particular cultural identities with which it would be more difficult for you to maintain an open attitude?

4. How much interaction have you had in the past month, outside of school or work, with people of cultural backgrounds different from your own?

One mark of a counselor who has made progress in this self-exploration is a higher level of emotional comfort with clients from other backgrounds. Another is a true appreciation for the richness and complexity of other cultural traditions and an openness to further growth in understanding one's own culture and those of clients. Detailed presentations of the counselor competencies necessary for culture-sensitive counseling is available in Arrendondo et al. (1996) and Jordan (1997). In addition, several of the books listed in the references at the end of this chapter will provide an excellent starting point for this process of self-exploration. It is important to note that self-exploration is required of all counselors, not just majority counselors. Virtually all Americans have been acculturated in a racist and elitist society, and all counselors, whatever their race or ethnicity, will work with increasing numbers of clients with different cultural backgrounds.

Knowledge Base for Effective Counseling of Culturally Diverse Clients

The next step in becoming a culturally effective counselor is to become educated about other cultures. Where should counselors start this sizable task? Counselors in Minneapolis will be likely to encounter clients of different cultural backgrounds than will counselors in Cleveland, Los Angeles, or Toronto. Given current population patterns, for example, one would expect to find a greater density of Latino and Asian-American clients in Los Angeles than in Minneapolis, but a greater proportion of Native American clients in Minneapolis. Thus, the other cultures that a counselor needs to understand best will depend somewhat on the geography of the work setting. Population projections, however, suggest that all counselors will need to become knowledgeable about Asian-American, Latino, and African-American cultural traditions because these cultures represent the largest, fastest-growing segments of the U.S. population.

To gain knowledge of other cultures, counselors should read the abundant literature on culturally diverse clients. (Again, the books on the reference list provide a good departure point.) Counselors need to focus this reading on understanding how each culture views language, nonverbal behavior, mental health and personality, and family and interpersonal dynamics.

Counselors should also study the worldview and values of each cultural group that is well represented in their service area. The multicultural counseling competencies endorsed by the Association for Multicultural Counseling (Arrendondo et al., 1996) also suggest that counselors become involved with the cultural group in the community so that their knowledge is more integrated and less academic. Counselors may attend festivals, political meetings, community events, and similar activities to develop this fuller sense of the culture. Counselors should be open to friendships with persons of different cultural backgrounds and actively seek out such personal connections. (The absence of friends from different cultural backgrounds may be one signal that a counselor has not yet succeeded in overcoming cultural elitism.) Such immersion also gives the counselor an appreciation of the contribution of the culture to the society, an appreciation that cannot be obtained in the classroom or counseling office (see Lee (1997), for more information on this topic).

The second aspect of a knowledge of the cultural heritage of one's clients involves understanding how racism and cultural elitism have negatively impacted them. Sue, Arrendondo, and McDavis (1992) call for understanding of "immigration issues, poverty, racism, stereotyping and powerlessness" because these issues affect clients' responses to counseling, to the majority culture, and to their own cultural heritage (p. 482). This awareness is particularly critical for counselors who have been fortunate enough to be spared such injustices; their background does not predispose them to understand the interrelationship between personal difficulties and the sociopolitical environment.

Third, there is a growing literature on cultural identity development that can be a valuable resource for counselors in understanding their own cultural identity and that of their clients. This literature posits that cultural identity development proceeds in levels or stages, just as others have theorized that personality development moves in stages. Atkinson, Morten, and Sue (1998) present a five-stage model of racial/cultural identity development, summarized in Table 12.1. This model focuses on identity development for people whose cultural or racial backgrounds have made them members of a minority or oppressed group in a dominant culture. Atkinson, Morten, and Sue propose that cultural identity development is manifest in one's attitudes toward self, toward one's own cultural group, toward other minorities, and toward the dominant group. The lower stages are characterized by negative or conflicted views about oneself and one's culture and the same views of other minorities but more positive evaluations of the dominant culture. At these stages, there is some self-hate or self-depreciation, a negative view of one's own culture, and an identification with the values of the dominant culture. At the middle stage, one seems to move to the other end of the continuum, developing self-pride and an appreciation for one's culture while depreciating the dominant culture and holding conflicted views of other minorities. At this stage, the person comes to identify with his or her own group and thus has empathy for the minority role of other groups, but still views his or her own culture as superior. Few of the positive attributes of the dominant culture or of individual members of it are

Table 12.1 Racial/cultural Identity Development

Stages of Development Minority Model	Attitude Toward Self	Attitude Toward Others of the Same Minority	Attitude Toward Others of Different Minority	Attitude Toward Dominant Group
Stage 1—Conformity	Self-depreciating	Group-depreciating	Discriminatory	Group-appreciating
Stage 2—Dissonance	Conflict between self-depreciating and appreciating	Conflict between group-depreciating and group-appreciating	Conflict between dominant-held views of minority hierarchy and feelings of shared experience	Conflict between group-appreciating and group-depreciating
Stage 3—Resistance and immersion	Self-appreciating	Group-appreciating	Conflict between feelings of empathy for other minority experiences and feelings of culturo-centrism	Group-depreciating
Stage 4—Introspection	Concern with basis of self-appreciation	Concern with nature of unequivocal appreciation	Concern with ethnocentric basis for judging others	Concern with the basis of group-depreciation
Stage 5—Synergetic articulation and awareness	Self-appreciating	Group-appreciating	Group-appreciating	Selective appreciation

From Donald R. Atkinson, George Morten, and Derald Wing Sue, *Counseling American Minorities: A Cross-Cultural Perspective*, 5th ed. Copyright 1998 by Wm. C. Brown Communications, Inc., Dubuque, IA. All rights reserved. Reprinted by permission.

acknowledged. At the higher stages, the person maintains the positive view of self and his or her culture and begins to develop a less culturally elite view of other minority cultures. At these levels, a more differentiated view of the dominant culture emerges with less depreciation of the culture as a whole and a more positive attitude, especially toward individuals who do not manifest cultural elitism.

Even though research evidence supporting this theory is meager and its hypotheses must be considered tentative until additional evidence is accumulated, it is a useful heuristic for approaching counseling with culturally diverse clients. Atkinson, Morten, and Sue (1998) recommend that counselors assess the stage of cultural identity that best characterizes their client's views and respond accordingly. For example, individuals at the lower stages may have little conscious discomfort with a majority counselor and little conscious rejection of the views of even a culturally encapsulated counselor. However, the client's negative views toward himself or herself and his or her culture of origin need to be taken into account if empathy is to be achieved. A client at Stage 3 of cultural identity development may mistrust a majority counselor. This client may respond to the counselor with challenging or nonrevealing comments and could be mislabeled as hostile or resistant if the counselor is unaware of the role of cultural identity in the interaction. Unless the counselor addresses that cultural mistrust, an effective counseling relationship may never develop. Sue and Sue (2003) suggest that it is possible for clients at this stage of cultural identity development to need more self-disclosure from the counselor about the cultural difference to allay fears and mistrust. They suggest direct responses to client statements questioning the counselor's ability to be helpful, such as "It sounds like you're wondering whether I can really help you because I am white and you are Latino." Counselors in the midst of becoming culturally sensitive may also find this model a useful gauge to measure their own progress in this task.

Skills for Effective Counseling of Culturally Diverse Clients

Not only do counselors need more self-awareness, understanding of other cultures, and knowledge of models of cultural identity development, they also need to develop a specific set of skills to work effectively with multicultural clients. Although the following is not an exhaustive list of the skills counselors need to serve a multicultural society, taken together, these recommendations describe fundamental competencies.

First, because a growing number of Americans do not have English as their first language, counselors who are bilingual will be able to serve their clients better. At the least, counselors need to be aware of the burden of using English for some clients and be open to including a translator (perhaps a family member) in counseling sessions. When language barriers are present, counselors should use methods that are somewhat less language dependent (behavioral techniques or expressive media such as art and music).

Second, counselors need more flexibility in the means by which they convey the core conditions of unconditional positive regard, empathy, and genuineness. Ivey and Authier (1978) suggest that the core conditions are indeed universally appropriate, but that the methods typically used to convey those core conditions (reflecting, paraphrasing, and letting the client lead the self-exploration) may be culture specific. For a client accustomed to authorities who direct and structure interaction, for example, a narrow response repertoire that is limited to clarifying, reflecting, and summarizing client comments may make the client so uncomfortable that he or she will not be able to tolerate the ambiguity. The flexibility to take into account the client's deep assumptions about the role of an expert counselor and the usual pattern of interpersonal relationships in the client's culture is critical to the success of the counseling enterprise. Specifically, counselors may need to engage in more extensive client orientation to counseling and a greater use of structuring and questioning techniques. Some use of affective exploration responses is natural and appropriate, but exclusive reliance on them in the early stages of counseling may not be prudent.

Third, counselors need to be adaptable in their attention to intrapsychic issues and affective material. Sue and Sue (2003) point out that for some culturally diverse clients, attention to career and educational needs has a higher priority than self-exploration or affective functioning. Unfortunately, the folklore of the counseling profession—and the hidden agenda in many training programs—is that career counseling and educational counseling are more superficial or less personal forms of counseling. The message has been that "real" counselors attend to affective content and intrapsychic dynamics. This message fails to acknowledge the centrality of career and educational choices to personal identity and the enormous distress career and educational problems can produce. Counselors need to be sensitive to their own bias about these forms of counseling and recognize different expectations for the counseling process for some clients. Once this new attitude is achieved, counselors need skills in career and educational counseling to be able to work effectively in these domains. Similarly, there is some evidence to suggest that culturally diverse clients respond better to more structured, directive, and behavioral counseling approaches than to affectively oriented sessions (Sue & Sue, 2003; Sue, Zane, & Young, 1994). Although no prediction can be made about what any individual client needs or expects from counseling, effective multicultural counselors are open to the use of more active and directive approaches and have the skills to employ them.

Fourth, counselors should include intervention strategies that not only involve the client's personal actions and feelings but also acknowledge institutional influences on the client's behavior or situation. Many of the difficulties for culturally diverse clients stem from racist or prejudiced actions by specific others or by institutions. Atkinson, Thompson, and Grant (1993) refer to this activity as identifying the *locus of the problem*. For example, an African-American woman may feel depressed and hopeless not because of low self-esteem, negative expectations for the future, or inadequate self-help methods, but because her boss may have actively impeded her promotion because of her race and sexually harassed her because of her gender. In this situation, a counselor must be open to identifying the central issues as external to the client's psychic functioning and helping the client to respond to the injustices in her life. Some intrapsychic factors may be operating in her depressive feelings, but the counselor must see the complexity of causes in this case. Otherwise, the counselor may inadvertently seem to "blame the victim" (Ryan, 1976) for the racism and sexism she is experiencing. Instead, the counselor needs to help the client develop the skills and sense of personal power she needs to address these injustices.

Fifth, because counselors' knowledge of other cultures cannot always be complete and current, counselors need to develop contacts with professionals of diverse cultural backgrounds who are willing to consult with them to make the counseling process more effective. These consultants can also serve as referral sources in situations where the counselor's gap in understanding is too great or the client's preference is for a counselor with a similar culture. A counselor who does not have access to such a consultant has an added responsibility to seek out written material on the client's culture.

Because there is no such thing as a culture-free test, counselors also must be skilled in using standardized assessment instruments appropriately with diverse clients. Standardized tests that do not have norms for minority groups should be used with great caution. Whenever a test is employed, the counselor bears the responsibility for ensuring that the test results are accurate and are employed in ways to promote the best interests of the client. Counselors should also familiarize themselves with newer assessment methods that are somewhat less culture dependent than earlier instruments. *The Handbook of Multicultural Assessment,* written by Suzuki, Ponterotto, and Meller (2000), is an excellent resource for counselors seeking culturally appropriate assessment tools.

Counselors who match the intervention strategies they use to the needs of the individual and the cultural tradition that impacts most strongly on that individual are more likely to be effective. As we mentioned previously, methods arising out of the Western tradition that emphasize individual autonomy as the prime value and personal responsibility for one's actions as a core assumption must be used cautiously with persons whose cultures give stronger weight to family or group needs. In these situations, greater involvement of the client's family in the selection of counseling goals and strategies is critical for the success of counseling.

Finally, counselors should develop skills in working with the traditional support persons that are part of the culture and an openness to cooperating with designated helpers in the community. Traditional support persons include religious leaders, family matriarchs or patriarchs, or others whom the client sees as culturally accepted sources of help.

Cautions About the Emic Cultural Perspective

There is one danger of taking culture into account in the counseling process—the danger of stereotyping individuals. Not all Asian Americans view family identically. Not all Native Americans resist eye contact with higher-status persons. Not all persons with disabilities place a strong value on independence. The examples are almost endless. The point is that the individuality of the person is not lost in the culture. Cultural traditions must be seen as a hypothetical influence on a particular individual until evidence accumulates that they have been embraced by that person. For example, discussing the African-American culture in the singular form is inaccurate. There are many subcultures within the broader African-American culture, and the diversity of experiences may be lost on a counselor who is overemphasizing culture or viewing it too narrowly. Thus, counselors should seek a balance: culture is not to be ignored, nor is it to substitute for understanding the particular experience of the individual who seeks counseling.

━━━━━━━━━━━━━━━━━━━ *Case: Lee* ━━━━━━━━━━━━━━━━━━━

Lee is a 30-year-old architecture student who immigrated to the United States from Southeast Asia 2 years ago, leaving his family behind. He had been a licensed architect in Cambodia, but his credentials are not recognized outside that country. He requests an emergency appointment at the university counseling service in the middle of the semester. As he enters the session, he appears outwardly calm and dignified, but his voice shakes and the expression on his face is pained. Three weeks ago, Lee received word that his mother became ill the day before she was to immigrate to the United States and then died one day later in the hospital there. His brother, the only remaining family member, is so lost in grief that he is saying that he no longer wants to come to the United States. Lee made the counseling appointment because he is having great difficulty studying and does not think he will be able to complete the midterm projects that are due soon. He is worried that he will flunk out of school. He says that his purpose for immigrating is now lost, but because he can't return to Cambodia, he must find a way to carry on. His eyes become moist as he speaks, but no tears fall from them. He responds fully and respectfully to probes about his loss and recent experience but seems more focused on his academic concerns. After they have talked for several minutes, the counselor, a white woman, asks Lee whether he would be more comfortable discussing this painful issue with a counselor at the international student advising office. Lee immediately declines, indicating that he is an American now and no longer an "international" student.

Think for a moment about how you would proceed in this situation. How much do you know about the cultural background of this client? What role does the client's ethnicity and your knowledge of it (or lack of knowledge) play in your decision making? How do you balance Lee's focus on academic issues with the reality of his grief and loss? What role, if any, do you think the gender difference between the counselor and the client plays in your decision making?

The approach we recommend in this situation depends, of course, on the counselor's degree of knowledge of the Cambodian culture. Because most American-born counselors are unlikely to have much understanding of this tradition, we will focus on that aspect. When confronted by a client whose background is culturally different and little known to the counselor, the best course of action is a conservative one that respects the client's wishes and expectations for counseling. In this case, Lee was most pressured about his academic performance, so counseling should first attend to this issue. The value of this emphasis is also indicated by his lack of experience with American universities and possible ignorance about the option of incompletes or withdrawals from courses because of medical and family emergencies. The counselor should first explain to Lee his alternatives for dealing with his courses for the semester and then discuss the advantages and disadvantages of each possibility. Practical information about how to handle the university bureaucracy and obtain course extensions may also be appropriate given Lee's newness to the system and his level of grief.

What about all that affective pain? Is it enough to attend only to educational issues? This is a difficult question. On the one hand, Lee is already isolated, and an empathic listener may be especially valuable at this juncture. The possibility that his grief may deteriorate into clinical depression at some point is real and should be considered. On the other hand, he is a Cambodian man who appears to have a strong investment in acting with dignity and self-control and encouraging affective expressions of grief may leave him feeling ashamed and unwilling to show his face to this counselor again. Given the tendency of Cambodian and other Asian cultures to have clearly defined gender roles (Atkinson, Morten, & Sue, 1998), the gender of the counselor may also make this client feel uncomfortable about open expressions of grief. Thus, the latter argument is more compelling, we think, given the possible negative implications of a "loss of dignity" for Lee. The prudent course of action is to assist Lee immediately with his academic concerns and follow up with a second appointment to be sure those issues are resolved.

The counselor should walk a fine line here, not cutting off Lee from expressing his pain but also avoiding a strong focus on the affective material. In the meantime, the counselor can consult with her resource person on Cambodian culture and get some supervision on how to proceed responsibly with Lee's grief and pain. With this course of action, the client has also received what he asked for, is likely to view the counselor as expert and credible, and thus is more likely to return should the depression or academic problems worsen.

COUNSELING WOMEN AND GIRLS

Why should counselors consider women to be a population with special counseling needs? Some experts have argued that women and girls have unique ways of experiencing the world (Estes, 1992), ways of thinking (Belenky, Clinchy, Goldberger, & Tarule, 1997), making moral judgments (Gilligan, 1993), and using language and processing information (Tannen, 1990). These scholars contend that this unique perspective is grounded in women's developmental experience and, perhaps, their biology. However, all of these theories are newly developed and, although they present intriguing hypotheses, need additional research before their validity is fully demonstrated. What is indisputable at this point, however, is the evidence that women and girls have experiences in American culture that give them mixed or negative signals about their gender. This narrow set of beliefs about what women and girls ought to be like regardless of their individual characteristics is called sexism. Specifically, women in this culture have been valued primarily for their appearance, their reproductive capacities, and their domestic capabilities. The message in the culture has been that women who are sexually attractive, able to reproduce and nurture children, and carry out domestic and caretaking functions skillfully are valuable. Conversely, women who do not hold these interests or attributes have been seen as less worthy and often dysfunctional. Obviously, not all men and women in this culture hold these views of women. The cultural message is common enough, though, that all counselors ought to examine whether they too have absorbed this narrow view of women. Similarly, counselors should be aware of the possible influence of these cultural messages on their male and female clients.

Research demonstrates that sexist attitudes in the culture have resulted in discriminatory practices toward girls in schools and colleges, which diminish their educational opportunities. For example, research suggests that girls are not encouraged to be skilled in math and science in school (American Association of University Women, 1992). Women in the workplace experience sexism through outright employment discrimination and the "glass ceiling," which interferes with their promotion to executive positions. In addition, a large body of evidence has accumulated that indicates that women in American society are at significant risk for victimization, an experience of physical, emotional, or sexual abuse by a person they know (American Psychological Association, 1990). The list of victimization experiences to which females are more vulnerable is long and includes sexual harassment at school or at the workplace; acquaintance, or "date," rape; physical and verbal battering by a spouse or significant other; rape by a marital partner; sexual abuse during development; and sexual exploitation by a therapist or other helping professional. For example, current statistics indicate that almost one-third of adult women have experienced sexual abuse by a person close to them during their lives. (One of every six adult men has had an experience of sexual victimization during development.) Also, more than 90% of those who are sexually exploited in counseling and therapy are female clients of male therapists (Welfel, 2002).

The following sections discuss how cultural attitudes toward women affect counselors' beliefs and values, the ways in which experience affects women's response to counseling, and the specific skills the counselor must have to be effective with women clients. Finally, we will attend to the issues for women who come from culturally diverse backgrounds (and thereby deal with both sexism and racism).

Counselor Attitudes Toward Women Clients

There is a large body of research that has examined the degree to which counselors and therapists share the sexist views of the culture. The landmark study that initiated this research was conducted by Broverman and her colleagues (Broverman, Broverman, Clarkson, Rosenkrantz, & Vogel, 1970). They found that therapists had different definitions of what constituted a healthy adult, a healthy man, and a healthy woman. They reported that the therapists in their study used adjectives such as submissive, emotional, excitable, easily hurt, less independent, less objective, and less competitive to describe the healthy woman but did not use any of these adjectives when defining a healthy adult or a healthy man. Broverman and her colleagues characterized their results as indicative of a double standard of mental health for women:

> Acceptance of an adjustment notion of health, then, places women in the conflictual position of having to decide whether to exhibit those positive characteristics considered desirable for men and adults, and thus have their "femininity" questioned, that is, to be deviant in terms of

being a woman; or to behave in the prescribed feminine manner, accept second-class adult status, and possibly live a lie to boot. (p. 6)

Although not all of the research to follow Broverman's study came to the same devastating conclusion about sexist attitudes, enough of a trend exists in the findings to cause experts to conclude that sexism of helping professionals, both male and female, is a continuing problem. Certainly, the rigidity of definitions of how women ought to behave has loosened since 1970, but the basic prejudice has not been erased entirely. The existence of these attitudes is not surprising, because counselors have been raised in a culture that stereotypes women. Thus, the first step in effective counseling with female clients is the process of self examination and self-knowledge that is also required for successful cross-cultural counseling. It is important to examine one's own development and explore the messages passed down about appropriate role behaviors for males and females. In some families, the sexist attitudes are overt and easily identifiable; in others, the messages are subtler and harder to detect. The following questions may be useful in the self-exploration:

Developmental Experiences

- How did your family react to activities of any member that were not consistent with the predominant gender role stereotypes?
- Did your family convey that appearance, nurturing capacities, and domestic skills were more important for women than men? Were girls in the family more often praised for looking pretty and boys more often praised for their accomplishments?
- How did the family react when dealing with a man or woman in a nontraditional role? Did any member of the family show discomfort or convey the message that there must be something wrong with the person for his or her career choice?
- What family messages were conveyed about emotional expression for males and females? For example, were boys discouraged from expressions of sadness, fear, or nurturing and girls discouraged from expressions of anger?
- If there were both male and female children in the family, were there different priorities about the importance of education for each gender?

Current Experiences

- How much of that developmental experience is still influencing your behavior today? Are you still discouraging males from crying or females from open expressions of anger?

- How much do you expect females to take responsibility for nurturing others and exclude men from such responsibility? For example, when fathers care for their young children, do you call that baby-sitting?
- How comfortable are you with persons in nontraditional career choices? If you get services from a plumber, surgeon, or nurse, do you respond differently if the person is male or female?
- If a woman remarks to you that she doesn't want to be married, is not interested in having children, and is not particularly concerned about appearing attractive, how does that statement strike you? Do you tend to think something must be wrong with her psychological or interpersonal functioning? Conversely, if a male indicates that he is not particularly ambitious, wants to place more emphasis on family than on career, and is sensitive and emotionally expressive, does that intuitively strike you as problematic? (Clearly, individuals who are denying any affiliative needs with other persons are not functioning at their highest possible level. A counselor should attend to such difficulties with intimacy regardless of gender. The point here is whether you look at the tendency to evaluate affiliative needs differently for males and females.)

Once an honest self-assessment has been completed and a counselor knows the degree to which he or she has internalized the cultural stereotypes about gender, the counselor can begin the attitude change process. For some attitudes, change will come almost simultaneously with the recognition of the existence of sexism. The "aha" experience of uncovering the stereotype will go a long way toward bringing change. For other attitudes, a longer process that includes reading about sexism, discussing attitudes with colleagues and supervisors, and even seeking out consultation with a therapist may be useful.

The Implications of Gender Bias for Females' Experience in Counseling

Unfortunately, sexist attitudes toward women are not limited to European-American culture. These beliefs characterize many other cultural groups. Although the specific form and expression of sex stereotyping are somewhat culture specific, the existence of some rigid gender role expectations is widespread across cultural groups. Thus, the majority of clients who enter counseling have been raised in cultures with some gender bias, and they will be continuing to experience it in their interactions with the majority culture. There are two particularly important considerations about working with women in counseling. First, they are likely to have internalized to some degree the view that women who are attractive, nurturing, emotionally expressive, and domestically competent are more valued or valuable to society. Second, they are likely to have experienced some form of discrimination or victimization because of their gender. (Note that these are probability statements; the experience of any individual female client may be different on either or both dimensions.)

The cultural definition of female attractiveness is frequently embedded in the concerns a woman brings to counseling, especially because the current standard for body shape can be attained by a very small minority of women. The thin body type with small waist and large breasts that characterizes models, actresses, and beauty contest participants is simply not genetically possible for most women. Thus, the standard against which women measure their attractiveness is as unattainable for most as running a 3-minute mile. Yet the culture places so much attention on physical attractiveness that many women feel they must keep trying to attain the standard anyway and, in the meantime, devalue themselves for their lack of success. Recent evidence suggests that the focus on thinness and appearance is affecting girls at younger and younger ages. In the face of these cultural messages, it is not surprising that body dissatisfaction and low self-esteem are common problems that females bring to counseling. Even for those few women whose body shape matches the cultural standard, appearance may still be a subtle or overt counseling issue because they may wonder whether their appearance is the only aspect that makes them valuable to other people.

Many experts have asserted that this emphasis on appearance plays a causal role in the high incidence of eating disorders among women. Women who buy into the cultural standard for thinness are at greater risk for untested diet schemes, injury to their health from repeatedly losing and gaining back weight, and the more serious problems of anorexia nervosa and bulimia nervosa. In addition, body satisfaction is one part of a person's self-esteem, and the loss of this satisfaction because of unattainable cultural norms for women means that global self-esteem may be at risk as well.

Thus, women clients can bring to counseling a good deal of body dissatisfaction, a greater risk of eating disorders, and a sense of self-worth inappropriately tied to appearance and sexual attractiveness. Women may also use the same standards the culture uses in measuring the worth of other women and have difficulties in their interpersonal relationships with both men and women. Adolescent girls who are adjusting to their rapidly changing bodies may be particularly affected by these cultural standards.

The second major impact of sexism on women's experience is their high risk of an experience of discrimination or victimization (American Psychological Association, 1990). This fact is disturbing in itself, but experts also suggest that an experience of victimization early in life, such as sexual or physical abuse, puts an individual at greater risk for future exploitive experiences. Several explanations have been presented for this phenomenon, but the essence of the arguments is that girls come to experience victimization as normal, unaware of how pathological such behavior is, and that women internalize the message they receive from their abusers—that the responsibility for the abusive behavior lies on the woman's shoulders. Thus, these women often carry enormous guilt and have low self-esteem and are therefore vulnerable to those who want to manipulate them. Frequently, these women repress the memories of victimization, but the scars of low self-esteem and guilt remain.

Even if a woman has escaped victimization during her development, she may have experienced discrimination or sexual harassment at her workplace or school. For example, some evidence suggests that as many as 70% of women in the workplace have been the victims of sexual harassment (APA, 1990). Although women who experience sexual harassment are less likely to blame themselves for their coworker's or boss's behavior, they still feel shame and embarrassment about the harassment and usually feel little power to make it stop. This sense of powerlessness can lead to depressed and angry feelings and sometimes to behaviors that seem counterproductive. Some scholars argue that victimization and discrimination experiences in which women feel powerless are major contributors to the high rate of depressive disorders among women (APA, 1990). Adolescent girls and women in Western societies have twice the rate of depressive disorders as adolescent boys and men. The risk of victimization can also lead many women to seek counseling for post-traumatic stress, either as an immediate response or as a delayed reaction.

In short, the victimization experience of females suggests vulnerability to low self-esteem, high amounts of guilt and shame, and symptoms of depression or post-traumatic stress. These feelings often bring a girl or woman to counseling.

The cultural expectations about women identified first in the Broverman study cited earlier suggest that there are also more subtle impacts of sexism on women's experience of the counseling process. Because traits of submissiveness, influenceability, sensitivity to others' feelings, and lower levels of independence have been valued in women, female clients who have internalized these cultural values may have greater difficulty in disagreeing with a counselor, in striking out independently, or in taking action that they think may offend the counselor. In other words, traditionally socialized women may be at risk for too much deference to the counselor or too much attention to a positive relationship with the counselor; as a result, their counseling needs may not be addressed. By the same token, counselors who have internalized these standards may be uncomfortable with assertive or independent women who do not work to nurture the relationship and may also be diverted from the important individual agenda by such stereo-types. In addition, counselors who expect women to be more emotional, more easily hurt, and less objective than men may also reinforce cultural stereotypes about women and may overlook opportunities to have a client process cognitive material or deal with material that may be painful but essential for future growth. It is important to remember, however, that these are general issues likely to be present for many women who enter counseling but not necessarily present for any particular woman who enters a counselor's office. The unique experience of the individual may or may not fit with the experiences of women in general. Counselors must hold these ideas as tentative hypotheses that need to be substantiated with evidence from the individual, not as blueprints that apply to all women.

Specific Counseling Skills Necessary for Women Clients

The best resource for identifying the essential counseling skills and attitudes for working with women clients is *Principles Concerning the Counseling and Psychotherapy of Women* (Fitzgerald & Nutt, 1986). The following comments rely heavily on this document.

Much of scientific knowledge of human development, human personality, and dysfunction is based on male subjects and male gender role definitions. Historically, the tendency was for scholars to assume that what was true for males could be directly applied to females. When theories of female development were proposed, they tended to use male experience as the starting point and therefore often greatly distorted female development. Freudian theory, for example, has been especially criticized for this practice. The male bias in psychology and human development has meant that the unique aspects of the female experience have been ignored or misunderstood. Many training programs in counseling and human service have educated their graduates to assume that male definitions of health, personality, and dysfunction can be directly applied to all human behavior. Currently, training programs are improving their curricula to have a more inclusive scope, but many counselors still lack information about the male bias of traditional human development theories and about the newer theories that are more inclusive. Thus, the first step in learning new skills is education about female development, female experience, and the role of gender bias in defining health and dysfunction. Those who have not been exposed to courses in the psychology of women or gender issues in counseling should seek out such courses. Books that familiarize counselors with basic concepts are readily available. Those listed in this chapter's references represent an excellent starting point.

Second, because the motivation of women to seek counseling is often related to experiences of discrimination, victimization, and prejudice, counselors need to have a repertoire of counseling interventions that includes strategies to help individuals deal with injustice. Models of dysfunction that assume that the whole problem is internal or intrapsychic ignore the experiences of women (and culturally diverse groups in the society). Feminist therapists use the term *empowering clients* and talk of the need to advocate on behalf of the client to address the injustices she is experiencing (Rosewater & Walker, 1985; Worell & Remer, 2003). They suggest that a major goal of therapy is to help the client use the power she does have to intervene against unjust treatment. The role of advocate is a controversial one, but the important point in this debate is the need for the counselor to acknowledge the social and political influences on the individual. Acknowledgment of social influences on human behavior is embraced by virtually all models of counseling and therapy, not just feminist ones. The recognition of social injustice as a barrier to effective functioning is especially important in light of two factors: the female client's tendency to blame herself for victimization experiences that are objectively not her responsibility at all and her risk for continued victimization if her inappropriate guilt and poor self-esteem are not addressed.

Third, counselors need to refrain from social and sexual dual relationships with female clients. The evidence indicates that many women are victims of unscrupulous therapists who use them to gratify their own needs (Welfel, 2002). The culture's message that submissiveness is equivalent to mental health for adult women is one contributor to this vulnerability. A second contributing factor is women's history of victimization by others in their lives. Counselors must also avoid creating other forms of dependency in any female client such that the autonomy of the woman is jeopardized. Counselors who find themselves instructing women clients about how to live their lives or making their decisions for them have violated this principle.

Just as counselors ought not to condone racist or culturally insensitive behavior by colleagues, they should not accept or condone sexist attitudes and behaviors toward women. Instead, counselors have a responsibility to educate colleagues, supervisors, and students about sexism and gender bias. They also have a responsibility to work with institutions and other professions to change policies and practices that are inherently unfair. Not only should counselors help clients realize their own power to respond to unjust practices by individuals and institutions, they also have an affirmative responsibility to get involved in combating sexist practices in institutions where they have some affiliation. For example, a counselor in a school or community agency has a responsibility to be helpful in the development and enforcement of sexual harassment policies.

The Experience of Culturally Diverse Women

Women from culturally diverse backgrounds are often victims of double discrimination. For example, girls get less teacher attention and reinforcement in math classes than their male counterparts, but when the ethnicity of female students is taken into account, African-American girls get the least attention and reinforcement of all math students (American Association of University Women, 1992). Thus, effective counseling requires that this double discrimination be taken into account in the definition of problems of a minority female client and in the therapeutic interventions designed to help her resolve those difficulties. Counselors must take into account the interplay between a woman's ethnicity and gender. For example, Saunders-Robinson (1991) argues that dealing with battering by a male partner can be especially difficult for an African-American woman because of her reluctance to expose her male partner to the risk of racist treatment by police and the courts. This reluctance is supported by the tendency of the African-American woman to see the discrimination and prejudice she does experience primarily as due to racism rather than sexism (Jordan, 1991). Similarly, when working with Latina women, counselors need to be sensitive to their clients' experience in the majority culture and the Latino culture's definitions of appropriate roles for males and females. Lopez-Baez (1997) presents an excellent discussion of this topic. In short, counselors who work with culturally diverse women need to be well informed about the client's culture, including specific cultural gender role definitions, and about the role of racism and sexism in the difficulties the client presents in counseling. In addition, counselors must be patient with the pace of developing trust and should be prepared to work hard to demonstrate credibility and trustworthiness.

Case: Doris

Doris is a 24-year-old accountant working for a law firm in a southern city. She came to the mental health center at the encouragement of her closest friend, who was very worried about Doris. Doris described feeling worthless and sad for several months and remembers that these feelings started all at once rather than gradually. However, she can't recall any specific event that triggered them. Along with those negative feelings have come periods of high anxiety and bouts of sleeplessness. She says she feels removed from other people and is having a hard time relating to anyone. Lately, she has taken many sick days from work and even visited her doctor because of these problems. Her physician also recommended counseling as a first step when Doris asked for tranquilizers. Doris says she has not had any suicidal thoughts but is getting discouraged by the fact that none of her usual coping strategies seem to be working. Typically, when she feels blue or jittery, she exercises more or distracts herself from the problems with friends or hobbies. Doris is a fourth child of an intact family who all live close to her. She has several close friends and has dated a lot since college but is not interested in a committed relationship now or at any time in the near future. Doris does not think she ever wants to become a parent because of her dedication to her career.

Given what you already know about Doris, think for a few minutes about what additional information you would find necessary to help this client. If possible, discuss this case with a classmate, and write down the additional areas you would like to explore. Then examine your rationale for those choices. Finally, suppose that Doris were a Donald. Does that change any of your thinking? Examine closely whether that affects your view of Doris's decision not to have children or her lack of interest in marriage. Again, talk with a partner if possible about the implications of gender. Did you take into account the possibility of an experience of victimization such as acquaintance rape or sexual harassment that could have triggered the depressed and anxious feelings? Even though she says she does not recall a trigger event, it is possible that one occurred but she is repressing it or simply did not label it as a victimization experience. This response is not uncommon among women and is perhaps made even more likely by Doris's usual degree of control over her life and future. Another possibility is that Doris may remember but feel ashamed about disclosing it to a stranger. The fairly sudden onset of these feelings in a female who otherwise functions well should be cause to explore that possibility along with other experiences of loss or disappointment.

COUNSELING MEN AND BOYS

Although the special counseling needs of girls and women have been acknowledged and articulated over a period of 40 or more years, the special counseling needs of men and boys have received serious attention primarily in the past 15 years. Early researchers and practitioners concerned with male issues were, in fact, scorned for their focus on the problems of "the privileged class in America" (Jolliff & Horne, 1999, p. 3). The attitude of their critics was that men not only experienced special privilege, but they also were seen as the cause of many of the problems in our society. Men were viewed by some feminists as the perpetrators of the subjugation of women and were seen as emotionally unresponsive and sometimes violent. It was initially through the eyes of the women's movement that attention was first drawn to the functionality and dysfunctionality of the stereotypical male role in the contemporary world (Joliff & Horne, 1999).

Construction of the Culturally Stereotyped Male Role in America

Brooks and Good (2001) question whether human males are predisposed toward aggression and dominance and conclude that, although there may be a biological tendency, it has been amplified and channeled by a "multithousand year layer of culture" (p. 285). Without resolving how much of the masculine "essence" may be inherent, Levant (1995), Levant and Pollack (1995), Pleck (1995), Pollack (1995), Jolliff and Horne (1999) and others take the constructionist view that boys learn both functional and dysfunctional ways of being men through their life experiences.

Levant (1995) is specific in breaking masculine role norms down into positive and negative attributes. He notes that it is valuable for men to be willing to set aside their own needs for the sake of family and to withstand hardship and pain to protect others. Effective men express love by doing things for others. They are loyal, dedicated, and committed to others. They have the ability to think logically, solve problems, take risks, and stay calm in the face of danger. Learning these aspects of the male stereotype helps boys grow into what Jolliff and Horne (1999) refer to as "mature masculinity."

On the other hand, Pollack (1995) notes that "Men are often found walling themselves off from their own feeling states, fending off sadness and depression as well as empathic intimate relationships—especially with women—in ways that cause their significant others to feel a great deal of pain and consternation, and . . . in ways that tend to hurt and confuse the men themselves" (pp. 33–34). Current thinking is that the "walling off" of the emotional side of life occurs as boys are taught to be tough, self-reliant, and independent. Spielberg (1999) says that boys in early childhood are taught to feel ashamed of their needs for support and nurturance. The message "Don't be a mama's boy" is soon followed by "Don't be a sissy" and "Don't throw like a girl" on the school playground. Though less a sanction than it was a few years ago, the message that "men don't cry" is sufficiently internalized by most dominant culture American males that they feel ashamed to let sorrow show publicly. Jolliff and Horne (1999) described that this process of repressing pain and sorrow "to be a boy/man" generalizes to the repression of more positive feelings of tenderness and joy as well. In the extreme, this socialization can result in a male who is "cold, narcissistic, unfeeling, and nonrelational" (Pollack, 1995).

Levant (1995) summarizes the outcomes of culturally sustained "walling off" to be inability of men to identify and express their own emotions, a relative inability to experience emotional empathy, a tendency to flip anger into rage resulting in violence, a tendency to experience sexuality as separated from relationships, difficulties with emotional intimacy, and difficulty in being a full partner in maintaining a household and raising children. Lacking skills for effective intimate relationships and possessing the cultural imperative that real men are productive, walled-off men often become workaholics.

Pleck (1995) proposes a gender role strain paradigm that specifies three ways in which males face shame and discomfort as they encounter the male gender role stereotype:

1. A significant proportion of males simply cannot meet the societal expectation of what it means to be a male (e.g., to be calm in the face of danger) and therefore feel inferior.
2. All males experience a certain amount of trauma in the shaming process used by parents and peers to teach male toughness.
3. Men who are successful in learning the stereotyped role often find that it does not lead to good working relationships with others in either domestic or work relationships. Domestic partners and children are distanced; work associates are dominated and harassed. As Levant (1995, p. 232) said, "for many men, the essential dilemma is that much of what they have been taught to value since childhood is under attack or fully discredited."

Spielberg's (1999) model of the "whole male" provides a goal for counseling males who have been ingrained with a dysfunctional male role ideal through this stressful process. As elaborated by Jolliff and Horme (1999), the goal in counseling is for men to "become fully developed in all human traits without selection on the basis of traditional gender roles. . . . The 'whole man' has synthesized those traits considered masculine and those considered feminine according to what is true for him as a fully functioning human being" (p. 17).

Implications of Gender Bias for Males' Experience in Counseling

The impetus to study the socialization of men came initially from what women's studies learned about the socialization process and perhaps even from the dissatisfaction of some women with the behavior of the men in their lives. However, it is important to identify that our purpose in elaborating on the counseling of men is governed neither by political correctness nor by the desire to mold men to the specifications of their women. Our focus is on the client himself, as is appropriate in all counseling. We believe that boys and men can be helped to avoid or can escape from the isolated and lonely lives that result from walling off caring and vulnerable feelings. Effective counseling allows the male client to explore satisfactions and dissatisfactions with his life and provides assistance that allows him to make new choices.

Still, fewer men than women seek counseling, and men who do seek counseling often are reluctant and resistant to the counseling process (see Chapter 9). Addis and Mahalik (2003) reviewed studies of man's help-seeking behaviors and concluded that "men of different ages, ethnicities, and social backgrounds are on the average less likely than women to seek professional help for physical and mental health problems" (p. 6). Men, more than women, regard participation in counseling as an admission of failure to master their life tasks and they see it as nonmasculine. Furthermore, based on the socialization process described in the previous section, some male clients will initially lack the ability to identify their own feelings and the feelings of others and will have little understanding that many of their difficulties in life stem from their insensitivity. If their behaviors are violent, controlling, or sexually exploitive, they are likely to be especially defensive. For all these reasons, fewer men than women are self-referred. Those who are self-referred have recognized the need to try to change their lives, but many men arrive in counseling at the insistence of wives and significant others or as mandated by some legal procedure. The experience of counseling will often challenge what the client has learned it means to be male and will therefore be unfamiliar and threatening (Addis & Mahalik, 2003; Cochran & Rabinowitz, 2003; Malakik, Good, & Englar-Carlson, 2003). The counselor will need to practice all the skills of relationship building described in Chapter 3 as well as the special skills for poorly motivated clients in Chapter 9. As always, the counselor must be respectful of the client's vulnerability moment to moment but must gently move toward identifying and working with the key issues.

Specific Issues and Counseling Skills for Male Clients

First, it is important to realize that many males who enter a counselor's office have been parented effectively and have acquired many of the instrumental and assertive behaviors of the societally transmitted male role while continuing to experience a normal range of affect. Many boys, with the help of the significant others in their lives, recognize that it is not necessary to be insensitive and aggressive to be masculine. Those boys and the men they become may need assistance from time to time in coping with stressful life situations, but they may be no more at risk for developing various mental health problems than anyone else.

The issues and strategies that follow emerge from the perspective of dysfunctional learning of a masculine role as developed in the previous discussion and apply only to males who fit the etiology. It is important to remember, however, that all males experience much pressure to conform to the stereotypical role, and most will have some conflict around issues of owning and expressing feelings of vulnerability versus presenting a tough façade. We will describe four of the most common presenting issues of men who enter counseling because of unsatisfying interpersonal experiences: emotional dissociation, inability to respond empathically, predisposition to abuse and violence, and the failure to link emotion and sexuality. We also present the bare outline of some strategies for helping with each of these issues, but we caution that a more thorough study of men's issues should be undertaken by reading the references suggested here and other literature on the subject.

A starting point in the assessment process is to determine whether the male client seems to be able to experience and label a full range of emotions. Levant (1995) has labeled a deficit in this area as *alexithymia,* where a = without, *lexi* = words, and *thymia* = feelings—thus, without words for feelings. Many boys and men as noted previously have been taught not to express their caring or their vulnerable feelings and over time become unable to identify these feelings in themselves. Once the client becomes aware of this emotional paucity, he and the counselor can plan a strategy that will help the client to develop a personal vocabulary of emotion. As in empathy training, it is useful first to develop an extensive list of human emotions with the client, with the counselor adding words that the client does not think of. This may be followed by the viewing of taped vignettes of emotional scenes to help the client recognize facial gestures, tone of voice, body language, and other expressions associated with the range of emotions. The client can then be sent out to observe emotions in real-life situations. Levant (1995) also suggests that the client keep an emotional response log, noting when he experiences a feeling he can identify or a bodily sensation of which he is aware (but cannot quite label). The log, used as a basis for discussion in follow-up sessions, becomes concrete evidence that the client has a richer emotional world than he realized and provides reinforcement to experience previously repressed feelings. The counselor can also encourage the client to express (caring and vulnerable) feelings to significant others and can role-play anticipated domestic scenes to help the client gain confidence in being expressive.

Once the client becomes aware of his own emotions, he then has the basic tools to begin to feel empathy for the emotions of others. This is particularly crucial in the ability to establish intimacy with others. Levant (1995) suggests that many boys learn "action empathy," where they observe others and learn to predict the action of those others—but without an awareness of the feelings of the others. As noted in Chapter 3, identifying the feelings of another is just the first step; the second step involves communicating one's understanding of the other's feeling. For one who has been unaccustomed to dealing with caring or vulnerable feelings, practice in formulating empathic responses to another person can be very effective. This can be done in role-play, in response to recorded vignettes, or as a part of a group process with other clients.

Management of anger proceeds from two assumptions: that males frequently react to feelings of vulnerability with the bravado of anger, and that many males with limited awareness of their own feelings fail to recognize incipient and mild stages of anger and build to an explosive response before they know they are irritated. The work described in the previous paragraphs gives males more effective ways of dealing with vulnerability; specific training in learning to recognize the progression of anger can help to head off explosions which, of course, can become violence directed at significant others (romantic partners and children).

The separation of sexuality from emotion is the final sequela of stereotyped socialization that we will discuss here. Brooks and Silverstein (1995) state that in a society where male conquest is encouraged, "Greater masculinity is bestowed upon young males who have frequent sex with multiple partners and with minimal regard for intimacy, tenderness, or compassion" (p. 286). There has been much discussion about women's greater need for tenderness in the sex act, and there is possibly an anthropological explanation of that need in the fact that it is the woman who carries and bears children and needs a partner's help in parenting. Men can more easily walk away from the consequences of the sex act. On the other hand, men who become good spouses and fathers are men who experience and value a full range of emotion. Therefore the theme of enhancing emotional awareness and expression that is developed throughout this section of counseling skills with male clients has the potential to promote more responsible sexual expression as well.

The counseling strategies presented are useful in helping adolescent and adult males to reclaim a fuller measure of their emotional lives and to improve their self-satisfaction as well as their relationships with others. With younger clients, the effort can be more preventive than remedial. School guidance programs can (and frequently do) include activities that allow children to identify and express their feelings and to have the experience of caring for the feelings and welfare of others. Group and individual counseling designed around the strategies of reinforcing the expression of personal feelings and empathy for others is much like the treatment suggested earlier for men and would be appropriate for boys who already show signs of peer- or parent-sustained "walling off." Programs for parents can provide them with techniques for supporting their sons in becoming more caring and more accepting of their vulnerability. Programming for boys should identify strong, complete male role models and avoid any connotation that the goal is to "feminize" men. Men are acknowledged to have some different needs and roles from women.

Brooks and Silverstein (1995) state that "Psychotherapy with men takes off when we infuse it with attention to the core issues of traditional male identity—work, violence, emotional dissociation, sexuality, patriarchal fathering, and risk-taking" (p. 317). Work and risk-taking are positive attributes of the male role that may require decision making and support during the counseling process. The other problems on Brooks's and Silverstein's agenda should be responsive to counseling that leads men and boys to the experience of a fuller emotional life.

══════════════ *Case: Michael* ══════════════

Michael is a 47-year-old white male who appeared for counseling the week after his wife of 28 years left him. Michael and Charlotte had met early in their freshman year of college and married the following spring. He described the intervening week as a "hellish" time during which he was lonely and angry at his wife for "leaving him in the lurch." He reported that it was a total surprise to him when he came home from work and found that his wife had moved out, leaving a note saying that living with him was like living alone "only worse."

Their 23-year-old daughter and 18-year-old son were out of the house, the son having left for a residential college weeks before. Michael described that life had been good when he and Charlotte were young and she had worked to help him finish his business degree before the children came along. After their daughter was born, Michael had insisted that "No wife of mine is going to work. A woman's place is at home with the children." Recently, the couple hardly talked at all, and when they did it was mostly about the routines of managing the household. They had sex regularly, but Michael said that it was repetitive, over quickly, and minimally satisfying. When asked whether he and his wife fought, Michael said that they did not—that it would have been too much trouble "to get that worked up over nothing." Michael, a mid-level manager in an insurance firm, worked many evenings and traveled some for his job.

When asked to describe his feelings about Charlotte, he repeated that he was angry that she had left and then added that he could not see himself as living singly for the rest of his life. He wanted Charlotte to return to him but could think of nothing he could do to cause her to want to return. After all, he was a good provider; Charlotte did not want for anything in his view. She had moved to an apartment in the same town where the couple owned their home and had filed for a no-fault divorce. She had declined Michael's repeated demands that they meet to talk out this "little bump in the road."

Questions for Further Thought

1. In what ways do you see Michael as exhibiting characteristics of one who has internalized? To what degree do you believe that he has an awareness that he has contributed to the failure of the relationship with his wife? Justify your answer.

2. Extrapolate what Charlotte's existence in this marriage might be like.
3. What would you like to try to accomplish in counseling with Michael?
4. How would you begin to enlist his cooperation in your work with him?
5. What is your prognosis about whether Michael and Charlotte's marriage can be saved? Do you see any basis for rebuilding their relationship? What else would you like to know to make this prognosis more reliable?
6. What is your prognosis about the likelihood of Michael developing a new zest for life and the capacity to enjoy the many remaining years of his life expectancy?

COUNSELING GAY, LESBIAN, AND BISEXUAL CLIENTS

Gay, lesbian, and bisexual individuals are sexual minorities, not only in terms of their numbers in society (from 5% to 10% of the population [Michaels, 1996]), but also in terms of their status. Research suggests that the majority of citizens in the United States, for example, subscribe to homophobic attitudes toward gay, lesbian, and bisexual people (Atkinson & Hackett, 1998; Barret & Logan, 2002). Homophobia refers to an irrational fear of anyone gay or lesbian, or perceived to be gay or lesbian (Dworkin & Guitierrez, 1992). Western cultures have long labeled these sexual orientations as deviant and have long permitted discrimination against sexual minorities. Indeed, they have often established laws declaring homosexual practices criminal (Atkinson & Hackett, 1998; Barret & Logan, 2002). Consequently, sexual minorities often suffer from discrimination in employment, housing, health insurance, and access to the other benefits of society if they are open about their sexual orientation. Gay, lesbian, and bisexual individuals are at greater risk for violence and family problems than heterosexual persons as well (Besner & Spungin, 1995). The depression and suicide risk of sexual minority youth is significantly higher than their heterosexual counterparts. Moreover, because a number of religious organizations find nonheterosexual practices unacceptable, sexual minorities often feel unaccepted by the religions they wish to practice (Toman, 1997).

The mental health system has not been immune from homophobic attitudes and oppression of sexual minorities. Until 1973, a same-sex sexual preference was officially labeled as a psychiatric disorder by the American Psychiatric Association. (In that year, the American Psychiatric Association voted to remove homosexuality from its list of mental and emotional disorders.) Even as recently as 1993, some practicing counselors still viewed it as a mental disorder, despite more than 20 years of official statements to the contrary (Gibson & Pope, 1993). The news is not all dismal, however, because research has shown that most counselors have more accepting attitudes toward sexual minorities than does the general public (Atkinson & Hackett, 1998). The majority seem to be disposed to providing good service to sexual minority clients. What they seem to lack is the specific knowledge and skill to do so (Atkinson & Hackett, 1998). The following paragraphs summarize the basic knowledge and skills essential for effective counseling with sexual minorities.

Knowledge and Skills Essential for Effective Counseling with Gay, Lesbian, and Bisexual Clients

Because negative attitudes toward sexual minorities are so pervasive in society, counselors need to first acknowledge that they probably have assimilated some of these attitudes, even if they themselves are sexual minorities. Homophobic attitudes can only be modified if counselors are aware of their presence and their scope. Counselors who do not have homophobic attitudes need to assess whether their reaction to sexual minorities is one of tolerance or acceptance. Tolerance is an attitude that still assumes that heterosexuality is preferable or more normal, whereas acceptance means understanding that homosexuality is simply different. We believe acceptance is the preferable attitude. When counselors' religious or moral beliefs indicate that homosexuality is improper, they need to find a way to provide responsible service in spite of those beliefs or, if that is not possible, to arrange for referral to other professionals when needed.

Counselors should also be aware that they may have a "heterosexist bias" (Atkinson & Hackett, 1998; Barret & Logan, 2002). In other words, they may indirectly express bias against sexual minorities when they approach all clients with the assumption that they are heterosexual. Rich (1980) refers to this as "compulsory heterosexuality." To illustrate, an adolescent counselor who asks every teenage boy she sees if he has a girlfriend is acting in a heterosexist way. Clients who are homosexual or bisexual are likely to be discomforted by such a question and would be discouraged from any discussion of same-sex relationships. Experienced counselors who say they have never had a homosexual client may in fact be identifying an inability to permit discussion of sexuality. Given the percentage of the population that are sexual minorities, it is highly unlikely that an experienced counselor has never had a homosexual client. It is possible, though, that sexual minority clients have been aware of the counselor's heterosexist bias and have not felt safe disclosing that information to the counselor.

Counselors with clients who self-identify as sexual minorities ought to be able to see the sexual orientation of those clients as simply one aspect of the self and not the central defining feature of personality. Most of the time, sexual minority clients come to counselors for other reasons than concerns about their sexuality. Sexual minority clients experience emotional, relationship, career, and educational problems to the same degree as other clients, and counselors should not assume that sexual orientation is a core piece of the problem the client is experiencing. For example, a college sophomore may see a counselor at a university counseling service with career indecision. She may be rethinking her lifelong ambition to be a physician. This career problem may be unrelated to her lesbian sexual identity. A counselor who insists that her career issues must be connected to her sexual orientation in the absence of evidence of such a connection is acting inappropriately. Sometimes, of course, sexual identity is the issue of concern or is a relevant factor in other problems, and in those cases, counselors are obligated to help the client examine its impact. In those cases, its relevance often derives from society's reaction to sexual minorities rather than to any fundamental connection to sexual orientation. The next section describes the problems that sexual minority clients may experience because of bias and discrimination.

Gay, lesbian, and bisexual clients frequently experience difficulty in "coming out" as sexual minorities. They have many reality-based concerns about how openly identifying themselves as gay, lesbian, or bisexual will affect their lives. Worries about being isolated from family and peers, about violence, and about career success are common. Because information about gay, lesbian, and bisexual identity development is not easily accessible, clients often have the task of sorting out what it means to be a sexual minority at their particular life stage. Effective counselors are equipped to assist clients in exploring these issues. They are knowledgeable about identity development issues for this population, informed about occupational and career issues, and skilled in helping clients decide about "coming out" to others. They explore with clients the risks of violence, discrimination, and rejection by loved ones and give clients a full measure of autonomy in making this important decision. Bradford and Ryan (1987) present a useful concept in this regard. They speak of *rational coming out,* a process of being as open as possible about oneself because it feels healthy and whole to be honest, but to be as closed as needed to be protected against violence and discrimination.

Effective counselors with sexual minorities also are cognizant of the influence of race, ethnicity, religion, and locale on the process of exploration of sexual identity. They assist clients of diverse cultural backgrounds in understanding the often complex relationship between culture and sexual orientation. For example, a gay Latino deciding whether to openly discuss his sexual orientation with his family and friends will need to explore the personal, familial, cultural, and religious issues in a population that places such high value on *machismo,* family, and traditional gender roles. Similarly, a lesbian client in a isolated rural area may wish to examine the effect of her locale on her coming-out process or her occupational or leisure pursuits.

Gay, lesbian, and bisexual individuals who make long-term commitments to partners do not experience the social supports that heterosexual couples take for granted. At this point, with the exception of the state of Vermont (which recognizes civil unions for nonheterosexual couples) and Massachusetts which allows marriage, legal marriage is not possible in the United States though current political activity may extend recognition of same sex unions to other states. Many religions refuse sexual minorities the right to a ceremony of marriage or commitment. Not all employers offer health insurance coverage to partners, and on many occasions, partners have been denied participation in medical decision making when their significant other is critically ill. In spite of these obstacles, many sexual minorities make long-term commitments to each other and remain in those relationships for decades (Mackey, O'Brien, & Mackey, 1997). These couples sometimes seek counseling for relationship difficulties that closely parallel those experienced by heterosexual couples, such as problems in managing dual careers. At other times, the realities of discrimination and marginalization of such couples are an important influence in their decision to enter counseling. Sometimes couples seek the support of a counselor because they have known few gay or lesbian couples who they identify as role models (Mackey, O'Brien, & Mackey, 1997). A gay couple who has adopted children may, for example, enter counseling to help cope more effectively with the stress of parenthood in a world that does not fully accept a gay couple's right to be parents. It is the responsibility of the counselor in each case to fairly and fully assess the sources of the problems and recommend appropriate interventions.

As with other diverse populations, the central task of the counselor with sexual minorities is to establish an effective therapeutic alliance, encourage the client to explore the issues in depth, and work with him or her to design and implement helpful interventions. The goals of the counselor can only be realized, however, when he or she is fully cognizant of the social, cultural, and political context in which the gay, lesbian, or bisexual client functions.

SUMMARY

Because of population changes and increased access to education and mental health services, counselors today must be prepared to work with an increasingly multicultural clientele. For the counseling process to be successful with culturally diverse clients, counselors must explore their own cultural traditions and attitudes to eliminate cultural elitism and gain a true appreciation for the value of cultural diversity in society. Knowledge of other cultures is also important so that counselors can accurately define client problems and choose appropriate intervention strategies. Furthermore, counselors must understand how racism and cultural oppression have affected the lives of clients and how these factors may affect the counseling relationship.

Specifically, culturally diverse clients faced with a counselor of a different background may be cautious, skeptical, or even openly mistrustful. In addition, counselors need specific skills to overcome these barriers and help the client solve the problems that led him or her to seek help. These skills include bilingualism, a broad repertoire of counseling strategies, appropriate use of assessment tools, a list of referral and consultation sources for multicultural clients, and the ability to work effectively with support persons in the community.

Women and girls are also considered a population for which effective counseling requires that counselors have special skills. Women have experienced gender role stereotyping that may affect the kinds of concerns they bring to counseling and their risk for victimization. Counselors need to understand the effects of sexism on female clients' development, the society's current values and norms for human behavior, and how sexism may interfere with the counseling process. Specifically, counselors need education in inclusive theories of human development and skills for helping girls and women who are currently experiencing victimization and discrimination.

Many men and boys are influenced by cultural role stereotyping as well. Growing boys are often shamed into denying feelings of vulnerability and caring, resulting in blunted emotional responding in adulthood. They are prone to poor relationships with significant others because of their emotional liability, and they sometimes resort to violence stemming from cultural learning that says aggression is masculine. Disturbances in sexual expression and the tendency to become workaholic are other manifestations. These negative consequences of exaggerated masculinity constitute an important part of the recent study of men's issues and an important new agenda for counseling with males. Boys and men can be helped to experience the joys of a full range of human emotions while retaining the positive stereotypes that men are expected to be strong, helpful, and productive.

Counselors who provide services to gay, lesbian, and bisexual clients have an obligation to understand the ways in which their own values, beliefs, and attitudes have been affected by homophobia and heterosexism. They must also be educated about the interactions between a minority sexual identity and the social, occupational, psychological, and educational functioning of this population.

≈≈≈ *DISCUSSION QUESTIONS* ≈≈≈

1. A culturally unaware counselor and a counselor with racial/ethnic prejudices would each have limitations in working with clients different from themselves. Describe the effects on counseling of each of these two conditions.
2. People are in some ways alike (*etic* perspective) and in some ways different (*emic* perspective). Discuss how the etic perspective underlies

a generic model of counseling, whereas the emic perspective influences how the model is applied with varied clients.

3. Values and behaviors typical of some minority cultures are not well received in the world of business as defined by the majority American culture. This can create a dilemma for minority clients (and their counselors) because it often generates negative economic consequences. What are the counselor's responsibilities in addressing this dilemma?

4. It has been argued that a well-trained professional counselor should be able to reach out to any client and to be an effective helper regardless of diversity issues. Does this generalization apply in extreme cases such as a male counselor working with a female who has been sexually assaulted? What policies do you think agencies or schools should have regarding the counselor–client match? Where there are few counselors and limited diversity in counseling staff, how can this issue be dealt with most effectively?

5. Gender socialization of both females and males teaches children about the roles they will play as women and men. In what ways is this socialization helpful to the maturation process? Under what circumstances might it be harmful as well? What is the counselor's responsibility in helping children with gender issues?

6. It may be true that traditional socialization limits women more in the instrumental endeavors of life and limits men more in their emotional experiencing. Do you agree with this generalization? Why or why not?

7. Gay, lesbian, and bisexual clients may not be identified as diverse by their appearance in the same way that race or gender is observable. They may also be reluctant to reveal their status to the counselor until well into a relationship. Why is this so? How can a counselor assure that sexual minority clients have as much freedom as other clients to discuss concerns they have? What may be done within the counseling sessions or in the environment where counseling takes place? What special problems may school counselors have in serving sexual minority clients?

8. Individual members of all minorities find ways of leading successful and fulfilling lives regardless of the discrimination or special circumstances they encounter. How do you account for the resilience of such individuals?

REFERENCES

Addis, M. E., & Mahalik, J. R. (2003). Men, masculinity and the contexts of help seeking. *American Psychologist, 58,* 5–14.

American Association of University Women. (1992). *How schools shortchange girls.* Washington, DC: Author.

American Psychological Association. (1990). *Women and depression.* Washington, DC: Author.

Arrendondo, P. M., Toporek, R., Brown, S. P., Jones, J., Locke, D., Sanchez, J., & Stadler, H. (1996). Operationalization of the multicultural counseling competencies. *Journal of Multicultural Counseling and Development, 24,* 42–78.

Atkinson, D. R., & Hackett, G. (1998). *Counseling diverse populations* (2nd ed.). Boston: McGraw Hill.

Atkinson, D. R., Morten, G., & Sue, D. W. (1998). *Counseling American minorities: A cross-cultural perspective.* (5th ed.). Dubuque, IA: Wm. C. Brown.

Atkinson, D. R., Thompson, C. E., & Grant, S. K. (1993). A three-dimensional model for counseling racial/ethnic minorities. *The Counseling Psychologist, 21,* 257–277.

Barret, B., & Logan, C. (2002). *Counseling gay men and lesbians: A practice primer.* Pacific Grove, CA: Brooks Cole.

Belenky, M. F., Clinchy, B. M., Goldberger, N. R., & Tarule, J. M. (1997). *Women's ways of knowing: The development of self, voice, and mind.* New York: Basic Books.

Besner, H. F., & Spungin, C. I. (1995). *Gay and lesbian students: Understanding their needs.* Washington, DC: Taylor and Francis.

Bradford, J., & Ryan, C. (1987). *National lesbian health care survey: Mental health implications.* Washington, DC: National Lesbian and Gay Health Foundation.

Brooks, G. R., & Good, G. E. (Eds.). (2001). *The new handbook of psychotherapy and counseling with men: A comprehensive guide to settings, problems, and treatment approaches* (Vols. 1 & 2). San Francisco: Jossey Bass.

Brooks, G. R., & Silverstein, L. B. (1995). Understanding the dark side of masculinity: An interactive systems model. In R. F. Levant & W. S. Pollack (Eds.), *A new psychology of men* (pp. 280–333). New York: Basic Books.

Broverman, I. K., Broverman, D. M., Clarkson, R. E., Rosenkrantz, P. S., & Vogel, S. R. (1970). Sex role stereotypes and clinical judgments of mental health. *Journal of Consulting Psychology, 34,* 1–7.

Cochran, S. V., & Rabinowitz, F. E. (2003). Gender-sensitive recommendations for assessment and treatment of depression in men. *Professional Psychology: Research and Practice, 34,* 132–140.

Dworkin, S. H., & Guitierrez, F. J. (Eds.). (1992). *Counseling gay men and lesbian women: Journey to the end of the rainbow.* Alexandria, VA: American Association of Counseling and Development.

Estes, C. P. (1992). *Women who run with the wolves.* New York: Ballantine.

Fischer, A. R., Jome, L. M., & Atkinson, D. R. (1998). Reconceptualizing multicultural counseling: Universal healing conditions in a culturally specific context. *The Counseling Psychologist, 26,* 525–588.

Fitzgerald, L. F., & Nutt, R. (1986). Division 17 principles concerning the counseling/ psychotherapy of women: Rationale and implementation. *The Counseling Psychologist, 14,* 180–216.

Gibson, W. T., & Pope, K. S. (1993). The ethics of counseling: A national survey of certified counselors. *Journal of Counseling and Development, 71,* 330–336.

Gilligan, C. (1993). *In a different voice: Psychological theory and women's development.* Cambridge, MA: Harvard University Press.

Ivey, A., & Authier, J. (1978). *Microcounseling: Innovations in interviewing training.* Springfield, IL: Charles C. Thomas.

Ivey, A., Ivey, M. B., & Simek-Morgan, L. (1997). *Counseling and psychotherapy: A multicultural perspective* (4th ed.). Boston: Allyn & Bacon.

Jolliff, D., & Horne, A. M. (1999). Growing up male: The development of mature masculinity. In A. M. Horne & M. S. Kiselica (Eds.), *Handbook of counseling boys and adolescent males: A practitioner's guide* (pp. 3–23). Thousand Oaks, CA: Sage.

Jordan, J. M. (1991). Counseling African-American women: "Sister-friends." In C. C. Lee and B. L. Richardson (Eds.), *Multicultural issues in counseling: New approaches to diversity* (pp. 51–63). Alexandria, VA: American Association for Counseling and Development.

Jordan, J. M. (1997). Counseling African American women from a cultural sensitivity perspective, In C. C. Lee (Ed.), *Multicultural issues in counseling: New approaches to diversity* (2nd ed., pp. 257–267), Alexandria, VA: American Counseling Association.

Lee, C. C (Ed.). (1997). *Multicultural issues in counseling: New approaches to diversity* (2nd ed.). Alexandria, VA: American Counseling Association.

Levant, R. F. (1995). Toward a reconstruction of masculinity. In R. F. Levant & W. S. Pollack (Eds.), *A new psychology of men* (pp. 229–251). New York: Basic Books.

Levant, R. F., & Pollack, W. S. (Eds.). (1995). *A new psychology of men.* New York: Basic Books.

Lopez-Baez, S. I. (1997). Counseling interventions with Latinas. In C. C. Lee (Ed.), *Multicultural issues in counseling: New approaches to diversity* (2nd ed., pp. 257–267). Alexandria, VA: American Counseling Association.

Mackey, R. A., O'Brien, B. A., & Mackey, E. F. (1997). *Gay and lesbian couples: Voices from lasting relationships.* Westport, CT: Praeger.

Mahalik, J. R., Good, G. E., & Englar-Carlson, M. (2003). Masculinity scripts, presenting concerns, and help seeking: Implications for practice and training. *Professional Psychology: Research and Practice, 34,* 123–131.

Michaels, S. (1996). The prevalence of homosexuality in the United States. In R. P. Cabaj & T. S. Stein (Eds.), *Textbook of homosexuality and mental health* (pp. 43–63). Washington, D.C.: American Psychiatric Press.

Pedersen, P. B. (Ed.). (1991). *Journal of Counseling and Development, 70* (1–250).

Pedersen, R. B. (2000). *A handbook for developing multicultural awareness* (3rd ed.). Alexandria, VA: American Counseling Association.

Pleck, J. H. (1995). The gender role strain paradigm: An update. In R. F. Levant & W. S. Pollack (Eds.), *A new psychology of men* (pp. 11–32). New York: Basic Books.

Pollack, W. S. (1995). No man is an island: Toward a new psychoanalytic psychology of men. In R. F. Levant & W. S. Pollack (Eds.), *A new psychology of men* (pp. 33–67). New York: Basic Books.

Rich, A. (1980). Compulsory heterosexuality and lesbian existence *Signs: Journal of Women in Culture and Society, 5,* 631–660.

Rosewater, L. B., & Walker, L. E. (Eds.). (1985). *Handbook of feminist therapy: Women's issues in psychotherapy.* New York: Springer.

Ryan, W. (1976). *Blaming the victim* (Revised). New York: Pantheon.

Saunders-Robinson, M. A. (1991). Battered women: An African-American perspective. *ABNF Journal, 2,* 81–84.

Spielberg, W. (1999). A cultural critique of current practices of male adolescent identity formation. In A. M. Horne & M. S. Kiselica (Eds.), *Handbook of counseling boys and adolescent males: A practitioner's guide* (pp. 25–34). Thousand Oaks, CA: Sage.

Sue, D. W. (1978). Eliminating cultural oppression in counseling: Toward a general theory. *Journal of Counseling Psychology, 25,* 419–428.

Sue, D. W., Arrendondo, R., & McDavis, R. J. (1992). Multicultural counseling competencies and standards: A call to the profession. *Journal of Counseling and Development, 70,* 477–486.

Sue, D. W., Ivey, A. E., & Pedersen, P. B. (1996). *A theory of multicultural counseling and therapy.* Pacific Grove, CA: Brooks/Cole.

Sue, D. W., & Sue, D. (2003). *Counseling the culturally diverse: Theory and practice* (4th ed.). New York: Wiley.

Sue, S., Zane, N., & Young, K. (1994). Research on psychotherapy with diverse populations. In A. Bergin & S. Garfield (Eds.), *Handbook of Psychotherapy and Behavior Change* (4h ed., pp. 78–817). New York: Wiley.

Suzuki, L. A., Ponterotto, J. G., & Meller, P. J. (2000). *Handbook of multicultural assessment* (2nd ed.). San Francisco: Jossey-Bass.

Tannen, D. (1990). *You just don't understand: Women and men in conversation.* New York: Morrow.

Toman, J. A. (1997). Dual identity: Being Catholic and being gay. *Dissertation Abstracts International, 58,* 1942A.

Welfel, E. R. (2002). *Ethics in counseling and psychotherapy: Standards, research, and emerging issues* (2nd ed.). Pacific Grove, CA: Brooks Cole.

Worell, J., & Remer, P. (2003). *Feminist perspectives in therapy* (2nd ed.). New York: Wiley.

Wrenn, C. G. (1962). The culturally encapsulated counselor. *Harvard Educational Review, 32,* 444–449.

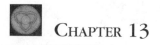 CHAPTER 13

WORKING WITH CHILDREN AND THEIR PARENTS

In the broadest sense, counseling with children involves the same process as counseling with older clients: a caring relationship with genuine empathic understanding that promotes disclosure, deeper-level empathy and confrontation with self that builds insight, and action planning that leads to better coping strategies. Nevertheless, the counselor who has worked only with adolescents and adults is likely to find that initial encounters with children in counseling require knowledge and skills he or she may not possess. Most books on the counseling process, and until recently most counselor education programs, have given scant attention to the special qualities that children bring to counseling.

This chapter presents an introduction to counseling children with the clear recognition that those seeking to specialize in working with children need to extend their study well beyond the scope found here. The purpose of this chapter is to apply the general principles of counseling to this population and to suggest some of the issues that form the fabric of a specialization in child counseling. Because all counselors work with children or with the parents and older siblings of young children, we believe that all counselors need a basic understanding of the helping process as it applies to young children.

For purposes of definition, we will refer to children as persons who have not yet reached puberty. However, it is obvious that there are big differences between 4-year-olds and 10-year-olds. As a general principle, the more mature the client, the less it is necessary to employ the special counseling procedures described in this chapter and the more applicable are the standard procedures described in earlier chapters of this book.

HOW CHILDREN DIFFER FROM ADULTS

The first quality of children that the counselor will notice is a limitation in verbal skills. The young child has a vocabulary that allows for labeling of persons and objects and for describing simple happenings but does not usually provide the ability to verbalize emotions. According to Nelson (1966), "In contrast with his older siblings who can verbalize frustrations, love, anger, and acceptance, the younger child acts out his feelings. He crashes cars together, he hugs his Mom, he shoots the enemy, and he hands another child a toy" (p. 24). Any child's statement of a problem is likely to be communicated in simple terms with little clue to the cause or surrounding circumstances. In fact, children who are brought to counseling (in contrast to mature clients) "may not agree or recognize that there are problems or concerns" (Prout, 1999, p. 9).

Verbal skill is, of course, intimately related to cognitive functioning, and if the counselor is able to sustain counseling with a young client long enough to encourage disclosure, immature cognitive processes will become apparent. "Children in their first few years of life think mainly in concrete terms and have not yet acquired the capacity for abstract thought" (Barker, 1990, p. 4). According to Piaget and Inhelder (1969), children do not become capable of problem solving through hypothesis testing until age 11 or later. Prior to that time, the child develops through several more basic stages that are characterized by initial acquisition of language, egocentrism, and problem solving focused on tangible objects. The understanding of problems of human interaction that have clear cause–effect components for the counselor may be beyond the comprehension of the child.

Two elements of cognitive development that often prove confounding to the efforts of an adolescent- or adult-oriented counselor who undertakes work with a child are the limited time perspective and the limited ways of viewing right and wrong. To appreciate the time perspective problem, one need only remember the last time one took a long automobile trip with a child or promised that his or her birthday party would be in one week. In both instances, the child probably began inquiring almost immediately about the culmination ("Are we there yet?" or "Is my birthday going to be here tomorrow?") No amount of explaining will convey accurately that "We will be at Grandmother's in three hours" or that "The sun must come up seven more times before your birthday." To a child, the world is eternal, and he or she is at the center of that world. To the counselor, time is finite, and one important responsibility is helping clients think about and plan for the future—a concept beyond the capacity of young children to understand.

The child's early conception of right and wrong, according to Kohlberg (1964, 1981) is focused on the avoidance of punishment and the satisfaction of immediately felt personal needs. The assumption (possibly correct for very young children) is that "others are in control, and I am not really responsible." At this stage of development, it is not yet really possible for the child to operate from an internal locus of control based on personal values or standards, because these have not yet developed. The young child will comply with demands from parents and teachers, or he or she will find ways to manipulate them to satisfy egocentric desires. Over time, children's moral decision making shifts to concern for how others will view them and how they view themselves (as good or bad children). By the end of childhood, the typical level of moral reasoning results in controls on behavior in order to abide by rules that contribute to the social good. (There are three further levels of moral development in Kohlberg's system that describe adults as exercising increasingly independent personal valuing in making decisions, though many adults never progress beyond the "law and order" stage.) Gilligan (1993) postulated that women and girls tend to be more concerned than males with how their behavior affects their relationships with others, whereas males tend to be more concerned with rights and justice.

The counselor working with children needs to appreciate how a newborn child begins with virtually no concepts about relating to others and no skills and then progresses through stages to greater and greater levels of competence. Erikson (1993) described eight stages of human psychosocial development, four of which occur during the childhood years. Aligning these stages with specific tasks, Thompson and Rudolph (1996) characterized children's first developmental task as "the need to develop trust in their environment and caregivers." Then, they "begin to develop some self-control and control over their environment" (p. 31), followed by a sense of initiative. During the elementary school years, their attention should shift to learning a variety of skills. According to Erikson, a child who does not at least partially accomplish the tasks of one stage cannot move to the next. Thus, to understand the origins of a child's failure to undertake the skills of second grade, the counselor may find it useful to explore that child's earlier experiences.

Finally, it is important for the counselor to consider the fact that children have limited freedom to change the conditions of their lives and little experience in devising solutions to life's problems (Nelson, 1991). Typically, children cannot choose to live with different parents, to attend a different school, or to change the environmental influences that result from being born into a particular family and culture. "Children are reactors to changes in their living situations rather than initiators of change. They have relatively little power to take action to eliminate or prevent environmental causes of stress" (Prout, 1999, p. 11). Although freedom to make choices gradually increases with age, children must often learn to live with things as they are or depend on adults to intervene to improve their circumstances. And because the child has had little life experience, his or her store of strategies and skills is limited. Nelson (1991) said, "There are a great many ways in which young children are incapable and feel that incapability. There are things they cannot reach, words they cannot read, tasks they cannot perform" (p. 289).

In summary, it is important to appreciate that children are not simply small adults. Their behaviors are not mediated by thoughts in the same way as those of adults, and they have life tasks to perform that are shaped by their dependent status and their need to acquire skills. Among the skills that remain incomplete is the use of language. As they try to manage stress, their coping mechanisms are immature. Right and wrong do not carry the same meanings as for adults, or indeed across the different ages of childhood. Yet young children do experience emotional distress, feelings of inadequacy and endangerment, frustration, and many other problems that mirror their more mature counterparts. Prevalence estimates suggest that approximately one-fifth of children and adolescents have an emotional, behavioral, or developmental problem serious enough to need intervention (Doll, 1996; Kazdin & Johnson, 1996). Fortunately, they can also be resilient in the face of the challenges they experience if given some support and guidance (Rak, 2002; Rak & Patterson, 1996). The remainder of this chapter addresses ways in which the counselor can help children, even though they do not possess all the capabilities of older clients.

COMMUNICATING

As with any client, the first counseling objective with a child is to establish communication. The counselor's goal is to learn how the young client views and interacts with the significant others in his or her world and to discover whether the client believes that he or she is loved, competent, and attractive. The counselor must also adjust counseling procedures to maximize the client's ability to communicate experiences, taking into account cognitive, emotional, physical, and behavioral immaturity.

Confidentiality

To encourage a free flow of information, counselors should discuss confidentiality (and its limits) early in counseling, even with young children (Barker, 1990; Thompson & Rudolph, 1996). Many counselors become confused about the issue of confidentiality with children both because of their dependency relationship with parents and because of parents' right to know what is happening with their children. Unless a statute exists that permits minors to obtain service without parental consent or unless parental involvement would be seriously harmful to the child, parents must provide informed consent for the counseling to take place (Welfel, 2002). Still, the child's ethical right to confidentiality must be balanced against the parents' legal right to know what is happening with their child (Orton, 1997). In fact, the criterion for breaking confidentiality with children parallels that with older clients: confidentiality must be suspended if the client discloses actions that involve danger to self or others or information related to abuse or neglect. Because of the child's inability to move about the world safely alone, running away is added to suicidal or homicidal ideation as threatening behavior.

Barker (1990) makes a useful distinction between two types of information that emerge from a counseling session. One type has to do with the child's condition (e.g., is he or she depressed, developmentally delayed, attention deficit disordered?) and how the child manages that condition. The other type of information is what the client actually says or reveals in other ways during the counseling sessions. The first type of information is usually discussed with the parents and may be shared with teachers or others who are responsible for assuring a favorable climate for the child's growth and learning (provided the parents and child are willing). Decisions about how much of this kind of information to share with whom should be based on considerations about the recipients' need to know and their ability to use the information for the client's benefit. The second type of information—the actual content of the counseling sessions—can and generally should be held in confidence. In instances when parents request knowledge of what actually transpired in a counseling session, the counselor should ask the client to help determine what will be communicated and how (Welfel, 2002). It is also important to explain the value of confidentiality to the parents and to secure their cooperation in creating as much privacy as possible (Orton, 1997; Taylor & Adelman, 2001). When information is to be shared, giving the child as much involvement as possible in the decision about what to share and with whom maximizes his or her feeling of confidentiality and thus safety in the counseling setting. In fact, even though a child's permission for such communications is not legally binding, obtaining a child's assent to such actions is ethically advisable. It communicates respect for the child and encourages his or her active participation in the counseling process.

Talking with Children

Young children are not oriented to approaching a counselor with a statement such as "Here is my problem" or "These are some of the things that have been happening to me." The counselor is initially an adult stranger, and many children are unaccustomed to talking with adults other than family members, friends of the family, or teachers. Some children have never talked to an adult who really listens and tries to understand. Because counseling is a new experience for most children, the counselor must structure what occurs in such a way that the young client is less anxious about talking, understands what to do, and is motivated to participate.

Many adults (including counselors who have not worked with children) are accustomed to talking *to* rather than *with* children, and even when they are trying to express concern and caring, they may be subtly condescending. We are reminded of a scene created by humorist Jean Kerr in which a doting relative walks into a room and exclaims, "My, look who is in the playpen!" The child is purported to be thinking, "Who do you think would be in the playpen?" All too often adults seem uncomfortable in a child's presence; they don't know what to say, so they comment on how the child has grown or changed. But growth and change are expected occurrences in childhood, and children are often embarrassed by these awkward attempts at communication. Other people seem to believe that they need to talk loudly to children, who, in fact, have better hearing than adults as a rule.

Counselors should begin counseling with a child as with any other client—holding respect for the child's dignity as a human being and maintaining an attitude of exploration. The initial goal is to get to know the individual. The counselor should speak in a well-modulated voice with a friendly manner, keeping in mind the vocabulary of the client and his or her level of cognitive maturity. Short sentences, using the client's terms and people's names rather than pronouns, are best (Garbarino & Stott, 1992). The counselor's task is to enter the child's world and understand his or her experience from his or her perspective. This is the same as entering the world of any client during the initial-disclosure and in-depth exploration stages of counseling, with the important exception that the counselor must now reach back into the world of childhood to establish empathic contact.

Thompson and Rudolph (1996) recommend frequent use of "Tell me about . . ." as a way of encouraging expansive responses. "Tell me about your family" or "Tell me about school this year" often result in stories that include both the happenings of importance to the child and his or her feelings about those happenings. Nelson (1991) notes that children benefit by hearing their feelings restated by the counselor, and that they need even more help than adults do in labeling their feelings. Thompson and Rudolph also caution, "Children easily fall into the role of answering adults' questions and then waiting for the next question" (p. 42); thus the pattern of a question and answer session is easily set. If an inquisition is allowed to begin, the counseling may self-destruct because the counselor loses the role of the listener and instead must devote all of his or her energy to generating more questions. "Counselors learn more by listening and summarizing than by questioning" (Thompson & Rudolph, 1996, p. 43).

Barker (1990) suggests two additional techniques for encouraging children to engage in revealing talk. The first taps into the client's fantasies by asking him or her to state three wishes. If one of the wishes is, for example, that Mommy and Daddy would not fight so much, the significance for the child's feelings of security is obvious. The second technique is to inquire whether the client ever has dreams. The majority of children acknowledge that they do and can then be encouraged to describe their dreams. If a client says that he or she does not dream, Barker sometimes uses the alternative of asking the client to make up a dream. Either of these approaches provides access to the child's private and even unconscious world.

Even though many children have not developed extensive facility with language, it is usually possible to establish some conversation if the counselor remembers what childhood is like and expresses a genuine interest in learning something of the client's world. In fact, Barker (1990) states that some children—those who are older, of above average intelligence, and with good verbal skills—enjoy conversation and engage eagerly in telling their stories. However, many other children are more at home with play and may become acclimated to counseling more readily if toys and other media are provided. The next section provides an introduction to using play to encourage children's communication.

Use of Play in Counseling

The use of play and art supplies in a counseling session with a child usually aids the communication process. Play has been linked to a number of cognitive phenomena, including problem solving, language learning, creativity, and the development of social roles (Brady & Friedrich, 1982). Therefore, observing a child play offers a window on the child's thoughts and feelings. As Hall, Kaduson, and Schaefer (2002) note, "For children, toys are their words, and play is their conversation" (p. 515). A little girl who is angry at her teacher can use crayons to draw her angry face or cast her teacher as dead during doll or puppet play. A little boy who is experiencing disorganization and abuse in his family can use a dollhouse and human figures to illustrate family life as he knows it. A child who is nervous and full of energy can let off steam by punching a punching bag. Given some things to play with, a child does not need to be told how to play. The counselor needs only to know how to encourage significant play, to observe what happens, and to talk with the child about it. "In the safety of the play therapy setting, children can act out traumatic life experiences that they may be only vaguely aware of, thus affording the therapist a glimpse of the children's unconscious thoughts and feelings" (Orton, 1997, p. 222).

The introduction of play into counseling sessions provides a mode of communication that is natural for children (Schaefer & Cangelosi, 2002). While playing, catharsis takes place: the child's nervous energy is expended in using a punching bag, the child's emotions can be expressed in a drawing, or the dynamics of the child's family become apparent through what happens in the dollhouse. Play provides a means for structuring time and a comfortable atmosphere in which neither the client nor the counselor feels obliged to maintain constant conversation.

Nevertheless, intermittent conversation about the play helps the counselor understand the meanings the child attaches to what he or she does. In time, as the client becomes comfortable with the counselor, he or she is likely to engage in more and more direct conversation that extends beyond the play activity. The counselor's participation includes a physical presence, involvement in the play, observation of activity, and verbal interaction with the client. As with older clients, counselor responses in early sessions should be nonintrusive (minimum degree of leading), and the length of lead can be extended as the relationship builds.

Brady and Friedrich (1982) have suggested four levels of intervention: physical presence, reflecting or paraphrasing the child's statements, third-person interpretations, and direct interpretations. In the first level, physical presence, the counselor limits his or her responses to encouraging or describing the child's explorations and play: "Let's see what's in here" or "The boy doll is hiding under the bed." At the second level, reflection of feeling might extend to a statement like this: "The boy doll is really afraid of something." The third level, third-person interpretation, the counselor describes what the child seems to be experiencing without any attribution of the feelings involved to the child: "Sometimes it is very frightening if a child is left all alone at home for a long time." The fourth level is the most direct, because the counselor attributes what has been displayed in the play to the child's actual experience: "You feel very frightened when you are left alone at home." Although a fourth-level response probably has the greatest potential for moving to discussion of the child's real-life concerns, it is safer for the child to begin talking about his or her concerns as though he or she were discussing someone else. A child who is acting out a scene where the mother is intoxicated may reveal much of what happens in his or her own family if the counselor simply comments on the experiences of the play figures. If the counselor prematurely says, "You get very concerned about your mother's drinking," the client may well deny that his or her mother drinks and may become frightened and reluctant to continue with the counseling.

In general, children probably do not reach sophisticated levels of insight about their problems through discussion of their play. As we indicated earlier, their cognitive skills, moral judgment, and experience all reflect immature capacities for coping with life. Nevertheless, catharsis—combined with exploration and problem solving through play—creates perceptual and behavior change, and the experience of being truly valued and listened to as a client helps build feelings of self-worth. For children, playing out their experiences and feelings is a natural and self-healing process (Landreth, 2001).

Some play materials are much more useful than others for promoting affective expression. Unstructured materials allow the young client to place his or her own meanings on the play and are therefore preferable to structured games. Lebo (1979) systematically studied several different kinds of play material to determine which prompted the greatest amount and variety of verbal expression by his clients. His review of the literature offered support for the view that children who talk during their play sessions make more rapid progress than those who do not. He found that a dollhouse, family, and furniture were most effective in eliciting conversation with his sample of average-intelligence boys and girls, ages 4 through 12. Poster paints, brushes, paper, and easels were nearly as good. Next in order, but somewhat less helpful, were a sandbox, chalkboard and colored chalk, cap gun and caps, coloring books, and hand puppets.

Dolls and puppets should be simple enough that the young client can use his or her imagination in playing. Among the dolls and puppets, there should be males and females and adults and children of various racial backgrounds. The child can use them to build the drama. Art supplies are valuable because they can be used to create anything the child needs to share.

Schaefer (2003) and Kottman (2001) provide excellent reviews of effective use of such techniques with preadolescent children.

We do not recommend using structured competitive games in counseling with young children. In the first place, these games require the counselor to enter into competition with the client, and there must be a winner and a loser. In most instances, if the counselor plays at his or her skill level, he or she will win, creating an experience of failure for the client. If the counselor lets the client win, there is the risk that the client will recognize the manipulation; then the genuineness of the relationship will be compromised. Second, such games are highly structured, so there is little opportunity for the client to infuse the interaction with material from his or her life. The initial advantages of high structure in getting the play started and in providing a familiar mode of interaction for the child are soon lost in the limitations that the structure places on communication. There are, however, some noncompetitive structured games designed for use in counseling (e.g., *The Talking, Feeling, and Doing Game* from Creative Therapeutics or *The Ungame* published by Ungame) that contain situations posing common concerns of children and create a basis for discussion. They are fairly easy to use even when a counselor is inexperienced in working with children.

A counselor who is using media with a child may also engage in direct conversation about the daily events of the child's life. The client will become more comfortable with direct conversation as the two people spend more time together, and this conversation can be interspersed with conversation about the play activity. We have found that materials can be useful in building communication with clients of all ages. As children mature and their verbal and cognitive abilities increase, more and more of the counseling is likely to be direct conversation. Even with adults, however, it is sometimes helpful to provide a pen and paper and suggest that clients draw how they feel about a situation they are having trouble verbalizing. See Schaefer (2003) for a detailed discussion of the use of play with adults in counseling. As children approach puberty and begin to leave toys behind, puppets and dolls will gradually drop out of the sessions. However, pillows can still be punched to express anger or frustration, and drawing or sculpting may be used to express other feelings. Verbal role-playing will gradually replace doll and puppet activities as a way of bringing interpersonal situations into the counseling room.

Summary of Communication Techniques

This section has focused on how the counselor encourages communication with a child about things that are important to the child. Direct conversation accompanied by observation and interaction about play are the two primary methods. An attitude of respect for the child underlies any successful interaction, and language should be tailored to the child's developmental level. Leads should be fashioned to encourage expansiveness of client responses rather than narrow answers to counselor questions; play materials should be selected for their value in promoting imaginative play reflective of real-life concerns. The counselor should construct the experience so that he or she can spend time listening and observing. Counselors, of course, play a role in assessing and socializing children as well. Subsequent sections of this chapter address these topics.

ASSESSMENT

The assessment question when working with a child is basically the same as with any other client: "How successfully is this person meeting the challenges of his or her life?" But the assessment process with children requires special knowledge and skill because the capabilities of children change markedly from year to year and the challenges of life depend in large measure on the significant adults in the child's life. The basic assessment question is therefore adapted: "How successfully is this child meeting challenges for a person of his or her age, compared to what the adults in the environment expect?" Problems occur because the child is in some way deficient in meeting age-appropriate challenges (such as assuming increasing responsibility for dressing himself or herself) or because adults are making unreasonable demands (such as demanding periods of concentration beyond the developmentally related attention span of the child).

The purpose of assessment, which commences with the first contact, is to begin setting goals and devising an action plan. As when working with older clients, the counselor attempts to identify arenas in which the child is not functioning effectively and to determine the factors contributing to the difficulty. With a child, it is often a significant adult who asserts that a deficit or difficulty exists, and the child may or may not perceive that there is a problem. In working with children, the counselor must take more responsibility for assessing the nature and source of dysfunction than is necessary with older clients. The counselor then works to set goals with the client and/or with significant others in the client's life.

Assessment Tools

A number of different procedures may be used in the assessment of a child's functioning:

- The counseling interview
- Observation of play in counseling sessions
- Observation in naturalistic settings
- Interviews with parents, teachers, and others
- School records, including anecdotal comments

- Incomplete sentence blanks
- Structured (clinical) interviews
- Standardized tests
- Analysis of children's drawings

All of these techniques can be enhanced through specialized training, but a counselor who has mastered the generic counseling process as presented in this book should be able to utilize the first six techniques at an initial level. We urge anyone who will work regularly with children to engage in extensive training on all of these techniques.

As with older clients, a principal source of information used in the assessment process is the client's self-disclosures in counseling sessions. However, because the child's cognitive and language skills are immature, the counselor should attend to nonverbal behaviors and develop experience in encouraging play and understanding the language of play, as described in the preceding section. In addition, the counselor may also choose to observe the child in a natural setting (such as a child care facility or classroom) to evaluate how well and how long the child is able to concentrate on assigned tasks, his or her success with assigned responsibilities, and his or her interactions with peers and authority figures.

Interviews with parents, teachers, siblings, and other adults who are responsible for supervising the child are a rich source of information. The inclusion of observations from several different people increases the total amount of the child's behavior that has been observed. Sometimes data gathered from different sources may be inconsistent and may indicate observer bias, depending on the circumstance or on the child's relationship with the observer. Direct discussion with parents and teachers about their expectations of the child is an important component of the diagnostic picture.

School is one of the major responsibilities of children, and there is much to be learned by reviewing the educational record. The record reveals whether the child is progressing satisfactorily, whether there are apparent strengths and weaknesses in different subjects, whether achievement seems congruent with measured ability, and how grades relate to results of achievement tests. Anecdotal entries in the record may provide clues as to how the child gets along with other children and staff.

Incomplete sentence blanks are structured written protocols, with stems of sentences to be completed by the client (for example, "I get frightened when . . ." or "My mother . . ." or "A favorite time was . . ."). A child who is old enough to do so may write out responses for later discussion in counseling, or the counselor may read the stems and record the client's responses. Inspection of the client's responses reveals areas where tension (or satisfaction) is expressed and provides an opening to discuss the issues identified. Many counselors find this technique useful in establishing conversation during the initial-disclosure stage of counseling, and little special expertise is required of the counselor who uses this means to stimulate discussion.

Clinical interviews with children and parents can be accomplished with the aid of published questionnaires such as *The Diagnostic Interview for Children and Adolescents* (Herjanic & Reich, 1982) or Achenbach's *Child Behavior Checklist* (1991). These instruments seek to identify particular symptoms and their frequency, duration, and severity. They are usually used as a part of an intake process in clinical settings and have one form for the child and another for the parents. The use of clinical interviews has increased in recent years (Nystul, 2003), paralleling the increased use of the diagnostic categories for children and adolescents in the *Diagnostic and Statistical Manual of Mental Disorders* (American Psychiatric Association, 2000).

Use of standardized tests and analysis of children's drawings are special areas of study beyond the scope of this presentation. (Swales, 2001, provides an excellent overview of structured approaches to assessing children's mental health problems for readers interested in gathering more information on this topic.) Usually a counselor who has a basic knowledge of child development can make some observations about drawings, including their completeness, facial expressions, and so on. However, there is an extensive literature on children's drawings and their interpretation (Cox, 1992; Orton, 1997) and specialized training greatly increases the counselor's ability to use drawings for assessment purposes.

Scope of Assessment

The assessment process should focus on the child's functioning in each of the important sectors of his or her life, using the typical performance of persons of the same age as a standard of effectiveness. One among many examples of multimodal assessment models is BASIC ID by Lazarus (1989, 1990). The acronym BASIC ID stands for seven areas of functioning that may become problem areas treated in counseling: behavior, affect, sensation/ school (e.g., headaches, school failure), imagery (e.g., self-concept, dreams, fantasies), cognition, interpersonal relationships, and drugs/diet.

Knowledge of age-appropriate functioning in each of these areas may be acquired through the study of child development and will become more familiar with experience. A convenient brief summary of many age-normed characteristics was developed by Muro and Dinkmeyer (1977). Their presentation includes two- to three-page descriptions of each age group from 5 to 12, complete with some implications for counseling arising from the developmental level of the child. The content covers a broad range—from a recognition that 5-year-olds are comforted and encouraged by structure but have only a 20-minute attention span, to the recognition that 12-year-olds are developing sexually and need the kind of understanding and information that can come from group counseling. However, no simple guide is a substitute for more extensive study and experience.

Children are born with different talents and capacities and to families that vary in their abilities to provide nurturance and to teach the ways of the world. This leads to differences in accomplishments and satisfactions as children grow. In addition, parents have diverse expectations for their children that reflect the parents' own needs and experiences. The majority of children who come to the attention of counselors are not progressing well because of the chances of nature and nurture. Most of these children are experiencing normal, even expected, difficulties with developmental tasks, and most respond to the caring attention and environmental manipulations that counselors can accomplish. Just as with older clients, some children experience serious difficulties for which specialized attention is needed to diagnose and treat the problem. Counselors should be alert to signs of child abuse, childhood depression, and severe forms of antisocial behavior that may lead a child to harm him or herself or others. Specialists should be consulted when these conditions prevail.

Case: Ryan

Ryan, age 7, was referred to a counselor at a university clinic because his behavior was disruptive at school, he was not accomplishing his schoolwork, and he was disobedient at home. He was brought to counseling by his mother, age 27, an articulate and concerned single parent who worked long hours. Ryan's parents were separated, and Ryan and his mother constituted the household. Ryan's father had been at home until about a year prior to the referral, but Ryan saw him only infrequently after the separation. There was no history of family violence, nor did the parents openly carry on their personal conflict in Ryan's presence.

The initial interview revealed that the mother had very high expectations for her son. When school was over each day, Ryan was required to take two public buses to get from the parochial school he attended to his home. He let himself into the house with a key and was alone for 3 to 5 hours before his mother arrived home. During that time, he was expected to do his homework, clean the house (including dusting and vacuuming), and make initial preparations for dinner. After dinner, he was required to help with the dishes, and then he was often alone again while his mother entertained her boyfriend.

The mother felt that she was fulfilling her obligations to Ryan to the best of her ability. She worked long hours to provide for him and to pay tuition to a good school. She couldn't understand why he was so resistant to doing what she expected of him and felt panicked when Ryan started acting out in school and refusing to do his work. An intervention by the school psychologist, isolating Ryan when he misbehaved, seemed to result in more rebellion. The mother's concern for Ryan was demonstrated by her seeking help at the university, even though this added an additional activity each week to an already busy schedule.

In a client–parent–counselor session, the counselor observed that many of the mother's communications to Ryan were critical and disapproving and focused on small issues. She chastised Ryan for fidgeting during the session, even though he was attentive and his behavior was reasonable for a 7-year-old boy. She repeatedly corrected his speech, using precise and formal language to do so. Discussion revealed that the mother and son had no "quality" time together: they did not talk with each other except about life maintenance activities, they did not read together, and they did not go anywhere for recreation. Furthermore, Ryan was not permitted to have friends in when his mother was not home. When she was home, it was too late. Thus, Ryan rarely played with children his age—for that matter, he rarely played at all.

When he met with the counselor alone, Ryan was initially reluctant to say much but was attentive and friendly. He appeared to like the full attention of an adult. As time passed, the counselor gave Ryan some crayons and paper and asked him to draw scenes of his daily life. Soon Ryan was picturing himself as a child who was often left alone or with only demanding adults in his environment. He was reluctant to express negative feelings about these adults, but finally began to tell how mean James, his mother's boyfriend, was. James did not physically abuse him, but he was firm in requiring certain behavior and was not "nice" like Ryan's father. As time passed, all the adults in Ryan's life were eventually described as demanding, rejecting, and not very affectionate. Ryan was enabled to express his anger about the way he was treated.

As Ryan talked more to the counselor about his angry feelings, his disruptive behavior at school disappeared. The teacher was persuaded to use some positive reinforcers rather than isolation, and within 2 months, Ryan was again doing well in school.

The problem at home was harder to solve. Ryan's mother had a difficult time accepting the suggestion that she should spend more time with Ryan doing things for fun. She was a busy woman and believed she was already doing all she could for him. She did come to realize, through consultation, that she was perhaps too demanding in her expectations about housework for a boy so young, and she eased up a bit on those demands. Ryan began to learn how to negotiate with his mother so that he could do some of his work when he wanted and could have time to himself part of each evening. He was permitted to visit friends after his mother came home in the evenings and began to get some playtime.

Counseling was terminated at that point because the mother had gotten what she wanted out of it. Her son was doing well in school and was more manageable at home. The counselor made every effort to continue the relationship with mother and son in order to accomplish a more positive relationship, but further counseling was refused.

Case Discussion

In this case, a variety of communication techniques were used to establish contact with Ryan's world. He was given the full attention and respect of the counselor. This was a marked contrast to the communication style of his mother, who was the most significant other in his life. Drawing was a comfortable activity that created material for projective understanding of Ryan's interactions with his mother, her boyfriend, his teacher, and other children. Physical activity was provided to permit release of energy. Finally, comfortable verbal communication increased as the counselor and the client came to know one another and built a trusting relationship.

The assessment process revealed that physical demands were being made on Ryan that he could not meet. Socially, his interactions were all with controlling adults, the most important of whom (his mother) had little idea what to expect of a 7-year-old. He was not permitted to express his opinion on anything—compliance was the behavior of a "good" boy. Emotionally, Ryan was lonely and angry but, fortunately, not yet bitter. With some support, he was able to express his feelings of anger and seek ways of alleviating some of his loneliness. His learning had been disrupted by physical and emotional overload, but he was a bright child who easily readjusted to school when other factors were moderated.

Note that the primary goals of counseling were to get Ryan to express and unload some of his negative feelings and to seek some ways of adding companionship and variety to his life. At the same time, work with his mother was directed toward encouraging her to express love, to reduce the demands she placed on Ryan, and to try to understand what his life was like. These goals emerged directly from using the kind of assessment process described in this section.

Questions for Further Thought

1. What factors contributed to Ryan's anger?
2. What elements of the mother's personality formed the fabric of a negative living routine for Ryan? Which of her personality attributes were helpful to Ryan?
3. Do you believe that counseling resulted in satisfactory outcomes for the client? What else might have been attempted? How feasible do you believe these additional goals might have been?

AUGMENTING THE SOCIALIZATION PROCESS

Many of the difficulties that children experience result from a lack of experience. As children gain experiences, they become socialized by observing and eventually modeling the behaviors of others. To "socialize," according to *The Random House Dictionary,* means "to make social; to make fit for life in companionship with others." Bandura's (1977) social learning theory describes a process by which children learn to deal with life by observing others.

One of the authors recalls an incident in which his son-in-law expressed frustration that his then 2-year-old son had "no judgment at all." The author observed that this was a normal state of affairs for a 2-year-old, and that was why Nathan had parents to help him develop better judgment. Remembering that a baby is born an unsocialized being a few short years before he or she first enters school brings into perspective how much growth and learning occur in a short time. It also clarifies why it is so likely that some valuable learning may be overlooked in the life of a particular child.

Orton (1997) points to the importance of socioeconomic and sociocultural factors as they influence the experience a particular child has as he or she learns how to live in companionship with others. Socioeconomic factors are important determinants of the child's richness of experience or the possibility of the stark deprivation of living in poverty. Sociocultural background teaches certain traditions essential to developing a sense of self, but those traditions may leave out information that is important to getting along in the world outside the family, perhaps something as pervasive as learning the majority language (see Chapter 12). Whereas Chapter 12 focused on sensitivity to cultural differences in relationship building and goal setting with multicultural clients, the focus here is on opportunities to learn fundamental life skills. Thompson and Rudolph (1996) observe that latchkey children (nearly half of upper elementary grade children) are thrust into self-care before they have the experience to assure their own safety or to make good choices about the use of time. Alone, children may resort to television as a source of socialization stimuli, or they may simply be deprived of needed stimuli altogether. Research suggests that unstructured and unsupervised time after school can be a risk factor for preteen involvement with substances and other high-risk behaviors (Goyette-Ewing, 2000; Stewart, 2001).

Ryan (a latchkey child) in the preceding case study has had limited opportunities to learn from others, either his mother or others of his own age, during casual interactions. Some children whose parents communicate few expectations may fail to learn such basic things as personal care and hygiene, to say nothing of more complex tasks. Children whose families are impoverished often have little contact with the world beyond a four- or five-block radius from their homes—territory that may be unvaried, ugly, and possibly dangerous. They have few books or other cultural artifacts in their homes. Children in these neighborhoods experience a limited range of role models, and those who are negative models (criminals, drug-dealers, persons without jobs) are often quite visible. Parents in such circumstances have a difficult task in coping with the enormous stresses that they and their children face each day.

Clearly, socialization is a complex lifelong process, and whole courses have been devoted to understanding its many facets. The counselor is probably *not* one of the primary socializing agents in a child's life; parents and teachers are in much more influential positions because of their daily opportunities for teaching and modeling. Nevertheless, the counselor is in a position to observe deficits in socialization and to develop remedial plans to be implemented within counseling or in conjunction with parents and teachers.

One advantage of working with young children is that such deficits are fairly easy to moderate if they are identified early. Sometimes small interventions such as helping a child learn how to come to school clean yields big dividends in his or her relationships with others and in building self-esteem. A counselor can also serve as a resource to parents and teachers who are looking for ways to enrich the lives of children.

In the case that follows, the client was experiencing significant problems in her peer relationships that had the potential to spill over into her ability to succeed in school and to affect her future options. Her home was culturally different from the community where she lived and socioeconomically deprived. Furthermore, it was a single-parent home, where the caregiver was of a different gender than the client, a generation older than a typical parent, and limited in experiences about which the client needed to know. Though the client's circumstance may seem unusual, the case, like all others in this text, is based on the true facts of a real client's life (though identifying information has been disguised). We have chosen this case to illustrate how easily a negative outcome can be averted by augmenting the socialization process of a child who has missed important experiences.

Case: Robina

Robina was an 11-year-old African-American girl who was attending a predominantly white, affluent, suburban junior high school. She was an average student but was regarded as a "curiosity" by students and faculty alike. She used foul, openly sexual language with everyone, and her appearance was often bizarre. Her use of makeup made her look like she had on a mask.

A female counselor at the junior high school decided to try to help Robina. Soon the counselor discovered a huge deficit in Robina's socialization experiences. Since birth, she had lived with her father in a small run-down dwelling at the edge of the community. He was in his late sixties and seemed to have no means of support. He cared for Robina and provided for her to the best of his ability. However, he obviously was not equal to the task of guiding a pubescent girl. (It is hard to say why the school system had never provided any special services to Robina, except that she was an average student who caused no trouble until she began to mature physically.)

Robina quickly began to relate positively to the counselor (who was an attractive and well-dressed woman), and her hunger for information was enormous. Many of her early questions focused on "what is beautiful." She seemed to have almost no aesthetic sense of what looks good in clothing or makeup. She also seemed confused because of her brown skin, which the other girls in school did not have. The counselor spent several sessions using magazines with primarily African-American models to help Robina establish some sense of how she could look, and the girl's appearance changed practically overnight. She was highly motivated to look good, and with the help of some donated clothing and some information, she was able to appear and feel much more attractive.

Not surprisingly, her language also reflected a knowledge deficit. She had little sense of the meaning of some words she used and had no overt desire to be sexually involved with the people in her school. As she learned from the counselor the meanings others attached to what she said, she quickly began to refrain from lewd comments that had made her a laughingstock among students.

Fortunately, Robina was helped at a crucial time and was able to develop a degree of acceptance among her peers through her subsequent education, even in a school where she was racially different. She left school with the ingredients for a productive life.

Questions for Further Thought

1. The reasons for Robina's information deficits rested with her father's inability to provide needed information. Do you think this is a common problem? To what extent is it limited to parents who have suffered the effects of poverty?
2. What strengths do you observe in Robina?
3. Try to place yourself in the role of the counselor. What feelings might you have had in trying to relate to Robina's unsocialized and seemingly crude behavior? What knowledge might you have needed that you don't possess now?
4. In addition to the magazines that were used to talk about grooming and fashion, what other materials might you have used with Robina?

WORKING WITH PARENTS

Earlier sections of this chapter established that children are profoundly affected by the adults in their lives, particularly their parents. However, traditional notions of who is parenting children must be revised, and counselors need to be prepared to reach out to many adults in the role of child caretaker. The family is changing, and according to recent U.S. Census Bureau data, 41% of American children do not live in two-parent households, and nearly 1.5 million American children reside with grandparents without either parent present in the home (Fields & Caspar, 2001). In many instances, it may be difficult or impossible to help a child change without enlisting the support and cooperation of the natural parents, custodial single parent, and/or foster parents, stepparents, or grandparents. We will use the word *parents* in this discussion to mean those adults who are serving the parenting role for a given child, regardless of their exact relationship to one another or to the child.

The initial contact with parents may occur in a variety of ways. Sometimes a parent will recognize the need for help with his or her parenting behavior and will consult a counselor, ready to consider change. Occasionally, a parent will contact a counselor and request that the counselor change the child in some way, but will not take any responsibility for the child's problem. Typically, particularly in school settings, a counselor will first have contact with the child and will decide to involve a parent only after having acquired the child's perspective on his or her interactions with parents. Regardless of how a parent arrives at a counselor's office the first time, he or she needs to be respected and cared about just as surely as the child needs understanding. With few exceptions, parents care about their children and are trying to do what's right.

The process of effective parenting is complex, and adult status alone does not assure competence. Few parents have any training in the art of parenting, and most have learned from their own parents some problematic patterns of interacting. Sometimes parents able to provide a nurturing environment under favorable conditions are under stress because of work, money problems, health problems, marital conflict, or substance abuse by the parent or partner. Under such conditions, the children's needs may be neglected, and frustration may be vented on them. In cases where stress exceeds a parent's capacity to cope effectively, emotional disturbance may significantly debilitate any parenting competence, and children may become fixtures in the parent's maladaptive lifestyle.

There are a number of procedures for helping parents improve their parenting effectiveness. Perhaps the simplest intervention is consultation with a parent on an occasional basis to encourage supportive efforts and learn about the progress a family is making toward positive interaction. Sometimes parent groups are established to provide parenting education and to encourage parents to share their concerns and solutions with one another. Packaged training programs such as *Systematic Training for Effective Parenting* (Dinkmeyer, McKay, & Dinkmeyer, 1997) are excellent resources for counselors seeking to develop skills for consulting with parents. The focus of much parent consultation is the improvement of parent–child, sibling, and peer relationships; the development of more effective means of supporting the child's schooling; and the management of troublesome behavior.

Counseling with parents moves beyond educational efforts aimed at improving the management of children and attempts to address some of the parents' own behavioral and emotional problems. Counseling interventions with parents can range from counseling about situational stress (e.g., caring for an ill and aging parent) to marital counseling to psychotherapy. Often the focus moves away from the children to debilitating problems in other sectors of the parents' lives. Although school counselors engage in extensive consultation with parents, they typically refer parents who need counseling to mental health facilities. The following section discusses contributions that consulting with parents can make to the counselor's work with children.

As indicated earlier, the first consideration in consulting effectively with parents is to accept each parent as a person in need of some kind of assistance, not as a "bad" parent. Second, it is important to remember that all children initially had two parents and most still do, even if divorce or separation has occurred. It is important to learn how each parent is functioning in the family. Third, parents who have suffered stress within the parenting process frequently become neglectful about expressing affection toward their children. Finally, parents often need help understanding what their children are trying to accomplish by their behavior so that they can help their children get what they want in more acceptable ways.

Commonly the initial contact occurs with only one parent, usually the mother or other female caregiver if self-initiated. If a child has interaction with both parents or other adults have significant responsibility for caregiving, it is almost always desirable to request that the other parent or caregiver become involved in the consultation. Frequently, the parents have differing perceptions of their child, and one may be defeating the parenting efforts of the other. The mother may see her son's behavior as unruly and aggressive, and the father may think he's "just being a boy." The grandmother may tolerate virtually any behavior, and the grandfather may believe in strict control. One or the other parent may simply not pay much attention to what the child does. It is important to determine whether the parents are sufficiently reinforcing prosocial behavior and effectively punishing antisocial behavior (Patterson, 1982) while allowing sufficient latitude for normal experimentation.

Sometimes children become expert in playing one parent against the other. It is best to see all major caregivers to determine how much support each is currently providing to the child and what each parent's strengths may be. The counselor may be acting on bias if he or she accepts the views of one parent and rejects or ignores those of the other. Families function as systems in which the behaviors of each member influence the behaviors of all others. Therefore, each parent needs the support of the other parent to initiate change in the family, and chances for success are enhanced if both become involved in the consultation. When one parent has total responsibility for a child or when grandparents are assuming exclusive responsibility for child rearing, counselors must be attuned to the enormous stress that child rearing can mean for these individuals who may have no adult support or who may be weary and overwhelmed by the physical and emotional demands of raising a second generation of children.

Parents in blended families often have extra difficulty settling on their appropriate roles with the children. Whether the children were born to just one or to each of the adults, there is often the feeling that the birth parent has more rights and responsibilities with a given child than the stepparent does. Blended families work best when the parents become full partners in their interactions with each other and with the children. Otherwise, concerns about one parent feeling undermined by the other one and/or children playing one parent against the other can become extremely troublesome. It naturally takes time for parents and children to develop comfort with their roles when a blended family is formed, and many schools currently offer support groups for children with stepparents. For a fuller discussion of stresses and strategies for working with blended families, see Goldenberg and Goldenberg (1998).

Many parents make a serious error in seeking to get their children to behave in a desired way by withholding expressions of their love for the child. The child, feeling hurt by the parents' apparent lack of caring, becomes resistant to the parents' wishes. This results in further withholding of statements of caring. In many families, no one can remember the last time someone said something caring to another. Ironically, these breaks in affectional communication are often based on caring: it matters to the parent what the child does; it matters to the child what the parent thinks. It is often useful to point out to parents that someone has to break the standoff. Plans can be made to assure that both parents participate in reassuring the child of their love.

Finally, it is useful to help parents understand that children's behavior always has a purpose. Dinkmeyer, McKay, and Dinkmeyer (1997) suggest that children's misbehavior occurs to serve one of four purposes: seeking attention, seeking to control another (power), seeking to get even (revenge), or seeking to be excused from responsibility (giving up). A counselor can work with parents to help determine what the child wants and how to help the child make a place for himself or herself in a positive way. Through such intervention, often combined with continued counseling with the child, significant elements of the family system can be manipulated to support the child.

In the consultation process, the counselor begins with the assumption that the parents want to improve the nurturing environment for their child and that they have the capacity to do so. (If the assumption of capacity proves false, then parent counseling or marriage and family counseling may be required.) The focus of the consultation process is usually on the parent–child sibling and peer relationships, schoolwork, and misbehavior. Consultation helps parents to express their caring and to understand their children's motivations so that they can provide positive ways for the children to fulfill their needs. Inconsistent and ineffective parenting behaviors are identified and alternatives are planned, rehearsed, and reinforced.

SUMMARY

Counseling with children is based on the same three-stage process that is described in the earlier chapters of this book. However, children are developmentally different from adolescents and adults, and they are not as free as older clients to act on their own. The counselor must establish communication on the child's terms and enter the child's world of experience. The use of play media tends to elicit information from the child that helps the counselor to understand the child's experience. Assessing the locus and extent of the child's problem requires an understanding of child development and can be enhanced by the use of such techniques as the clinical interview, incomplete sentence blanks, and standardized tests. A child's dysfunction is often caused in part by lack of experience and deficits in abilities that are maturationally determined. Deficits can sometimes be reduced through socialization experiences that are planned as a part of counseling. In many instances, parents' help should be enlisted, and they often need consultation about how to be more supportive with their children while providing structure and setting expectations. Counselors also need to show empathy for the difficulties parenting presents, especially for the many adults who are raising children alone, in a blended family, or for a second time, and they need to be aware of community resources to support these adults' efforts to be effective parents.

≈≈≈ *DISCUSSION QUESTIONS* ≈≈≈

1. Most children become more comfortable with counseling once they get to know a counselor and get a better understanding of why they have been asked to attend counseling sessions. However, some children remain resistant to counseling even after several meetings with competent professionals and even when parents are interested in having their children come to counseling. How do you think counselors should respond in such situations? How would you balance the child's desires against the parents' wishes?

2. A few child counselors take exception to the view that structured competitive games are not appropriate for counseling children. If you were discussing this issue with a counselor who held that minority perspective, what position would you take? In other words, do you find the authors' arguments on this point convincing?

3. Counselors in schools and community settings are often pressured by time and budget to make assessments in the first sessions and to conduct counseling as briefly as possible. What unique difficulties do these pressures pose when working with young children?

4. Because children's problems often stem from deficits in parenting, from others' inadequacies rather than their own temperaments, child counselors often feel strong emotions about parents who are incompetent and bring suffering to children even if unintentional. Do child counselors need special skills or styles to cope with these strong emotions? Do you think child counselors are more vulnerable to burnout than adult counselors?

5. Barker recommends sharing information about diagnosis, progress, and length of counseling with parents but advises counselors to keep the

actual content of sessions with children confidential from parents. Do you agree with his recommendation? How would you respond to a parent who is demanding to have a full disclosure of all content in counseling with his or her child?

6. Describe which material in this chapter might be useful in counseling with a mentally retarded or developmentally delayed adult. Think about similarities and differences.

REFERENCES

Achenbach. T. M. (1991). *Manual for the Child Behavior Checklist/4–18 and 1991 Profile.* Burlington, VT: University of Vermont Department of Psychiatry.

American Psychiatric Association. (2000). *Diagnostic and statistical manual of mental disorders* (4th rev. ed.). Washington, DC: Author.

Bandura, A. (1977). *Social learning theory.* Englewood Cliffs, NJ: Prentice Hall.

Barker, P. (1990). *Clinical interviews with children and adolescents.* New York: W. W. Norton.

Brady, C. A., & Friedrich, W. N. (1982). Levels of intervention: A model for training in play therapy. *Journal of Clinical Child Psychology, 11,* 39–43.

Cox, M. V. (1992). *Children's drawings.* New York: Penguin Books.

Dinkmeyer, D., Sr., McKay, G. D., & Dinkmeyer, D., Jr. (1997). *The parent's handbook: Systematic training for effective parenting.* Circle Pines, MN: American Guidance Service.

Doll, B. (1996). Prevalence of psychiatric disorders in children and youth: An agenda for advocacy in school psychology. *School Psychology Quarterly, 11,* 20–47.

Erikson, E. H. (1993). *Childhood and society* (4th ed.). New York: W. W. Norton.

Fields, J., & Caspar, L. M. (2001). *America's families and living arrangements: March 2000.* Current Populations Reports, P20-537. U.S. Census Bureau Washington, DC.

Garbarino, J., Stott, F., & Faculty of the Erikson Institute. (1989). *What children can tell us: Eliciting, interpreting, and evaluating critical information from children.* San Francisco: Jossey-Bass.

Gilligan, C. (1993). *In a different voice: Psychological theory and women's development.* Cambridge, MA: Harvard University Press.

Goldenberg, H., & Goldenberg, I. (1998). *Counseling today's families.* Pacific Grove, CA: Brooks/Cole.

Goyette-Ewing, M. (2000). Children's after-school arrangements: A study of self-care and developmental outcomes. *Journal of Prevention and Intervention in the Community, 20,* 55–67.

Hall, T. M., Kaduson, H. G., & Schaefer, C. E. (2002). Fifteen effective play therapy techniques. *Professional Psychology: Research and Practice, 33,* 515–522.

Herjanic, B., & Reich, W. (1982). Development of a structured psychiatric interview for children: Agreement between child and parent of individual symptoms. *Journal of Abnormal Child Psychology, 10,* 307–324.

Kazdin, A. E., & Johnson, B. (1996). Advances in psychotherapy for children and adolescents: Interrelations of adjustment, development, and intervention. *Journal of School Psychology, 32,* 217–246.

Kohlberg, L. (1964). Development of moral character and moral ideology. In M. L. Hoff & L. W. W Hoffman (Eds.), *Review of child development research* (Vol. 1, pp. 383–342). New York: Russell Sage Foundation.

Kohlberg, L. (1981). *The philosophy of moral development: Moral stages and the idea of justice* (Vol. 1). San Francisco: Harper & Row.

Kottman, T. (2001). *Play therapy: Basics and beyond.* Alexandria, VA: American Counseling Association.

Landreth, G. L. (2001). *Play therapy: The art of the relationship.* Muncie, IN: Accelerated Development.

Lazarus, A. (1989). *The practice of multimodal therapy.* New York: McGraw-Hill.

Lazarus, A. (1990). Multimodal applications and research: A brief overview and update. *Elementary School Guidance and Counseling, 24,* 243–247.

Lebo, D. (1979). Toys for nondirective play therapy. In C. Schaefer (Ed.), *The therapeutic use of child's play.* Northvale, NJ: Jason Aronson.

Muro, J. J., & Dinkmeyer, D. C. (1977). *Counseling in the elementary and middle schools: A pragmatic approach.* Dubuque, IA: Wm. C. Brown.

Nelson, R. (1966). Elementary school counseling with unstructured play media. *Personnel and Guidance Journal, 45,* 24–27.

Nelson, R. (1991). Effective helping with young children. In S. Eisenberg & L. Patterson (Eds.), *Helping clients with special concerns* (pp. 287–305). Prospect Hts., IL: Waveland Press.

Nystul, M. S. (2003). *Introduction to counseling: An art and science perspective* (2nd ed.). Boston: Allyn & Bacon.

Orton, G. L. (1997). *Strategies for counseling with children and their parents.* Pacific Grove, CA: Brooks/Cole.

Patterson, G. R. (1982). *Coercive family process.* Eugene, OR: Castalia.

Piaget, J., & Inhelder, B. (1969). *The psychology of the child.* New York: Basic Books.

Prout, H. T. (1999). Counseling and psychotherapy with children and adolescents: An overview. In D. T. Brown & H. T. Prout (Eds.), *Counseling and psychotherapy with children and adolescents* (3rd ed., pp. 1–36). Brandon, VT. Child Psychology Publishing.

Rak, C. F. (2002). Heroes in the nursery: Three case studies in resilience. *Journal of Clinical Psychology, 58,* 247–260.

Rak, C. F., & Patterson, L. E. (1996). Promoting resilience in at-risk children. *Journal of Counseling and Development, 74,* 368–373.

Schaefer, C. E. (Ed.). (2003). *Play therapy with adults.* New York: Wiley.

Schaefer, C. E., & Cangelosi, D. (Eds.). (2002). *Play therapy techniques* (2nd ed.). Northvale, NJ: Jason Aronson.

Stewart, R. (2001). Adolescent self-care: Reviewing the risks. *Families in Society, 82,* 119–126.

Swales, T. (2001). Diagnostic evaluation of mental and emotional disorders of childhood. In E. R. Welfel & R. E. Ingersoll (Eds.), *Mental Health Desk Reference* (pp. 162–169). New York: Wiley.

Taylor, L., & Adelman, H. S. (2001). Enlisting appropriate parental cooperation and involvement in children's mental health treatment. In E. R. Welfel & R. E. Ingersoll (Eds.), *Mental health desk reference* (pp. 219–225). New York: Wiley.

Thompson, C. L., & Rudolph, L. B. (1996). *Counseling children* (4th ed.). Pacific Grove, CA: Brooks/Cole.

Welfel, E. R. (2002). *Ethics in counseling and psychotherapy: Standards, research, and emerging issues.* Pacific Grove, CA: Brooks/Cole.

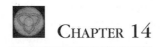 CHAPTER 14

WORKING WITH OLDER ADULTS

For purposes of this chapter, we have arbitrarily defined those over the age of 60 as older adults. Currently, the average life expectancy for U.S. residents at birth is 77.2 years (80.0 for European-American women, 74.8 for European-American men, 74.9 for African-American women, 66.2 for African-American men) (National Center for Health Statistics, 2002). On average men who reach the age of 60 can expect to live another 18.7 years, women, another 22.1 years (National Center for Health Statistics, 2002). Thus, our focus in this chapter will be directed toward the last one-quarter to one-third of the adult years. Daniel Levinson (Levinson, 1994; Levinson, Darrow, Klein, Levinson, & McKee, 1978) whose germinal studies of men's and women's lives stimulated and signaled new interest in the study of adult development, designated ages 60 to 65 as a boundary between middle and late adulthood. Age 60 is the time in life when many American adults are seriously considering or implementing retirement from active employment, and consequently they are establishing a new life structure for their remaining years. Warnick (1995) chooses age 60 as the demarcation for clients referred to as "third-age" clients.

Because life expectancies are based on an estimated median age at death, it is apparent the oldest of the old live much longer, into their 90s and beyond, and, of course, they face different issues from those who are 30 years younger. Finally, because of the differences in life expectancy by gender and race, the older adult population becomes increasingly female and European-American with advancing age.

We decided to include a chapter on working with older adults in this text because we recognize that older adults are an ever-increasing proportion of our population. The percentage of the population over 65 has increased from 5% in 1900 to 13% in 2001 and is projected to be 20% by the year 2030 (Qualls, Segal, Norman, Niederehe, & Gallagher-Thompson, 2002). The oldest-old (those over 75) constitute the fastest growing segment of the U.S. population with a projected increase to 8.9 million people by 2030 (U.S. Bureau of the Census, 2000). One in eight Americans is now an older adult, and that proportion will rise to one in four. In part the projected increase will occur when the "baby boom" cohort born between 1947 and 1967 arrives at the mature adult years early in the 21st century.

The increase in life expectancy has also created a profound change in the life experiences of the typical adult at age 60 compared to earlier times when this age meant limited life remaining. Put simply, there is another 25 years of living to do for most people. This life segment now includes an extended span of life after children are grown and a lengthy period of retirement. The systems of our society were built on the assumption of a shorter life span, and we are therefore still in the process of learning how to make the most of longer lives.

The counseling profession has recognized the need for special competencies in counseling older adults through the founding in 1986 of the Association for Adult Development and Aging as a division of the American Counseling Association, a national certification in gerontological counseling (by the National Board for Certified Counselors) in 1990, and a specialty emphasis in the preparation of counselors (by the Council for the Accreditation of Counseling and Related Educational Programs) in 1992 (Myers & Schwiebert, 1996). A fairly comprehensive literature (see references) on counseling with older adults has also developed over the past 20 years. Counseling for older adults is becoming increasingly available in senior centers, assisted living facilities, and community mental health centers. Because of problems of mobility, it is often necessary for counselors to travel to the home of the oldest and most infirm clients. Unfortunately, in spite of progress this population is still underserved by mental health professionals (Robb, Chen, & Haley, 2002). Nearly 20% of those in this age bracket have a diagnosable cognitive or psychological disorder (Gatz & Smyer, 2001), but they represent less than 2% of those seen by mental health professionals in private practice and less than 7% of those seen in community mental health settings (Robb et al., 2002). It is important to note, however, that when cognitive impairments are excluded from consideration, older adults experience fewer mental disorders than any other age group (American Psychological Association [APA] Working Group on the Older Adult, 1998).

In this chapter we address the content and process of counseling with older adults. First we consider the characteristics of older adults as clients, then the experiences of older adults that may create the need for counseling. Next we examine the "fit" of the generic model of counseling presented in Chapters 2 through 6 to the task of working with older adults and highlight counselor characteristics and counseling procedures that have particular value in working with older adults. Finally, we discuss the counselor's role in working with significant others in the lives of this population.

CHARACTERISTICS OF OLDER ADULTS AS CLIENTS

Willingness to Seek Counseling

At present, it can be stated that many older adults are a special case of the reluctant client. Warnick (1995) attributed the reluctance to participate to an "I can do it myself" attitude and the perception that going to counseling is a sign of weakness. Ganikos, Grady, and Olson (1979) stated that older adults "May believe their willingness to take part in the counseling process reveals to others a mental illness or a need to be told how to live their lives" (p. 177). Older adults may be particularly reluctant to discuss sexuality, finances, and personal inadequacies.

A brief review of the experiences of older adults reveals the origins of the reluctance of the current population of older people to seek counseling. First, counseling originated as a service for the young, those starting out in life and needing to find their way. Certainly one should not need such help at the mature age of 60 or 70 or beyond! Furthermore, in the world of older adults as they matured, people were far less likely to see professionals for help with health, emotional, financial, or other problems. People "toughed it out" on their own, perhaps with a little help from family or friends. Sex and finances were not usually discussed even with family and friends, and the only people who found their way into mental health situations were those with debilitating pathology. Finally, one of the anxious concerns of older people is the possibility of becoming incapable of managing for themselves and eventually losing their independence. Not surprisingly third-agers are reluctant to acknowledge inevitable age-related problems as they arise, and they may employ the defense of denial to assure themselves and others that everything is fine. When they do acknowledge problems, they tend to define them in medical rather than psychological terms and thereby may perceive the counselor as an extension of the physician and expect that he or she will approach the issues in ways similar to their physician. Frequently they are genuinely surprised at the suggestion of regular meetings for extensive discussion of the problem (Nordhus, Nielson, & Kvale, 1998).

In the near future, baby boomers, who have experienced a different world of social services throughout their lives, will be entering the third-age phase of their lives. Although a person's fear of losing independence by admitting problems is unlikely to change, it is reasonable to assume that members of this cohort will be more willing to participate in counseling and have a more accurate understanding of its dimensions and functions because they have been more willing to seek counseling in prior stages of their lives.

When older adults make the commitment to see a counselor and begin to understand the difference between speaking with a counselor and visiting a physician's office, they usually shed their reluctance rapidly and show tangible progress in resolving their concerns (APA Working Group on the Older Adult, 1998; Warnick, 1995). One factor accounting for the progress may be that our oldest clients become involved in microenvironments that include little contact with other people (Ganikos et al., 1979). Involvement with a caring counselor may be experienced as a welcome relief to a life of comparative solitude.

Physiological Changes That Affect Counseling

Among other characteristics to which counselors of older clients should attend are possible sensory, physical, and mental losses that are age related. Of particular importance are changes in hearing, vision, and memory. "Hearing impairment in older adults is often mild or moderate, but it is widespread. In 1990 48% of men and 37% of women had problems with hearing" (APA Working Group on the Older Adult, 1998, p. 415). For the younger old, the need for corrective lenses becomes nearly universal, and cataracts are experienced by 20 to 25% of those over 70. Typical visual changes include decreases in reading speed, difficulties in deciphering print in dim light, and problems in reading scrolling as on a computer screen (APA Working Group on the Older Adult, 1998). Even in instances where physical health is not the focus of counseling, counselors should provide for a comfortable environment and good acoustics, should make referrals if needed for sight and hearing aids, and may need to provide transportation or go to clients' homes. Barring serious illness, especially cardiovascular illness and Alzheimer's disease, most older adults maintain good mental ability until very late in life (Schaie & Willis, 1996) and can be expected as any other client to assume responsibility for the agenda of counseling and the decisions they need to make. They experience some decline in the speed with which they process information or divide attention between multiple simultaneous tasks but demonstrate no change in short-term memory or language ability. Long-term memory may show some change, but older adults experience no deficits in recognition of information when cued (APA Working Group on the Older Adult, 1998).

Variability of Individuals Within the Life-Stage

In Chapter 12 on counseling clients of diverse backgrounds, we cautioned that clients who belong to an identifiable group must still be understood as individuals who may exhibit only selected characteristics of the target group. This is especially true of older adult clients. We have already alluded to the difference between a 62-year-old employed person who may be active in community life, healthy, and mobile as contrasted with a 95-year-old in marginal health in a nursing home. Beyond these differences, Warnick (1995, p. 11) points out that "Because of the inequalities of life, how a person enters the third age varies tremendously." With the concise formula, "Difficult Childhood + Dysfunctional Adulthood = Vulnerable Third Age" (p. ii), he provides a basis for understanding that some people reach older adulthood far more equipped to deal with what life has to offer than others.

Change Potential

The theory of Erik Erikson (1963) describes eight stages of life, with tasks that must be at least partly accomplished at each stage for the person to function effectively at the next stage. During adolescence and early adulthood, effectively functioning people develop a sense of identity, an understanding of who they are and what they can do, and then affiliate with the love and work issues of the adult world during the intimacy stage. Those who are successful in accomplishing these two stages then reach the *generativity* stage of adulthood where their productivity peaks and where they focus on nurturing the next generation, both in their domestic and their public lives. According to Erikson, people who accomplish all these stages successfully can then move on to older adulthood, with a sense of *ego integrity*—a sense of peace in the perception that one has lived a worthy life. Erikson believed that those who do not succeed at least to some degree in each of the earlier stages (including those of childhood) will experience despair rather than ego integrity in their later years. Some older adults will still be finishing generativity tasks, as others will be moving toward ego integrity if their accomplishments earlier in life support such a transition.

The writings of Erikson and Warnick lend substance to the adage that "Old age is a reflection of young age" and lead to the conclusion that older clients possess varying amounts of what may be called "change potential" (Warnick, 1995, p. 21). Although it is the counselor's role to assess the change potential of each client as a part of the process of setting achievable goals with clients, we encourage counselors to remember the humanistic perspective that "older individuals have the capacity to develop psychologically right up to death, provided there is no mental deterioration. The older individuals get, the more self-actualized they become. Life is a dynamic, ever-changing and richly expanding experience" (O'Leary, 1996, p. 103). The myth that older adults cannot profit from counseling has long been laid to rest; counseling and psychotherapy have been consistently demonstrated as equally effective interventions for older adults as for those in other stages of life (Smyer, Zarit, & Qualls, 1990; Zarit & Knight, 1996). Counseling interventions can even substantially improve the quality of life for older adults with overwhelming problems such as Alzheimer's disease (Zarit & Zarit, 1998).

EXPERIENCES AND COUNSELING AGENDAS OF OLDER ADULTS

Normative Events

Across the period of 30 years or so (60–90+) that we refer to as older adulthood or the third age, there is a fairly predictable set of experiences that all of us encounter. These experiences come as the inevitable and irreversible consequence of biological, sociological, and psychological aging. A review of the current literature on the counseling issues of older adults, when summarized, produced essentially the same list that Robert Havighurst (1972) created and called the developmental tasks of late life:

- *Adjusting to decreasing physical strength and health.* By middle age most adults begin to notice that certain activities (like moving furniture or planting the garden) are not as easy as they once were and that recovery after strenuous activity takes longer. In older adulthood, declines in physical agility and sensory acuity accumulate so that simple tasks such as climbing stairs become a challenge for some. Sexual capacities decline, even though sexual functioning remains important to most. As systems of the body decline, we become more subject to acute illnesses such as colds and the flu and also acquire chronic afflictions such as cardiovascular disease, diabetes, and osteoporosis. As physical strength declines and illnesses accumulate, the older person's attention is inevitably drawn to contemplation of his or her own death.

- *Adjusting to retirement and reduced income.* Employment provides for a sense of accomplishment, an identity in the world of commerce, an arena for social discourse, a basis for structuring time into a daily routine, and money. It may also be physically and emotionally stressful and limit one's time and energy for other pursuits. In an idealized view, retirement may be seen as having completed life's work, freedom from required toil, opportunity to be free of a major responsibility and to pursue other interests, a time to reap the benefits of a life of working and saving. For some, many of these benefits, along with improved health and an opportunity to invest anew in relationships with spouse, children, and grandchildren, do in fact materialize and the period of adjustment is satisfying and produces growth. For others, the end of employment signals a sense of uselessness, a loss of personal identity that was intertwined with occupation, a feeling of having nothing of consequence to do and of time languishing, and a sense of loss of valued human contact. Needless to say, retirement is a life transition of major import that requires at the least a period of adjustment. For those unable to retire because of finances, or those forced to retire by action of an employer, a different but still important set of issues arises.

- *Adjusting to the death of a life partner or spouse.* For most older adults, this experience means the loss of a longtime companion who has chosen to share both bed and all existence. A household that was organized around the needs and interests of two individuals must now be reconfigured, with new daily routines and the absence of an in-house partner for social and sexual intercourse. Patterns of friendship that were previously configured around activities for couples do not work when one becomes single—and isolation from friends (after the funeral is over) adds to a profound sense of loneliness. All these changes in life routines are superimposed on and exacerbate the experience of grief that comes from the loss of the one person who has usually been the most important in one's life. Needless to say, in cases of second marriages, the duration of relationship is often shorter and there is not as much shared history. Still, many of the same adjustments are required, though perhaps to a lesser extent.

- *Establishing an explicit association with one's age group.* Throughout life, it is probably true that most of our friends are near our own age—at least roughly in the same cohort. However, with the withdrawal from work, and perhaps community involvements of one kind or another, opportunities to interact with younger people outside the family decrease. It is often helpful for older persons to seek new opportunities for social interaction with other seniors, sharing a common hobby, working on political issues of value to older citizens, or simply sharing recreational time together. Even so, it is a typical experience of the oldest of the old that their social circle of people their age diminishes, especially if they are still living in the community.

- *Adopting and adapting societal roles in a flexible way.* As older adults give up the roles of the generative period of midlife and younger old age, each person must decide what new roles are rewarding and what changes may be made in roles that will continue. One person may take on new responsibilities in a church, assume a role as an officer in his or her condominium association, or join a book club to expand intellectual horizons and gain social interaction. Another may assume an active role in grandparenting. Still others seem satisfied to devote their energies to the simple tasks of maintaining the comfort and quality of home life.

- *Establishing satisfactory practical living arrangement.* A major goal of most senior adults is to maintain the maximum independence possible in their living arrangements. For some, this means remaining in the home in which they have spent the majority of their adult lives. Others are ready to shed the responsibilities of maintaining a home that now has unused

and unwanted space. Still others recognize the need for
assistance with living that can be acquired only by moving in
with family or going to an assisted living facility. According to
APA's Working Group on the Older Adult (1998), only 1.4% of
adults ages 65 to 74 lived in nursing homes, only 6% of those
between 75 and 84 years did so, but nearly 24% of those over
85 resided in nursing homes. A small percentage lived with
relatives who are not spouses. Beginning with the young old,
most are living with their spouses, and moving to the oldest-
old, more than half of women are living alone, while most
men still have their spouses (due do the differences in life
span). Oftentimes, the need for a change in living
arrangements occurs as a result of an accident or catastrophic
illness of an older person, and the decision about where to
live adds to the stress of the event.

Predictable Counseling Agendas

Given these normative events of the third age, certain counseling agendas can also be expected to occur in response to these events. According to
McDonald and Haney (1988), Warnick (1995), and Sherman (1981), frequent
counseling agendas are as follows:

- *Decision making around adjustment problems associated with
  the transition events just described.* In some instances, clients
  will appear for counseling in a state of crisis, and the methods
  of crisis intervention presented in Chapter 11 will prevail.
  Elvira, age 86, who has been living alone in the home where
  she raised her family, contracts pneumonia and is hospitalized.
  Upon release from the hospital, she requires some care and
  her two children live in other states. Does she go temporarily
  to a nursing home with the hope of returning to her own
  home, or does she respond to her daughter's wish for her to
  enter an assisted living facility near the daughter's home?
- *Issues of search for identity and meaning.* Older adults may
  need to build satisfying new identities as older persons, and
  they often need help in understanding and accepting the value
  of their earlier life accomplishments. Harvey, who was a
  maintenance supervisor in a steel mill, was forced to retire at
  age 62 due to a reorganization at the plant. Because his job
  had been central to his identity, he initially felt that he had
  been "cast out like yesterday's newspaper." He quickly took a
  part-time job as a school bus driver, but soon found that the
  work seemed "trivial" and that the schedule was inconvenient.

After a discussion with a counselor at the senior center, Harvey decided to volunteer as a Meals-on-Wheels deliverer. Though this still required a fixed schedule, it did not include early morning work, and it provided for meaningful contact with other older adults. Harvey also began to take an active mentoring role with his grandchildren, especially a learning-disabled preadolescent grandson. Over time, with occasional discussions with a counselor, he transferred the generativity of his job to generativity in these new roles. Eventually, he gave up the Meals-on-Wheels activity, as his own aging made it more difficult, and moved into a life review process where his new role as the family elder was seen as a satisfying outgrowth of his move from his career.

- *Issues of anxiety and stress, related to the losses of later life, particularly the sense of losing control over one's life.* John, at age 80, lived with his wife in a small town where he was able to drive his car to church, business, and shopping, until he failed his eye test for his driver's license renewal. Initially he was fearful that he and his wife would have to enter a senior living facility because his wife did not drive and he had no idea how to acquire the services he needed. The anxiety was so consuming that he was unable to even consider that he could get help. With a counselor's help, he was able to find stores that would deliver groceries, mail-order alternatives for some of the couple's shopping needs, and friends who would provide transportation to church and for special needs that he could not meet on his own (e.g., medical appointments).

- *Depression and demoralization.* Dorothea, aged 70, lived in a quality senior living facility with nice surroundings and a well-designed program of activities. However, she engaged in few of the activities and said she "didn't care about all the fancy decoration." Because she was nearly blind she felt little interest in her physical surroundings. Except for one friend, on whom she depended for many small services (like making her bed and keeping track of her clothes), Dorothea minimized her contact with other residents. When her children visited, she went into angry tirades about why they had abandoned her to "strangers" and thus gained no pleasure from their visits. She spent many hours crying and sitting in her room alone. Always a person who saw the glass as "half empty" rather than "half full," Dorothea regarded her loss of vision as an "ultimate insult" and sank into an extended depression from which she has not recovered.

- *Substance abuse, which may be a pattern carried over from midlife or may be a new maladaptive response to the pressures of old age.* Alcohol is probably the most frequent problem, but abuse of prescription medication (or erroneous dosages of needed medication) can result in blunting both affect and cognition in older adults, creating a condition that resembles senile dementia. Anne was typical of many older adults. She had always been a social drinker and was basically a happy and sociable person. As it became harder for her to do such things as preparing food for guests, she became anxious when she would have people in. She found that she could ease her anxiety and feel more competent if she had some wine while preparing a meal. As time progressed, she used alcohol to medicate her anxiety more and more, until finally she would be drunk when her guests arrived on many occasions. Though not addicted to alcohol, it was interfering with her life, and she needed help in managing the problem. A frequent pattern in the abuse of medication (not Anne's problem) emerges from the fallacy that if one pill makes you feel better, two or three might make you feel really well. This is particularly problematic with medications that have psychoactive main effects or side effects like sedation, anxiety reduction, or mood enhancement.

It is apparent from the description of the life experiences of older adults that counselors working with these clients will face different issues than counselors of younger persons. Although issues of problem solving, meaning and identity, and the affective disorders are not unique to older adults, these issues include new fabric that is particular to the experiences of third-age adults.

COUNSELING PROCEDURES WITH OLDER ADULTS

Working with the Generic Model

Several authors (Ganikos, Grady, & Olsen, 1979; McDonald & Haney, 1988; Myers & Schwiebert, 1996; Sherman, 1981; Thorman, 1995; Warnick, 1995; Wolinsky, 1990) described supportive counseling that emphasizes coping strategies, essentially the generic model presented in this text, to be a primary approach for working with the adult over the age of 60. As with younger clients, the core conditions of the counseling relationship create an environment that encourages the client to disclose concerns and to explore the bases for those concerns as well as the margins of freedom the client has to initiate change. Planfulness and decision making address the variety of adjustment problems that are precipitated by the aging process. The generic model helps older clients to stabilize self-esteem, sustain morale, and master their problems.

To be effective when counseling older adults, counselors must first be clear about their attitudes toward third-agers. Before continuing with this chapter, take a few minutes to consider the following exercise.

Exercise

The purpose of this exercise is for you to take stock of your experiences with older adults and to surface attitudes and beliefs toward older adults that might help or hinder you in counseling with this population:

1. Write down the names of up to five people over age 60 with whom you have regular contact or a somewhat intimate relationship (e.g., a parent or grandparent whom you don't see all the time but who is important in your life). What relationship do you have with each? If you do not have five such relationships, reflect on why that might be so.
2. Granting that certain individuals may provoke different attitudes and feelings, do you have generally positive or negative responses as you think about the third-agers on your list. Write down a list of adjectives that would best describe this population. If there is a person (or persons) who are different from your general description, write down a list of adjectives that describes him or her. Why do you think this person is different?
3. When you think of your experiences with older adults, do you find that you admire their accomplishments and wisdom? Do you become impatient with their plodding pace and caution? Both? Do you have other reactions?
4. When was the last time that you engaged in a one-on-one activity with an older adult? What did you do? Who initiated the activity? Did you enjoy it?
5. Would you see it as a positive if your caseload in a counseling position included adults in this age group? Why or why not?

If you found that you admire older adults and enjoy spending time with them, it is likely that you will be interested in adapting counseling methods to work with this group. If you found that you have some negative attitudes about older adults, you are not alone in that perspective, but it raises questions about whether you can be effective with this population unless your attitudes change. Warnick (1995) observed that "Some therapists believe that third-age clients cannot be counseled effectively. . . . They question expending energy on clients whose life expectancy is so short. They believe that working with this age group is not only difficult but senseless" (p. 3). Clearly persons with such negative attitudes about third-agers would fail the test of having positive regard for their clients. If they spent time with older clients, they would discourage their clients and undermine their ability to cope with life. Sherman (1981) emphasized that counseling must be "optimistic about the innate capacity of older persons to prevent or overcome the demoralization that comes from these losses and traumas" (p. 2) of aging, without denying the inevitability of such losses taking place. Ageism can be defined as an attitude toward older adults that stereotypes them as rigid, slow, incapable, and cranky. Clearly a counselor with ageist attitudes is as destructive with older clients as a racist would be with ethnically diverse populations.

Familiarity with the experiences of older adults serves as a basis for empathic responding by the counselor. One's sensitivity to the life events of third-age clients can be enhanced by studying the adult development and gerontology literature, and personal experience with older individuals is good preparation for working with older persons as clients. As with other special populations of clients, one need not have actually "walked in the shoes" as an older person to respond with empathy, but one must make an effort to learn what it is like to be in "those shoes." In our ageist society, it is not uncommon for young people to disregard third-agers, to avoid circumstances where they will spend time with old people, and even to ignore the older people in their own families. A counselor who wants to work with the older adults is not likely to have such attitudes in the first place, but it is still desirable to spend time with the oldest members in one's own family and to arrange field experiences and internships where exposure to the full range of aging issues can be observed. Unintentional ageism can be just as destructive as deliberate acts of discrimination.

Remembering that many older adults are initially reluctant to participate in counseling, it is especially important for the counselor to offer them a genuine welcome to the counseling process, to show respect for privacy keeping the length of lead comfortable for the client, and to provide clear structure about the nature of counseling. For many, counseling will not have been a part of their earlier experiences and their readiness to engage in personal conversation will depend on the effectiveness of the orientation provided by the counselor. Warnick (1995) observed that older clients tend to be cooperative and to work hard on their issues once they get beyond an initial reticence, perhaps a function of habits of cooperation with authority figures that were ingrained in their generation.

The multitheoretical integrative model of counseling may be seen as a primary tool for addressing the many adjustment issues that older people face due to the transitions of aging—changes in health status, problems with mobility and transportation, needs to alter living arrangements, losses of partner and age mates, altered relationships (increasing dependency) with adult children and other family members, financial worries, and so on. Often the catharsis occurring in the initial disclosure stage of counseling provides some relief of anxieties, based on the notion that a problem shared is a problem halved. The caring attention of the counselor who accepts the problems as real and important validates the experience of the older client.

During the in-depth exploration phase of counseling, both the counselor and the client gain insight into the duration and causes of the presenting problems and begin to develop goals for solving them. In setting goals, it becomes important to recognize that lifelong dysfunctional patterns (e.g., diagnosed emotional and personality disorders, the tendency to catastrophize about manageable and predictable life events, quarrelsome interpersonal relationships) are difficult to change in response to late-life counseling. Goals are best focused on specific decision-making and relationship issues and their affective corollaries, where the counselor's powers of analysis (ego function) can be "loaned to" the client and serve as the model for addressing present and future dilemmas. According to Sherman (1984),

> The techniques of interpretation and confrontation are played down in favor of supportive techniques so as to help the older person sustain remaining strengths and relieve inner and outer stress. The supportive techniques, therefore, consist of encouragement, warmth, positive reinforcement of coping efforts, promotion of realistic hope, and acceptance of some regressive and dependent behavior. (p. 71)

Because many of the situational problems of third-agers may be ameliorated by access to housing, health care, financial, transportation, and other community services, counselors working with older people also need knowledge of sources of such assistance. In the third stage of counseling, when action plans are at the top of the agenda, this knowledge provides alternatives for consideration in the solution of practical problems. Older clients who engage in a process that helps them manage their lives better, even with the losses associated with aging, gain an increased sense of an internal locus of control over their lives and greater satisfaction that their behaviors are appropriate for their time in life.

Given the desire to work with older adults, an awareness of any age bias, familiarity with the experiences of aging in the last third of life, and knowledge of community resources, counselors should be able to employ the generic model of counseling to the benefit of older clients. The next section describes additional procedures or particular emphases that may be of particular special assistance to older clients.

Special Emphases and Useful Techniques for Third-Age Clients

Challenging Self-Defeating Myths. Many people arrive at the door to later life with incorrect (and ageist) expectations about what is to come (Thorman, 1995). The inevitability myth "assumes that all older people are destined to be physically and mentally impaired, and the changes that accompany old age are inevitable and cannot be reversed" (p. 50). Counselors can provide the correct alternative picture that most older adults have adequate health and physical stamina to enjoy life, retain their ability to learn, and adapt well to the real changes that occur. It is also untrue that "people withdraw from active pursuits in old age and await the end of life" or that they become asexual. Withdrawal from all active pursuits and loss of sexual interest are more correctly seen as dysfunctional responses to aging. Although it is true that some disengagement from social interactions may be seen as normal, especially with the oldest individuals (Cumming & Henry, 1961), seniors who remain active tend to retain their physical, mental, and sexual capacities. "Use it or lose it" is a useful cliché in working to reframe older people's views about their potentials. Of course, all people of any age have periods when things may not be going well, and it is important to pay attention to real difficulties. The purpose of debunking myths is to reduce the negative potential of a self-fulfilling prophecy.

Clarifying Identity and Bolstering Self-Esteem. Identity and self-esteem issues for older adults can be seen to include perceptions of their present experiences and retrospective assessment of their lives to date. Some older adults have difficulty seeing value in their current lives because our culture places major emphasis on our function (occupation and useful activities) as a basis for identity and meaning, so much so that one of the first elements of introducing oneself to others is by stating one's occupation. Sherman (1981) has observed that a functionalistic self-evaluation is not "seen as a valid or an emotionally sound standard for self-evaluation, particularly for older adults" (p. 5). Beginning with an alternative view that the purpose of life is to gain enjoyment and satisfactions for oneself and loved ones, third-age clients can be helped to build new life structures around activities that fulfill aesthetic and familial goals. Acceptance of the idea that ones required work in life is over and that pleasures have been earned is the first step for many.

According to Erikson (1963), life review, where one looks back over life to gain a sense of closure, of ego integrity, is a spontaneous activity of older adults. Norris (1986) suggests that reminiscing with older clients facilitates the life review process. Reminiscencing tends to highlight older peoples' assets rather then their disabilities and helps them to recognize and value their individuality and identity. "Counselors using life review may (also) be able to help older persons identify events that have been remembered negatively, and to reframe those events in a positive manner so that a positive sense of ego integrity can be achieved" (Myers & Schwiebert, 1996). Reminiscing is usually an enjoyable and stimulating process for those over 60, who become reaffirmed in the meanings of their lives as they recount the past. Scrutton (1989) pointed out that there is also a diagnostic value in reminiscence that "can provide the counselor with invaluable insight into the nature and quality of the counselee's early formative years, which can, to a large extent, determine the way people live their later lives" (p. 103).

Reframing Dysfunctional Thoughts. It is a fact that later adulthood is a period of *senescing,* where a series of incremental losses is a normative human experience. Some inconveniences and heartaches inevitably accompany such losses, and a sense of regret is a normal response. A certain percentage of third-agers, however, lose a sense of proportion about their experiences and begin to catastrophize. Instead of viewing the changes as predictable obstacles or expected inconveniences, they see them as awful, unfair, and possibly even the fault of family members who are seen as intentionally contributing to their demise. Anxiety responses, including full-blown anxiety attacks and phobias, may result from feelings of loss of control. Approximately 6% of older adults appear to suffer from anxiety disorders with generalized anxiety as the most common of these problems (APA Working Group on the Older Adult, 1998). More often, depression and a deep sense of demoralization sets in, extinguishing most of the pleasure in life. Depression is the single most common problem that can emerge in late life, but it is more likely to be expressed in symptoms of anxiety, agitation, memory problems, and bodily complaints than as sadness (APA Working Group on the Older Adult, 1998). At its deepest levels, depression in the older person shares many symptoms with dementia (a loss of mental acuity and personality definition due to brain cell loss). Diagnosis of which condition exists can be difficult. Both are characterized by sadness, failure to engage in meaningful activity, and sleep and eating disturbances. A detailed description of the process of reframing negative thoughts is beyond the scope of this chapter, but it consists of helping clients recognize the errors in their thought processes and substitute more effective beliefs. It is a process of helping the client see a half-full rather than a half-empty glass. The cognitive and behavioral methods referenced in Chapter 10 provide an introduction to cognitive reframing strategies. Antidepressant medications and tranquilizers are sometimes an adjunct to counseling in the treatment of depression and anxiety disorders with aging clients. The risk of suicide is high for older adults with depression, especially high for older European-American men who live alone (APA Working Group on the Older Adult, 1998).

Substance Abuse. With older adults, substance abuse may be a continuing problem carried on from midlife, or it may be a new problem resulting from attempts to self-medicate the stresses of old age. Approximately 1% of older women and 2% to 5% of older men abuse substances or are chemically dependent (APA Working Group on the Older Adult, 1998). Alcohol is the most commonly abused substance as is true with younger people, but sedating medications are also a problem, especially when they are used in combination with alcohol. The effects of substance abuse can blunt the motivation, senses, and coping behaviors of older adults. Counselors should seek specific training in substance abuse work or have ready referral resources at their disposal. The abuse of prescription medications presents some special considerations, but at the fundamental level, the issue is still that a substance ingested to promote better feelings can result in disabling main and side effects, as well as addiction.

Grief Work. Although it is true that anyone at any age will experience grief at the loss of loved ones, grieving is an especially important concern in the third age. According to Wolinsky (1990, p. 56), "There is a tendency to underestimate the distress and disability caused by grief reactions, as well as their duration." With older adults, the problem is compounded by multiple losses of age mates, and, of course, the loss of spouse or life partner is increasingly likely with increasing age. "As people grow older, the ego gradually loses its capacity to refuel itself, and multiple losses limit opportunities for refueling" (Wolinsky, 1990, p. 56).

Kubler-Ross (1969), who has been one of the most influential writers about the grieving process, indicated that there are fairly predictable responses that a dying person has to the knowledge of his or her own impending death: denial, anger, attempts to bargain, depression, and finally acceptance. Grieving persons are thought to mirror these reactions, but to lag behind the dying person in the timing of the reactions. It is also true that individuals will skip some of the responses, or that they may be in a slightly different order. The important point is that these are defensive responses to ease the impact of the death that must be experienced before the death is accepted and integrated into the client's history. Defenses are normal and recovery time is necessary; attempting to rush it to closure is likely to be counterproductive.

According to Warnick (1995), there are several tasks a client must complete in order to deal with grief:

- Accept the reality of the loss
- Experience the pain and grief
- Adjust to an environment in which the deceased is missing
- Withdraw emotional energy from the old relationship and reinvest it in another relationship or other activities

Many older individuals go through a normal grieving process without professional counseling, simply taking their time and interacting with other caring individuals who are a part of their lives. Those who seek counseling can be helped to understand what is known about the grieving process as a way of normalizing their own feelings and beginning to think about the steps they need to take to move on. Warnick (1995) lists several thoughts about grief that may encourage the client to face and adjust to the loss:

- Grief is the price we pay for loving
- To bury grief, take little steps forward
- The laws of nature do not protect good people
- Vulnerability to death is one of life's conditions
- After living through the death of a loved one, we fear the future less

In time the grieving person's fond memories of the lost person will begin to overtake the sense of loss. Periods of sadness persist, but the ability to go on with living is restored. Normal grieving usually requires 1 to 2 years and probably should not be considered exceptional until after the second anniversary of the death.

WORKING WITH FAMILIES OF OLDER CLIENTS

Some older adults, especially the oldest of the old, become sufficiently disabled, physically or emotionally, that they require caretaking from others, usually a spouse or adult children, but sometimes more distant relatives or other interested parties. Just as is true with children, there are dependencies on the caretakers, and fostering positive interactions with the caretakers is desirable. There are important differences, though, between the dependencies with children and with older adults. We know from the beginning that an infant will be dependent and that we will have major responsibilities to ensure his or her safety and development. With third-agers, neither the adult nor the caretaker is sure that help will be needed, and there is a fine line in determining when an older adult is no longer competent to handle safety and quality of life questions for himself or herself. "Ethical dilemmas occur most often when an older person's choices or wishes are significantly different from choices proposed as the 'best option' by the counselor and or the older person's family or service providers" (Myers & Schweibert, 1996, p. 192). With the goal of achieving the best quality of life possible for the client, the counselor should consider the capacity of significant others to help, their coping skills when balanced against other responsibilities (often including their own dependent children), and the wishes of the older client himself or herself. There are never easy answers to ethical dilemmas, but the material in Chapter 6 on ethics can by applied in working with older adults.

Elder abuse, unfortunately, must be taken into consideration when working with older, and particularly infirm, clients (Welfel, Danzinger, & Santoro, 2000). Forms of abuse can include all those perpetrated against children, including neglect, physical abuse, psychological abuse, and sexual abuse, as well as financial exploitation. Often the abuse is an ineffective and inappropriate act of desperation on the part of an overstressed care-taker, who may be trying to control disruptive or inconvenient behaviors of the older person. More sinister motives are also possible. On the one hand, the counselor ethically should attempt to consult with caregivers and create the best possible conditions for the safety and care of the older client; on the other hand, legally, most states have compulsory laws that require reporting of elder abuse to the authorities. When working with older adults and their families, this obligation to report should become a part of the limit to confidentiality discussed with the client at the beginning of a relationship (Welfel, Danzinger, & Santoro, 2000). Nevertheless, older adults have a right to confidential communication, which precludes disclo-sure to family of information the client wishes to keep private as long as the client's safety is protected.

Case of Marie

Marie, an 84-year-old widow, lived alone in the apartment to which she had moved when her husband died 17 years ago. The apartment had been chosen because it was close to shopping and church, to which Marie was able to walk in good weather. Her support system included a nephew who lived in a neighboring town and a daughter of a former neighbor, each of whom visited Marie about twice a month. The nephew or his wife provided transportation for medical care and assured that necessary shopping was done, especially in bad weather. A friend who lived in the same apartment building died in the fall before Marie began to experience problems.

As the winter progressed, Marie had several respiratory ailments, and she began having difficulty with eating and sleeping. A person who had always been quietly accepting of the losses of old age, Marie was now often tearful when visited by the nephew and the former neighbor. Finally, late one evening, Marie called her nephew and asked to be taken to the hospital because she felt too ill to be alone. Marie was hospitalized for observation of her digestive ailment, and during her hospital stay she broke her hip while going to the restroom.

Following surgery to repair the hip, Marie showed little interest in recovery, was uncharacteristically rude to caretakers and visitors, complained of nausea and intestinal cramping, and ate very little. Her internist requested a psychiatric consultation, and major depression was diagnosed. Marie was transferred to the psychiatric unit of the hospital for recovery where treatment consisted of the antidepressant medication and daily counseling sessions.

At first Marie was unmotivated to talk with the counselor, but as the medication began to elevate her mood, she became more welcoming of the counselor and began the initial disclosure of her fears. The loss of her last friend from her age cohort had saddened her and caused her to realize her own frailty. When she began experiencing routine symptoms of a cold, she became convinced that she would not recover, and her lack of interest in food and her digestive problems soon followed. Marie recognized that she was approaching the end of her capacity to live independently, and this had further diminished her already depressed mood. The crisis of fear, physical illness, and loneliness had prompted her call for help to go to the hospital. Her crisis was only exacerbated by her fall and the loss of mobility.

Marie seemed to be encouraged by the counselor's persistent interest in her dilemma and began to think again about a future. Counseling continued when Marie was moved from the psychiatric unit to the nursing care unit to begin physical rehabilitation of her ability to walk. At about the same time, Marie began to talk about the importance of eating well to regain her strength and even ate things she had never particularly liked if she thought they would be good for her. Periodic contact between the counselor and her nephew occurred with Marie's consent and participation, as the nephew was her financial adviser.

When Marie recovered enough to be released from the nursing unit, she did not feel ready to return to her apartment. She decided to move to an assisted living unit that was attached to the hospital and nursing facility where she had now resided for 6 months, but still retained possession of her apartment with the intent of eventually returning there. At about this same time, her antidepressant medication was tapered off, and her mood remained stable. The counselor continued to provide supportive conversations, now on a weekly basis, for the next 3 months. At the end of that time, Marie reluctantly decided to give up her apartment and began to see a satisfactory future in the assisted living facility. She decided with her nephew's help that she could afford a private room and would eat in the common dining facility. Marie is now living stably, has resumed reading and needlework, and participates in planning activities for residents of her community. She enjoys new friendships with the other aging residents. Her health is good, and she is now able to walk without the assistance of a cane or walker. She proudly describes herself as one of the most capable of the residents. The counselor has discontinued treatment but makes a periodic brief visit when she is in the building to see other clients.

Questions for Further Thought

1. Marie's crisis seems to have resulted from cumulative losses that eventually overcame her coping abilities. Enumerate the losses you believe she experienced.
2. Based on the limited information you have available, what personality characteristics do you believe may have contributed to Marie's difficulties?
3. Can you envision ways in which Marie's crisis might have been prevented?
4. Besides the antidepressant medication, Marie's treatment consisted mainly of a supportive relationship and help with making some difficult decisions. What else might have been done to assist Marie?
5. What would be your prognosis for Marie's degree of satisfaction over the course of her remaining years?

SUMMARY

Older adults are an ever-increasing presence in our society due to increases in human longevity. Many of the institutions and customs of our society were built around the expectation that old age would be an exceptional experience, and thus we are still learning how to accommodate an average length of life of 77 years or more. There are predictable transitions that occur in late life and certain predictable counseling agendas as a result: adjustment problems, meaning and identity issues, affective disorders, and substance abuse. The generic model of counseling is applicable to older adults, and several specialized skills dealing with meaning in current living, life review, grieving, and cognitive restructuring are presented. Counselors are encouraged to maintain positive collaborations with families of older clients when those families are in a caretaking role. Though gerontological counseling is an emerging specialty, counselors in general practice will likely see increasing numbers of adults at this stage of life as their numbers in the population continue to increase and as new cohorts more accustomed to using human services enter the ranks of the third age. Getting older is getting better.

≈≈≈ *DISCUSSION QUESTIONS* ≈≈≈

1. The reluctance toward seeking counseling felt by many in the current generation of older adults is likely to be less prominent as baby boomers reach the third age. What new challenges do you think this next cohort of older adults will present to counselors?
2. Based on your own experience, how true do you believe the formula Difficult Childhood + Dysfunctional Adulthood = Vulnerable Third Age is for identifying older adults who may be at risk for mental health problems? Do you think the third-agers in this group would also be more vulnerable to elder abuse or neglect?
3. Older adults are coping with many issues of loss, both of people whom they have valued and of some of their physical capabilities, which present them with stressors. We also know that as a group older adults who escape dementia and other cognitive problems are less likely to be counted among those who are diagnosed with psychological disorders. How do you reconcile these seemingly contradictory experiences?
4. What do you think makes older European-American males who have been widowed so vulnerable to late-life depression when their female counterparts experience no increase in depressive episodes late in life even though they are more likely to survive a life partner's death?
5. Reminiscing and life review have been demonstrated to be effective counseling approaches with older adults? What value, if any, might these approaches hold in working with adults at midlife or even at younger ages?
6. Because the population of those over 60 is increasing so substantially, should all counselors be mandated to obtain training in effective counseling with older adults?

REFERENCES

American Psychological Association Working Group on the Older Adult. (1998). What practitioners should know about working with older adults. *Professional Psychology: Research and Practice, 29,* 413–427.

Cumming, E., and Henry, W. (1961). *Growing old: The process of disengagement.* New York: Basic Books.

Erikson, E. (1963). *Childhood and society* (2nd ed.). New York: W. W. Norton.

Ganikos, M. L., Grady, K. A. & Olson, J. B. (1979). *Counseling the aged: A training syllabus for educators.* Falls Church, VA: American Personnel and Guidance Association.

Gatz, M., & Smyer, M. (2001). Mental health and aging at the onset of the 21st century. In J. E. Birren & K. W. Schaie (Eds.), *Handbook of the psychology of aging* (5th ed., pp. 523–544). San Diego, CA: Academic Press.

Havighurst, R. J. (1972). *Developmental tasks and education* (3rd ed.). New York: McKay.

Kubler-Ross, E. (1969). *On death and dying.* New York: Macmillan.

Levinson, D. J. (1994) *The seasons of a woman's life.* New York: Knopf.

Levinson, D. J., Darrow, C., Klein, E., Levinson, M., & McKee, B. (1978). *The seasons of a man's life.* New York: Knopf.

McDonald, P. A., & Haney, M. (1988). *Counseling the older adult.* New York: Lexington Books.

Myers, J. E., & Schweibert, V. L. (1996). *Competencies for gerontological counseling.* Alexandria, VA: American Counseling Association.

National Center for Health Statistics. (2002). *National vital statistics reports: Vol. 51, No. 3.* Hyattsville, MD: U.S. Department of Health and Human Services, Center for Disease Control and Prevention.

Nordhus, I. H., Nielson, G. H., & Kvale, H. (1998). Psychotherapy with older adults. In I. H. Nordhus, G. R. VandenBos, S. Berg, & P. Fromholt (Eds.), *Clinical geropsychology* (pp. 289–313). Washington, DC: American Psychological Association.

Norris, A. (1986). *Reminiscences with elderly people.* London: Winslow Press.

O'Leary, E. (1996). *Counseling older adults: Perspectives, approaches, and research.* London: Chapman and Hall.

Qualls, S. H., Segal, D. L., Norman, S., Niederehe, G., & Gallagher-Thompson, D. (2002). Psychologists in practice with older adults: Current patterns, sources of training and need for continuing education. *Professional Psychology: Research and Practice, 33,* 435–442.

Robb, C., Chen, H., & Haley, W. E. (2002). Ageism in mental health and health care: A critical review. *Journal of Clinical Geropsychology, 8,* 1–12.

Schaie, W. K., & Willis, S. L. (1996). *Adult development and aging* (4th ed.). New York: Harper Collins.

Scrutton, S. (1989). *Counseling older people: A creative response to ageing.* London: Edward Arnold.

Sherman, E. (1981). *Counseling the aging: An integrative approach.* New York: The Free Press.

Sherman, E. (1984). *Working with older adults: Cognitive and phenomenological approaches.* Boston: Kluwer-Nijhoff Publishing.

Smyer, M. A., Zarit, S. H., & Qualls, S. H. (1990). Psychological intervention with the aging individual. In J. E. Birren and K. W. Schaie (Eds.), *Handbook of the psychology of aging* (pp. 375–403). New York: Academic Press.

Thorman, G. (1995). *Counseling older adults.* Springfield, IL: Charles C. Thomas.

U.S. Bureau of the Census. (2000, September 7). *National population projections.* Retrieved June 17, 2002, from www.census.gov/populations/www/projections/natproj.html.

Warnick, J. (1995). *Listening with different ears: Counseling people over sixty.* Fort Bragg, CA: QED Press.

Welfel, E. R., Danzinger, P., & Santoro, S. (2000). Mandated reporting of maltreatment of older adults: A primer for counselors. *Journal of Counseling and Development, 78,* 284–292.

Wolinsky, M. A. (1990). *A heart of wisdom: Marital counseling with older and elderly couples.* New York: Bruner/Mazel.

Zarit, S. H., & Knight, B. G. (1996). *A guide to psychotherapy and aging: Effective clinical interventions in a life-stage context.* Washington, DC: American Psychological Association.

Zarit, S. H., & Zarit, J. (1998). *Mental disorders in older adults: Fundamentals of assessment and treatment.* New York: Guilford.

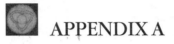

APPENDIX A

AMERICAN COUNSELING ASSOCIATION CODE OF ETHICS AND STANDARDS FOR PRACTICE (1995)

PREAMBLE

The American Counseling Association is an educational, scientific and professional organization whose members are dedicated to the enhancement of human development throughout the life span. Association members recognize diversity in our society and embrace a cross-cultural approach in support of the worth, dignity, potential, and uniqueness of each individual.

The specification of a code of ethics enables the association to clarify to current and future members, and to those served by members, the nature of the ethical responsibilities held in common by its members. As the code of ethics of the association, this document establishes principles that define the ethical behavior of association members. All members of the American Counseling Association are required to adhere to the Code of Ethics and the Standards of Practice. The Code of Ethics will serve as the basis for

processing ethical complaints initiated against members of the association.

SECTION A: THE COUNSELING RELATIONSHIP

A.1. Client Welfare

a. Primary Responsibility.
The primary responsibility of counselors is to respect the dignity and to promote the welfare of clients.

b. Positive Growth and Development.
Counselors encourage client growth and development in ways that foster the clients' interest and welfare; counselors avoid fostering dependent counseling relationships.

c. Counseling Plans.
Counselors and their clients work jointly in devising integrated, individual counseling plans that offer reasonable promise of success and are consistent with abilities and circumstances of clients. Counselors

and clients regularly review counseling plans to ensure their continued viability and effectiveness, respecting clients' freedom of choice. (See A.3.b.)

d. Family Involvement
Counselors recognize that families are usually important in clients' lives and strive to enlist family understanding and involvement as a positive resource, when appropriate.

e. Career and Employment Needs
Counselors work with their clients in considering employment in jobs and circumstances that are consistent with the clients' overall abilities, vocational limitations, physical restrictions, general temperament, interest and aptitude patterns, social skills, education, general qualifications, and other relevant characteristics and needs. Counselors neither place nor participate in placing clients in positions that will result in damaging the interest and the welfare of clients, employers, or the public.

A.2. Respecting Diversity

a. Nondiscrimination
Counselors do not condone or engage in discrimination based on age, color, culture, disability, ethnic group, gender, race, religion, sexual orientation, marital status, or socioeconomic status. (See C.5.a., C.5.b., and D.1.i.)

b. Respecting Differences
Counselors will actively attempt to understand the diverse cultural backgrounds of the clients with whom they work. This includes, but is not limited to, learning how the counselor's own cultural/ethnic/racial identity impacts her/his values and beliefs about the counseling process. (See E.8. and F.2.i.)

A.3. Client Rights

a. Disclosure to Clients
When counseling is initiated, and throughout the counseling process as

necessary, counselors inform clients of the purposes, goals, techniques, procedures, limitations, potential risks and benefits of services to be performed, and other pertinent information. Counselors take steps to ensure that clients understand the implications of diagnosis, the intended use of tests and reports, fees, and billing arrangements. Clients have the right to expect confidentiality and to be provided with an explanation of its limitations, including supervision and/or treatment team professionals; to obtain clear information about their case records; to participate in the ongoing counseling plans; and to refuse any recommended services and be advised of the consequences of such refusal. (See E.5.a. and G.2.)

b. Freedom of Choice
Counselors offer clients the freedom to choose whether to enter into a counseling relationship and to determine which professional(s) will provide counseling. Restrictions that limit choices of clients are fully explained. (See A.1.c.)

c. Inability to Give Consent
When counseling minors or persons unable to give voluntary informed consent, counselors act in these clients' best interests. (See B.3.)

A.4. Clients Served by Others

If a client is receiving services from another mental health professional, counselors, with client consent, inform the professional persons already involved and develop clear agreements to avoid confusion and conflict for the client. (See C.6.c.)

A.5. Personal Needs and Values

a. Personal Needs
In the counseling relationship, counselors are aware of the intimacy and

responsibilities inherent in the counseling relationship, maintain respect for clients, and avoid actions that seek to meet their personal needs at the expense of clients.

b. Personal Values
Counselors are aware of their own values, attitudes, beliefs, and behaviors and how these apply in a diverse society, and avoid imposing their values on clients. (See C.5.a.)

A.6. Dual Relationships

a. Avoid When Possible
Counselors are aware of their influential positions with respect to clients, and they avoid exploiting the trust and dependency of clients. Counselors make every effort to avoid dual relationships with clients that could impair professional judgment or increase the risk of harm to clients. (Examples of such relationships include, but are not limited to, familial, social, financial, business, or close personal relationships with clients.) When a dual relationship cannot be avoided, counselors take appropriate professional precautions such as informed consent, consultation, supervision, and documentation to ensure that judgment is not impaired and no exploitation occurs. (See F.1.b.)

b. Superior/Subordinate Relationships
Counselors do not accept as clients superiors or subordinates with whom they have administrative, supervisory, or evaluative relationships.

A.7. Sexual Intimacies with Clients

a. Current Clients
Counselors do not have any type of sexual intimacies with clients and do not counsel persons with whom they have had a sexual relationship.

b. Former Clients
Counselors do not engage in sexual intimacies with former clients within a minimum of two years after terminating the counseling relationship. Counselors who engage in such relationships after two years following termination have the responsibility to thoroughly examine and document that such relations did not have an exploitative nature, based on factors such as duration of counseling, amount of time since counseling, termination circumstances, client's personal history and mental status, adverse impact on the client, and actions by the counselor suggesting a plan to initiate a sexual relationship with the client after termination.

A.8. Multiple Clients

When counselors agree to provide counseling services to two or more persons who have a relationship (such as husband and wife, or parents and children), counselors clarify at the outset which person or persons are clients and the nature of the relationships they will have with each involved person. If it becomes apparent that counselors may be called upon to perform potentially conflicting roles, they clarify, adjust, or withdraw from roles appropriately. (See B.2. and B.4.d.)

A.9. Group Work

a. Screening
Counselors screen prospective group counseling/therapy participants. To the extent possible, counselors select members whose needs and goals are compatible with goals of the group, who will not impede the group process, and whose well-being will not be jeopardized by the group experience.

b. Protecting Clients
In a group setting, counselors take reasonable precautions to protect clients from physical or psychological trauma.

A.10. Fees and Bartering

(See D.3.a. and D.3.b.)

a. Advance Understanding
Counselors clearly explain to clients, prior to entering the counseling relationship, all financial arrangements related to professional services including the use of collection agencies or legal measures for nonpayment. (A.11.c.)

b. Establishing Fees
In establishing fees for professional counseling services, counselors consider the financial status of clients and locality. In the event that the established fee structure is inappropriate for a client, assistance is provided in attempting to find comparable services of acceptable cost. (See A.10.d., D.3.a., and D.3.b.)

c. Bartering Discouraged
Counselors ordinarily refrain from accepting goods or services from clients in return for counseling services because such arrangements create inherent potential for conflicts, exploitation, and distortion of the professional relationship. Counselors may participate in bartering only if the relationship is not exploitive, if the client requests it, if a clear written contract is established, and if such arrangements are an accepted practice among professionals in the community. (See A.6.a.)

d. Pro Bono Service
Counselors contribute to society by devoting a portion of their professional activity to services for which there is little or no financial return (pro bono).

A.11. Termination and Referral

a. Abandonment Prohibited
Counselors do not abandon or neglect clients in counseling. Counselors assist in making appropriate arrangements for the continuation of treatment, when necessary, during interruptions such as vacations, and following termination.

b. Inability to Assist Clients
If counselors determine an inability to be of professional assistance to clients, they avoid entering or immediately terminate a counseling relationship. Counselors are knowledgeable about referral resources and suggest appropriate alternatives. If clients decline the suggested referral, counselors should discontinue the relationship.

c. Appropriate Termination
Counselors terminate a counseling relationship, securing client agreement when possible, when it is reasonably clear that the client is no longer benefiting, when services are no longer required, when counseling no longer serves the client's needs or interests, when clients do not pay fees charged, or when agency or institution limits do not allow provision of further counseling services. (See A.10.b. and C.2.g.)

A.12. Computer Technology

a. Use of Computers
When computer applications are used in counseling services, counselors ensure that (1) the client is intellectually, emotionally, and physically capable of using the computer application; (2) the computer application is appropriate for the needs of the client; (3) the client understands the purpose and operation of the computer applications; and (4) a follow-up of client use of a computer application is provided to correct possible misconceptions, discover inappropriate use, and assess subsequent needs.

b. Explanation of Limitations
Counselors ensure that clients are provided information as a part of the counseling relationship that adequately explains the limitations of computer technology.

c. Access to Computer Applications
Counselors provide for equal access to computer applications in counseling services. (See A.2.a.)

SECTION B: CONFIDENTIALITY

B.1. Right to Privacy

a. Respect for Privacy
Counselors respect their clients' right to privacy and avoid illegal and unwarranted disclosures of confidential information. (See A.3.a. and B.6.a.)

b. Client Waiver
The right to privacy may be waived by the client or their legally recognized representative.

c. Exceptions
The general requirement that counselors keep information confidential does not apply when disclosure is required to prevent clear and imminent danger to the client or others or when legal requirements demand that confidential information be revealed. Counselors consult with other professionals when in doubt as to the validity of an exception.

d. Contagious, Fatal Diseases
A counselor who receives information confirming that a client has a disease commonly known to be both communicable and fatal is justified in disclosing information to an identifiable third party, who by his or her relationship with the client is at a high risk of contracting the disease. Prior to making a disclosure the counselor should ascertain that the client has not already informed the third party about his or her disease and that the client is not intending to inform the third party in the immediate future. (See B.1.c. and B.1.f.)

e. Court Ordered Disclosure
When court ordered to release confidential information without a client's permission, counselors request to the court that the disclosure not be required due to potential harm to the client or counseling relationship. (See B.1.c.)

f. Minimal Disclosure
When circumstances require the disclosure of confidential information, only essential information is revealed. To the extent possible, clients are informed before confidential information is disclosed.

g. Explanation of Limitations
When counseling is initiated and throughout the counseling process as necessary, counselors inform clients of the limitations of confidentiality and identify foreseeable situations in which confidentiality must be breached. (See G.2.a.)

h. Subordinates
Counselors make every effort to ensure that privacy and confidentiality of clients are maintained by subordinates including employees, supervisees, clerical assistants, and volunteers. (See B.1.a.)

i. Treatment Teams
If client treatment will involve a continued review by a treatment team, the client will be informed of the team's existence and composition.

B.2. Groups and Families

a. Group Work
In group work, counselors clearly define confidentiality and the parameters for the specific group being entered, explain its importance, and discuss the difficulties related to confidentiality involved in group work. The fact that confidentiality cannot be guaranteed is clearly communicated to group members.

b. Family Counseling
In family counseling, information about one family member cannot be disclosed to another member without permission. Counselors protect the privacy rights of each family member. (See A.8., B.3., and B.4.d.)

B.3. Minor or Incompetent Clients

When counseling clients who are minors or individuals who are unable to give voluntary, informed consent, parents or guardians may be included in the counseling process as appropriate. Counselors act in the best interests of clients and take measures to safeguard confidentiality. (See A.3.c.)

B.4. Records

a. Requirement of Records
Counselors maintain records necessary for rendering professional services to their clients and as required by laws, regulations, or agency or institution procedures.

b. Confidentiality of Records
Counselors are responsible for securing the safety and confidentiality of any counseling records they create, maintain, transfer, or destroy whether the records are written, taped, computerized, or stored in any other medium. (See B.1.a.)

c. Permission to Record or Observe
Counselors obtain permission from clients prior to electronically recording or observing sessions. (See A.3.a.)

d. Client Access
Counselors recognize that counseling records are kept for the benefit of clients, and therefore provide access to records and copies of records when requested by competent clients, unless the records contain information that may be misleading and detrimental to the client. In situations involving multiple clients, access to records is limited to those parts of records that do not include confidential information related to another client. (See A.8., B.1.a., and B.2.b.)

e. Disclosure or Transfer
Counselors obtain written permission from clients to disclose or transfer records to legitimate third parties unless exceptions to confidentiality exist as listed in Section B.1. Steps are taken to ensure that receivers of counseling records are sensitive to their confidential nature.

B.5. Research and Training

a. Data Disguise Required
Use of data derived from counseling relationships for purposes of training, research, or publication is confined to content that is disguised to ensure the anonymity of the individuals involved. (See B.1.g. and G.3.d.)

b. Agreement for Identification
Identification of a client in a presentation or publication is permissible only when the client has reviewed the material and has agreed to its presentation or publication. (See G.3.d.)

B.6. Consultation

a. Respect for Privacy
Information obtained in a consulting relationship is discussed for professional purposes only with persons clearly concerned with the case. Written and oral reports present data germane to the purposes of the consultation, and every effort is made to protect client identity and avoid undue invasion of privacy.

b. Cooperating Agencies
Before sharing information, counselors make efforts to ensure that there are defined policies in other agencies serving the counselor's clients that effectively protect the confidentiality of information.

SECTION C: PROFESSIONAL RESPONSIBILITY

C.1. Standards Knowledge

Counselors have a responsibility to read, understand, and follow the Code of Ethics and the Standards of Practice.

C.2. Professional Competence

a. Boundaries of Competence

Counselors practice only within the boundaries of their competence, based on their education, training, supervised experience, state and national professional credentials, and appropriate professional experience. Counselors will demonstrate a commitment to gain knowledge, personal awareness, sensitivity, and skills pertinent to working with a diverse client population.

b. New Specialty Areas of Practice

Counselors practice in specialty areas new to them only after appropriate education, training, and supervised experience. While developing skills in new specialty areas, counselors take steps to ensure the competence of their work and to protect others from possible harm.

c. Qualified for Employment

Counselors accept employment only for positions for which they are qualified by education, training, supervised experience, state and national professional credentials, and appropriate professional experience. Counselors hire for professional counseling positions only individuals who are qualified and competent.

d. Monitor Effectiveness

Counselors continually monitor their effectiveness as professionals and take steps to improve when necessary. Counselors in private practice take reasonable steps to seek out peer supervision to evaluate their efficacy as counselors.

e. Ethical Issues Consultation

Counselors take reasonable steps to consult with other counselors or related professionals when they have questions regarding their ethical obligations or professional practice. (See H.1.)

f. Continuing Education

Counselors recognize the need for continuing education to maintain a rea-

sonable level of awareness of current scientific and professional information in their fields of activity. They take steps to maintain competence in the skills they use, are open to new procedures, and keep current with the diverse and/or special populations with whom they work.

g. Impairment

Counselors refrain from offering or accepting professional services when their physical, mental, or emotional problems are likely to harm a client or others. They are alert to the signs of impairment, seek assistance for problems, and, if necessary, limit, suspend, or terminate their professional responsibilities. (See A.11.c.)

C.3. Advertising and Soliciting Clients

a. Accurate Advertising

There are no restrictions on advertising by counselors except those that can be specifically justified to protect the public from deceptive practices. Counselors advertise or represent their services to the public by identifying their credentials in an accurate manner that is not false, misleading, deceptive, or fraudulent. Counselors may only advertise the highest degree earned which is in counseling or a closely related field from a college or university that was accredited when the degree was awarded by one of the regional accrediting bodies recognized by the Council on Postsecondary Accreditation.

b. Testimonials

Counselors who use testimonials do not solicit them from clients or other persons who, because of their particular circumstances, may be vulnerable to undue influence.

c. Statements by Others

Counselors make reasonable efforts to ensure that statements made by others about them or the profession of counseling are accurate.

d. Recruiting through Employment

Counselors do not use their places of employment or institutional affiliation to recruit or gain clients, supervisees, or consultees for their private practices. (See C.5.e.)

e. Products and Training Advertisements

Counselors who develop products related to their profession or conduct workshops or training events ensure that the advertisements concerning these products or events are accurate and disclose adequate information for consumers to make informed choices.

f. Promoting to Those Served

Counselors do not use counseling, teaching, training, or supervisory relationships to promote their products or training events in a manner that is deceptive or would exert undue influence on individuals who may be vulnerable. Counselors may adopt textbooks they have authored for instruction purposes.

g. Professional Association Involvement

Counselors actively participate in local, state, and national associations that foster the development and improvement of counseling.

C.4. Credentials

a. Credentials Claimed

Counselors claim or imply only professional credentials possessed and are responsible for correcting any known misrepresentations of their credentials by others. Professional credentials include graduate degrees in counseling or closely related mental health fields, accreditation of graduate programs, national voluntary certifications, government issued certifications or licenses, ACA professional membership, or any other credential that might indicate to the public specialized knowledge or expertise in counseling.

b. ACA Professional Membership

ACA professional members may announce to the public their membership status. Regular members may not announce their ACA membership in a manner that might imply they are credentialed counselors.

c. Credential Guidelines

Counselors follow the guidelines for use of credentials that have been established by the entities that issue the credentials.

d. Misrepresentation of Credentials

Counselors do not attribute more to their credentials than the credentials represent, and do not imply that other counselors are not qualified because they do not possess certain credentials.

e. Doctoral Degrees from Other Fields

Counselors who hold a master's degree in counseling or a closely related mental health field, but hold a doctoral degree from other than counseling or a closely related field do not use the title "Dr." in their practices and do not announce to the public in relation to their practice or status as a counselor that they hold a doctorate.

C.5. Public Responsibility

a. Nondiscrimination

Counselors do not discriminate against clients, students, or supervisees in a manner that has a negative impact based on their age, color, culture, disability, ethnic group, gender, race, religion, sexual orientation, or socioeconomic status, or for any other reason. (See A.2.a.)

b. Sexual Harassment

Counselors do not engage in sexual harassment. Sexual harassment is defined as sexual solicitation, physical advances, or verbal or nonverbal conduct that is sexual in nature, that occurs in connection with professional activities or roles, and that either: (1) is unwelcome, is offensive, or creates a hostile workplace environment, and counselors know or are told this; or (2) is sufficiently severe or intense to be perceived as harassment to a reasonable person in the context. Sexual harassment can consist of a single intense or severe act or multiple persistent or pervasive acts.

c. Reports to Third Parties
Counselors are accurate, honest, and unbiased in reporting their professional activities and judgments to appropriate third parties including courts, health insurance companies, those who are the recipients of evaluation reports, and others. (See B.1.g.)

d. Media Presentations
When counselors provide advice or comment by means of public lectures, demonstrations, radio or television programs, prerecorded tapes, printed articles, mailed material, or other media, they take reasonable precautions to ensure that (1) the statements are based on appropriate professional counseling literature and practice; (2) the statements are otherwise consistent with the Code of Ethics and the Standards of Practice; and (3) the recipients of the information are not encouraged to infer that a professional counseling relationship has been established. (See C.6.b.)

e. Unjustified Gains
Counselors do not use their professional positions to seek or receive unjustified personal gains, sexual favors, unfair advantage, or unearned goods or services. (See C.3.d.)

C.6. Responsibility to Other Professionals

a. Different Approaches
Counselors are respectful of approaches to professional counseling that differ from their own. Counselors know and take into account the traditions and practices of other professional groups with which they work.

b. Personal Public Statements
When making personal statements in a public context, counselors clarify that they are speaking from their personal perspectives and that they are not speaking on behalf of all counselors or the profession. (See C.5.d.)

c. Clients Served by Others
When counselors learn that their clients are in a professional relationship with another mental health professional, they request release from clients to inform the other professionals and strive to establish positive and collaborative professional relationships. (See A.4.)

SECTION D: RELATIONSHIPS WITH OTHER PROFESSIONALS

D.1. Relationships with Employers and Employees

a. Role Definition
Counselors define and describe for their employers and employees the parameters and levels of their professional roles.

b. Agreements
Counselors establish working agreements with supervisors, colleagues, and subordinates regarding counseling or clinical relationships, confidentiality, adherence to professional standards, distinction between public and private material, maintenance and dissemination of recorded information, workload, and accountability. Working agreements in each instance are specified and made known to those concerned.

c. Negative Conditions
Counselors alert their employers to conditions that may be potentially disruptive or damaging to the counselor's professional responsibilities or that may limit their effectiveness.

d. Evaluation

Counselors submit regularly to professional review and evaluation by their supervisor or the appropriate representative of the employer.

e. In-Service

Counselors are responsible for inservice development of self and staff.

f. Goals

Counselors inform their staff of goals and programs.

g. Practices

Counselors provide personnel and agency practices that respect and enhance the rights and welfare of each employee and recipient of agency services. Counselors strive to maintain the highest levels of professional services.

h. Personnel Selection and Assignment

Counselors select competent staff and assign responsibilities compatible with their skills and experiences.

i. Discrimination

Counselors, as either employers or employees, do not engage in or condone practices that are inhumane, illegal, or unjustifiable (such as considerations based on age, color, culture, disability, ethnic group, gender, race, religion, sexual orientation, or socioeconomic status) in hiring, promotion, or training. (See A.2.a. and C.5.b.)

j. Professional Conduct

Counselors have a responsibility both to clients and to the agency or institution within which services are performed to maintain high standards of professional conduct.

k. Exploitive Relationships

Counselors do not engage in exploitive relationships with individuals over whom they have supervisory, evaluative, or instructional control or authority.

l. Employer Policies

The acceptance of employment in an agency or institution implies that counselors are in agreement with its general policies and principles. Counselors strive to reach agreement with employers as to acceptable standards of conduct that allow for changes in institutional policy conducive to the growth and development of clients.

D.2. Consultation (See B.6.)

a. Consultation as an Option

Counselors may choose to consult with any other professionally competent persons about their clients. In choosing consultants, counselors avoid placing the consultant in a conflict of interest situation that would preclude the consultant being a proper party to the counselor's efforts to help the client. Should counselors be engaged in a work setting that compromises this consultation standard, they consult with other professionals whenever possible to consider justifiable alternatives.

b. Consultant Competency

Counselors are reasonably certain that they have or the organization represented has the necessary competencies and resources for giving the kind of consulting services needed and that appropriate referral resources are available.

c. Understanding with Clients

When providing consultation, counselors attempt to develop with their clients a clear understanding of problem definition, goals for change, and predicted consequences of interventions selected.

d. Consultant Goals

The consulting relationship is one in which client adaptability and growth toward self-direction are consistently encouraged and cultivated. (See A.1.b.)

D.3. Fees for Referral

a. Accepting Fees from Agency Clients

Counselors refuse a private fee or other remuneration for rendering services to persons who are entitled to such services through the counselor's employing agency or institution. The policies of a particular agency may make explicit provisions for agency clients to receive counseling services from members of its staff in private practice. In such instances, the clients must be informed of other options open to them should they seek private counseling services. (See A.10.a., A.11.b., and C.3.d.)

b. Referral Fees

Counselors do not accept a referral fee from other professionals.

D.4. Subcontractor Arrangements

When counselors work as subcontractors for counseling services for a third party, they have a duty to inform clients of the limitations of confidentiality that the organization may place on counselors in providing counseling services to clients. The limits of such confidentiality ordinarily are discussed as part of the intake session. (See B.1.e. and B.1.f.)

SECTION E: EVALUATION, ASSESSMENT, AND INTERPRETATION

E.1. General

a. Appraisal Techniques

The primary purpose of educational and psychological assessment is to provide measures that are objective and interpretable in either comparative or absolute terms. Counselors recognize the need to interpret the statements in this section as applying to the whole range of appraisal techniques, including test and nontest data.

b. Client Welfare

Counselors promote the welfare and best interests of the client in the development, publication, and utilization of educational and psychological assessment techniques. They do not misuse assessment results and interpretations and take reasonable steps to prevent others from misusing the information these techniques provide. They respect the client's right to know the results, the interpretations made, and the bases for their conclusions and recommendations.

E.2. Competence to Use and Interpret Tests

a. Limits of Competence

Counselors recognize the limits of their competence and perform only those testing and assessment services for which they have been trained. They are familiar with reliability, validity, related standardization, error of measurement, and proper application of any technique utilized. Counselors using computer-based test interpretations are trained in the construct being measured and the specific instrument being used prior to using this type of computer application. Counselors take reasonable measures to ensure the proper use of psychological assessment techniques by persons under their supervision.

b. Appropriate Use

Counselors are responsible for the appropriate application, scoring, interpretation, and use of assessment instruments, whether they score and interpret such tests themselves or use computerized or other services.

c. Decisions Based on Results

Counselors responsible for decisions involving individuals or policies that are based on assessment results have a thorough understanding of educational and psychological measurement, including validation criteria, test research, and guidelines for test development and use.

d. Accurate Information

Counselors provide accurate information and avoid false claims or misconceptions when making statements about assessment instruments or techniques. Special efforts are made to avoid unwarranted connotations of such terms as IQ and grade equivalent scores. (See C.5.c.)

E.3. Informed Consent

a. Explanation to Clients

Prior to assessment, counselors explain the nature and purposes of assessment and the specific use of results in language the client (or other legally authorized person on behalf of the client) can understand, unless an explicit exception to this right has been agreed upon in advance. Regardless of whether scoring and interpretation are completed by counselors, by assistants, or by computer or other outside services, counselors take reasonable steps to ensure that appropriate explanations are given to the client.

b. Recipients of Results

The examinee's welfare, explicit understanding, and prior agreement determine the recipients of test results. Counselors include accurate and appropriate interpretations with any release of individual or group test results. (See B.1.a. and C.5.c.)

E.4. Release of Information to Competent Professionals

a. Misuse of Results

Counselors do not misuse assessment results, including test results, and interpretations, and take reasonable steps to prevent the misuse of such by others. (See C.5.c.)

b. Release of Raw Data

Counselors ordinarily release data (e.g. protocols, counseling or interview notes, or questionnaires) in which the client is identified only with the consent of the client or the client's legal representative. Such data are usually released only to persons recognized by counselors as competent to interpret the data. (See B.1.a.)

E.5. Proper Diagnosis of Mental Disorders

a. Proper Diagnosis

Counselors take special care to provide proper diagnosis of mental disorders. Assessment techniques (including personal interview) used to determine client care (e.g., focus of treatment, type of treatment, or recommended follow-up) are carefully selected and appropriately used. (See A.3.a. and C.5.c.)

b. Cultural Sensitivity

Counselors recognize that culture affects the manner in which clients' problems are defined. Clients' socio-economic and cultural experience is considered when diagnosing mental disorders.

E.6. Test Selection

a. Appropriateness of Instruments

Counselors carefully consider the validity, reliability, psychometric limitations, and appropriateness of instruments when selecting tests for use in a given situation or with a particular client.

b. Culturally Diverse Populations

Counselors are cautious when selecting tests for culturally diverse populations to avoid inappropriateness of testing that may be outside of socialized behavioral or cognitive patterns.

E.7. Conditions of Test Administration

a. Administration Conditions

Counselors administer tests under the same conditions that were established in their standardization. When tests are not administered under standard conditions or when unusual behavior or irregularities occur during the testing session, those conditions are noted in interpretation, and the results may be designated as invalid or of questionable validity.

b. Computer Administration

Counselors are responsible for ensuring that administration programs function properly to provide clients with accurate results when a computer or other electronic methods are used for test administration. (See A.12.b.)

c. Unsupervised Test-Taking

Counselors do not permit unsupervised or inadequately supervised use of tests or assessments unless the tests or assessments are designed, intended, and validated for self administration and/or scoring.

d. Disclosure of Favorable Conditions

Prior to test administration, conditions that produce most favorable test results are made known to the examinee.

E.8. Diversity in Testing

Counselors are cautious in using assessment techniques, making evaluations, and interpreting the performance of populations not represented in the norm group on which an instrument was standardized. They recognize the effects of age, color, culture, disability, ethnic group, gender, race, religion, sexual orientation, and socioeconomic status on test administration and interpretation and place test results in proper perspective with other relevant factors. (See A.2.a.)

E.9. Test Scoring and Interpretation

a. Reporting Reservations

In reporting assessment results, counselors indicate any reservations that exist regarding validity or reliability because of the circumstances of the assessment or the inappropriateness of the norms for the person tested.

b. Research Instruments

Counselors exercise caution when interpreting the results of research instruments possessing insufficient technical data to support respondent results. The specific purposes for the use of such instruments are stated explicitly to the examinee.

c. Testing Services

Counselors who provide test scoring and test interpretation services to support the assessment process confirm the validity of such interpretations. They accurately describe the purpose, norms, validity, reliability, and applications of the procedures and any special qualifications applicable to their use. The public offering of an automated test interpretations service is considered a professional-to-professional consultation. The formal responsibility of the consultant is to the consultee, but the ultimate and overriding responsibility is to the client.

E.10. Test Security

Counselors maintain the integrity and security of tests and other assessment techniques consistent with legal and contractual obligations. Counselors do not appropriate, reproduce, or modify published tests or parts thereof without acknowledgment and permission from the publisher.

E.11. Obsolete Tests and Outdated Test Results

Counselors do not use data or test results that are obsolete or outdated for the current purpose. Counselors make every effort to prevent the misuse of obsolete measures and test data by others.

E.12. Test Construction

Counselors use established scientific procedures, relevant standards, and current professional knowledge for test design in the development, publication, and utilization of educational and psychological assessment techniques.

SECTION F: TEACHING, TRAINING, AND SUPERVISION

F.1. Counselor Educators and Trainers

a. Educators as Teachers and Practitioners

Counselors who are responsible for developing, implementing, and supervising educational programs are skilled as teachers and practitioners. They are knowledgeable regarding the ethical, legal, and regulatory aspects of the profession, are skilled in applying that knowledge, and make students and supervisees aware of their responsibilities. Counselors conduct counselor education and training programs in an ethical manner and serve as role models for professional behavior. Counselor educators should make an effort to infuse material related to human diversity into all courses and/or workshops that are designed to promote the development of professional counselors.

b. Relationship Boundaries with Students and Supervisees

Counselors clearly define and maintain ethical, professional, and social relationship boundaries with their students and supervisees. They are aware of the differential in power that exists and the student's or supervisee's possible incomprehension of that power differential. Counselors explain to students and supervisees the potential for the relationship to become exploitive.

c. Sexual Relationships

Counselors do not engage in sexual relationships with students or supervisees and do not subject them to sexual harassment. (See A.6. and C.5.b.)

d. Contributions to Research

Counselors give credit to students or supervisees for their contributions to research and scholarly projects. Credit is given through coauthorship, acknowledgment, footnote statement, or other appropriate means, in accordance with such contributions. (See G.4.b. and G.4.c.)

e. Close Relatives

Counselors do not accept close relatives as students or supervisees.

f. Supervision Preparation

Counselors who offer clinical supervision services are adequately prepared in supervision methods and techniques. Counselors who are doctoral students serving as practicum or internship supervisors to master's level students are adequately prepared and supervised by the training program.

g. Responsibility for Services to Clients

Counselors who supervise the counseling services of others take reasonable measures to ensure that counseling services provided to clients are professional.

h. Endorsement

Counselors do not endorse students or supervisees for certification, licensure, employment, or completion of an academic or training program if they believe students or supervisees are not qualified for the endorsement. Counselors take reasonable steps to assist students or supervisees who are not qualified for endorsement to become qualified.

F.2. Counselor Education and Training Programs

a. Orientation

Prior to admission, counselors orient prospective students to the counselor education or training program's expectations, including but not limited to the following: (1) the type and level of skill acquisition required for successful completion of the training, (2) subject matter to be covered, (3) basis for evaluation, (4) training components that encourage self-growth or self-disclosure as part of the training process, (5) the type of supervision settings and requirements of the sites for required clinical field experiences, (6) student and supervisee evaluation and dismissal policies and procedures, and (7) up-to-date employment prospects for graduates.

b. Integration of Study and Practice

Counselors establish counselor education and training programs that integrate academic study and supervised practice.

c. Evaluation

Counselors clearly state to students and supervisees, in advance of training, the levels of competency expected, appraisal methods, and timing of evaluations for both didactic and experiential components. Counselors provide students and supervisees with periodic performance appraisal and evaluation feedback throughout the training program.

d. Teaching Ethics

Counselors make students and supervisees aware of the ethical responsibilities and standards of the profession and the students' and supervisees' ethical responsibilities to the profession. (See C.1. and F.3.e.)

e. Peer Relationships

When students or supervisees are assigned to lead counseling groups or provide clinical supervision for their peers, counselors take steps to ensure that students and supervisees placed in these roles do not have personal or adverse relationships with peers and that they understand they have the same ethical obligations as counselor educators, trainers, and supervisors. Counselors make every effort to ensure that the rights of peers are not compromised when students or supervisees are assigned to lead counseling groups or provide clinical supervision.

f. Varied Theoretical Positions

Counselors present varied theoretical positions so that students and supervisees may make comparisons and have opportunities to develop their own positions. Counselors provide information concerning the scientific bases of professional practice. (See C.6.a.)

g. Field Placements

Counselors develop clear policies within their training program regarding field placement and other clinical experiences. Counselors provide clearly stated roles and responsibilities for the student or supervisee, the site supervisor, and the program supervisor. They confirm that site supervisors are qualified to provide supervision and are informed of their professional and ethical responsibilities in this role.

h. Dual Relationships as Supervisors

Counselors avoid dual relationships such as performing the role of site supervisor and training program supervisor in the student's or supervisee's training program. Counselors do not accept any form of professional services, fees, commissions, reimbursement, or remuneration from a site for student or supervisee placement.

i. Diversity in Programs

Counselors are responsive to their institution's and program's recruitment and retention needs for training program administrators, faculty, and students with diverse backgrounds and special needs. (See A.2.a.)

F.3. Students and Supervisees

a. Limitations

Counselors, through ongoing evaluation and appraisal, are aware of the academic and personal limitations of students and supervisees that might impede performance. Counselors assist students and supervisees in securing remedial assistance when needed, and dismiss from the training program supervisees who are unable to provide competent service due to academic or personal limitations. Counselors seek professional consultation and document their decision to dismiss or refer students or supervisees for assistance. Counselors assure that students and supervisees have recourse to address decisions made, to require them to seek assistance, or to dismiss them.

b. Self-Growth Experiences

Counselors use professional judgment when designing training experiences conducted by the counselors themselves that require student and supervisee self-growth or self-disclosure. Safeguards are provided so that students and supervisees are aware of the ramifications their self-disclosure may have on counselors whose primary role as teacher, trainer, or supervisor requires acting on ethical obligations to the profession. Evaluative components of experiential training experiences explicitly delineate predetermined academic standards that are separate and not dependent on the student's level of self-disclosure. (See A.6.)

c. Counseling for Students and Supervisees

If students or supervisees request counseling, supervisors or counselor educators provide them with acceptable referrals. Supervisors or counselor educators do not serve as counselor to students or supervisees over whom they hold administrative, teaching, or evaluative roles unless this is a brief role associated with a training experience. (See A.6.b.)

d. Clients of Students and Supervisees

Counselors make every effort to ensure that the clients at field placements are aware of the services rendered and the qualifications of the students and supervisees rendering those services. Clients receive professional disclosure information and are informed of the limits of confidentiality. Client permission is obtained in order for the students and supervisees to use any information concerning the counseling relationship in the training process. (See B.1.e.)

e. Standards for students and Supervisees

Students and supervisees preparing to become counselors adhere to the Code of Ethics and the Standards of Practice. Students and supervisees have the same obligations to clients as those required of counselors. (See H.1.)

SECTION G: RESEARCH AND PUBLICATION

G.1. Research Responsibilities

a. Use of Human Subjects

Counselors plan, design, conduct, and report research in a manner consistent with pertinent ethical principles, federal and state laws, host institutional regulations, and scientific standards governing research with human subjects. Counselors design and conduct research that reflects cultural sensitivity appropriateness.

b. Deviation from Standard Practices

Counselors seek consultation and observe stringent safeguards to protect the rights of research participants when a research problem suggests a deviation from standard acceptable practices. (See B.6.)

c. Precautions to Avoid Injury

Counselors who conduct research with human subjects are responsible for the subjects' welfare throughout the experiment and take reasonable precautions to avoid causing injurious psychological, physical, or social effects to their subjects.

d. Principal Researcher Responsibility

The ultimate responsibility for ethical research practice lies with the principal researcher. All others involved in the research activities share ethical obligations and full responsibility for their own actions.

e. Minimal Interference

Counselors take reasonable precautions to avoid causing disruptions in subjects' lives due to participation in research.

f. Diversity

Counselors are sensitive to diversity and research issues with special populations. They seek consultation when appropriate. (See A.2.a. and B.6.)

G.2. Informed Consent

a. Topics Disclosed

In obtaining informed consent for research, counselors use language that is understandable to research participants and that: (1) accurately explains the purpose and procedures to be followed; (2) identifies any procedures that are experimental or relatively untried; (3) describes the attendant discomforts and risks; (4) describes the benefits or changes in individuals or organizations that might be reasonably expected; (5) discloses appropriate alternative procedures that would be advantageous for subjects; (6) offers to answer any inquiries concerning the procedures; (7) describes any limita-

tions on confidentiality; and (8) instructs that subjects are free to withdraw their consent and to discontinue participation in the project at any time. (See B.1.f.)

b. Deception

Counselors do not conduct research involving deception unless alternative procedures are not feasible and the prospective value of the research justifies the deception. When the methodological requirements of a study necessitate concealment of deception, the investigator is required to explain clearly the reasons for this action as soon as possible.

c. Voluntary Participation

Participation in research is typically voluntary and without any penalty for refusal to participate. Involuntary participation is appropriate only when it can be demonstrated that participation will have no harmful effects on subjects and is essential to the investigation.

d. Confidentiality of Information

Information obtained about research participants during the course of an investigation is confidential. When the possibility exists that others may obtain access to such information, ethical research practice requires that the possibility, together with the plans for protecting confidentiality, be explained to participants as a part of the procedure for obtaining informed consent. (See B.1.e.)

e. Persons Incapable of Giving Informed Consent

When a person is incapable of giving informed consent, counselors provide an appropriate explanation, obtain agreement for participation and obtain appropriate consent from a legally authorized person.

f. Commitments to Participants

Counselors take reasonable measures to honor all commitments to research participants.

g. Explanations After Data Collection

After data are collected, counselors provide participants with full clarification of the nature of the study to remove any misconceptions. Where scientific or human values justify delaying or with-holding information, counselors take reasonable measures to avoid causing harm.

h. Agreements to Cooperate

Counselors who agree to cooperate with another individual in research or publication incur an obligation to cooperate as promised in terms of punctuality of performance and with regard to the completeness and accuracy of the information required.

i. Informed Consent for Sponsors

In the pursuit of research, counselors give sponsors, institutions, and publication channels the same respect and opportunity for giving informed consent that they accord to individual research participants. Counselors are aware of their obligation to future research workers and ensure that hose institutions are given feedback information and proper acknowledgment.

G.3. Reporting Results

a. Information Affecting Outcome

When reporting research results, counselors explicitly mention all variables and conditions known to the investigator that may have affected the outcome of a study or the interpretation of data.

b. Accurate Results

Counselors plan, conduct, and report research accurately and in a manner that minimizes the possibility that results will be misleading. They provide thorough discussions of the limitations of their data and alternative hypotheses. Counselors do not engage in fraudulent research, distort data, misrepresent data, or deliberately bias their results.

c. Obligation to Report Unfavorable Results

Counselors communicate to other counselors the results of any research judged to be of professional value. Results that reflect unfavorably on institutions, programs, services, prevailing opinions, or vested interests are not withheld.

d. Identity of Subjects

Counselors who supply data, aid in the research of another person, report research results, or make original data available take due care to disguise the identity of respective subjects in the absence of specific authorization from the subjects to do otherwise. (See B.1.g. and B.5.a.)

e. Replication Studies

Counselors are obligated to make available sufficient original research data to qualified professionals who may wish to replicate the study.

G.4. Publication

a. Recognition of Others

When conducting and reporting research, counselors are familiar with and give recognition to previous work on the topic, observe copyright laws, and give full credit to those to whom credit is due. (See F.1.d. and G.4.c.)

b. Contributors

Counselors give credit through joint authorship, acknowledgment, footnote statements, or other appropriate means to those who have contributed significantly to research or concept development in accordance with such contributions. The principal contributor is listed first and minor technical or professional contributions are acknowledged in notes or introductory statements.

c. Student Research

For an article that is substantially based on a student's dissertation or thesis, the student is listed as the principal author. (See F.1.d. and G.4.a.)

d. Duplicate Submission

Counselors submit manuscripts for consideration to only one journal at a time. Manuscripts that are published in whole or in substantial part in another journal or published work are not submitted for publication without acknowledgment and permission from the previous publication.

e. Professional Review

Counselors who review material submitted for publication, research, or other scholarly purposes respect the confidentiality and proprietary rights of those who submitted it.

SECTION H: RESOLVING ETHICAL ISSUES

H.1. Knowledge of Standards

Counselors are familiar with the *Code of Ethics* and the *Standards of Practice* and other applicable ethics codes from other professional organizations of which they are members, or from certification and licensure bodies. Lack of knowledge or misunderstanding of an ethical responsibility is not a defense against a charge of unethical conduct. (See F.3.e.)

H.2. Suspected Violations

a. Ethical Behavior Expected

Counselors expect professional associates to adhere to the *Code of Ethics*. When counselors possess reasonable cause that raises doubts as to whether a counselor is acting in an ethical manner, they take appropriate action. (See H.2.d. and H.2.e.)

b. Consultation

When uncertain as to whether a particular situation of course of action may be in violation of the *Code of Ethics*, counselors consult with other counselors who are knowledgeable about ethics, with colleagues, or with appropriate authorities.

c. Organization Conflicts

If the demands of an organization with which counselors are affiliated pose a conflict with the *Code of Ethics*, counselors specify the nature of such conflicts and express to their supervisors or other responsible officials their commitment of the *Code of Ethics*. When possible, counselors work toward change within the organization to allow full adherence to the *Code of Ethics*.

d. Informal Resolution

When counselors have reasonable cause to believe that another counselor is violating an ethical standard, they attempt to first resolve the issue informally with the other counselor if feasible, providing that such action does not violate confidentiality rights that may be involved.

e. Reporting Suspected Violations

When an informal resolution is not appropriate or feasible, counselors, upon reasonable cause, take action such as reporting the suspected ethical violation to state or national ethics committees, unless this action conflicts with confidentiality rights that cannot be resolved.

f. Unwarranted Complaints

Counselors do not initiate, participate in, or encourage the filing of ethics complaints that are unwarranted or intend to harm a counselor rather than to protect clients or the public.

H.3. Cooperation with Ethics Committees

Counselors assist in the process of enforcing the *Code of Ethics*. Counselors cooperate with investigations, proceedings, and requirements of the ACA Ethics

Committee or ethics committees of other duly constituted associations or boards having jurisdiction over those charged with a violation. Counselors are familiar with the ACA Policies and Procedures and use it as a reference in assisting the enforcement of the *Code of Ethics.*

STANDARDS OF PRACTICE

All members of the American Counseling Association (ACA) are required to adhere to the *Standards of Practice* and the *Code of Ethics.* The *Standards of Practice* represent minimal behavioral statements of the *Code of Ethics.* Members should refer to the applicable section of the *Code of Ethics* for further interpretation and amplification of the applicable Standard of Practice.

SECTION A: THE COUNSELING RELATIONSHIP

Standard of Practice One (SP-1)

Nondiscrimination
Counselors respect diversity and must not discriminate against clients because of age, color, culture, disability, ethnic group, gender, race, religion, sexual orientation, marital status, or socioeconomic status. (See A.2.a.)

Standard of Practice Two (SP-2)

Disclosure to Clients
Counselors must adequately inform clients, preferably in writing, regarding the counseling process and counseling relationship at or before the time it begins and throughout the relationship. (See A.3.a.)

Standard of Practice Three (SP-3)

Dual Relationships
Counselors must make every effort to avoid dual relationships with clients that could impair their professional judgment or increase the risk of harm to clients. When a dual relationship cannot be avoided, counselors must take appropriate steps to ensure that judgment is not impaired and that no exploitation occurs. (See A.6.a. and A.6.b.)

Standard of Practice Four (SP-4)

Sexual Intimacies with Clients
Counselors must not engage in any type of sexual intimacies with current clients and must not engage in sexual intimacies with former clients within a minimum of two years after terminating the counseling relationship. Counselors who engage in such relationship after two years following termination have the responsibility to thoroughly examine and document that such relations did not have an exploitative nature.

Standard of Practice Five (SP-5)

Counselors must take steps to protect clients from physical or psychological trauma resulting from interactions during group work. (See A.9.b.)

Standard of Practice Six (SP-6)

Advance Understanding of Fees
Counselors must explain to clients, prior to their entering the counseling relationship, financial arrangements related to professional services. (See A.10.a.–d. and A.11.c.)

Standard of Practice Seven (SP-7)

Termination
Counselors must assist in making appropriate arrangements for the continuation of treatment of clients, when necessary, following termination of counseling relationships. (See A.11.a.)

Standard of Practice Eight (SP-8)

Inability to Assist Clients
Counselors must avoid entering or immediately terminate a counseling relationship if it is determined that they are unable to be of professional assistance to a client. The counselor may assist in making an appropriate referral for the client. (See A.11.b.)

SECTION B: CONFIDENTIALITY

Standard of Practice Nine (SP-9)

Confidentiality Requirement
Counselors must keep information related to counseling services confidential unless disclosure is in the best interest of clients, is required for the welfare of others, or is required by law. When disclosure is required, only information that is essential is revealed and the client is informed of such disclosure. (See B.1.a.–f.)

Standard of Practice Ten (SP-10)

Confidentiality Requirements for Subordinates
Counselors must take measures to ensure that privacy and confidentiality of clients are maintained by subordinates. (See B.1.h.)

Standard of Practice Eleven (SP-11)

Confidentiality in Group Work
Counselors must clearly communicate to group members that confidentiality cannot be guaranteed in group work. (See B.2.a.)

Standard of Practice Twelve (SP-12)

Confidentiality in Family Counseling
Counselors must not disclose information about one family member in counseling to another family member without prior consent. (See B.2.b.)

Standard of Practice Thirteen (SP-13)

Confidentiality of Records
Counselors must maintain appropriate confidentiality in creating, storing, accessing, transferring, and disposing of counseling records. (See B.4.b.)

Standard of Practice Fourteen (SP-14)

Permission to Record or Observe
Counselors must obtain prior consent from clients in order to electronically record or observe sessions. (See B.4.c.)

Standard of Practice Fifteen (SP-15)

Counselors must obtain client consent to disclose or transfer records to third parties, unless exceptions listed in SP-9 exist. (See B.4.e.)

Standard of Practice Sixteen (SP-16)

Data Disguise Required
Counselors must disguise the identity of the client when using data for training, research, or publication. (See B.5.a.)

SECTION C: PROFESSIONAL RESPONSIBILITY

Standard of Practice Seventeen (SP-17)

Boundaries of Competence
Counselors must practice only within the boundaries of their competence. (See C.2.a.)

Standard of Practice Eighteen (SP-18)

Continuing Education
Counselors must engage in continuing education to maintain their professional competence. (See C.2.f.)

Standard of Practice Nineteen (SP-19)

Impairment of Professionals

Counselors must refrain from offering professional services when their personal problems or conflicts may cause harm to a client or others. (See C.2.g.)

Standard of Practice Twenty (SP-20)

Accurate Advertising

Counselors must accurately represent their credentials and services when advertising. (See C.3.a.)

Standard of Practice Twenty-one (SP-21)

Recruiting Through Employment

Counselors must not use their place of employment or institutional affiliation to recruit clients for their private practices. (See C.3.d.)

Standard of Practice Twenty-two (SP-22)

Credentials Claimed

Counselors must claim or imply only professional credentials possessed and must correct any known misrepresentations of their credentials by others. (See C.4.a.)

Standard of Practice Twenty-three (SP-23)

Sexual Harassment

Counselors must not engage in sexual harassment. (See C.5.b.)

Standard of Practice Twenty-four (SP-24)

Unjustified Gains

Counselors must not use their professional positions to seek or receive unjustified personal gains, sexual favors, unfair advantage, or unearned goods or services. (See C.5.e.)

Standard of Practice Twenty-five (SP-25)

Clients Served by Others

With the consent of the client, counselors must inform other mental health professionals serving the same client that a counseling relationship between the counselor and client exists. (See C.6.c.)

Standard of Practice Twenty-six (SP-26)

Negative Employment Conditions

Counselors must alert their employers to institutional policy or conditions that may be potentially disruptive or damaging to the counselor's professional responsibilities, or that may limit their effectiveness or deny clients' rights. (See D.1.c.)

Standard of Practice Twenty-seven (SP-27)

Personnel Selection and Assignment

Counselors must select competent staff and must assign responsibilities compatible with staff skills and experiences. (See D.1.h.)

Standard of Practice Twenty-eight (SP-28)

Exploitive Relationships with Subordinates

Counselors must not engage in exploitive relationships with individuals over whom they have supervisory, evaluative, or instructional control or authority. (See D.1.k.)

SECTION D: RELATIONSHIP WITH OTHER PROFESSIONALS

Standard of Practice Twenty-nine (SP-29)

Accepting Fees from Agency Clients

Counselors must not accept fees or other remuneration for consultation with persons entitled to such services through the counselor's employing agency or institution. (See D.3.a.)

Standard of Practice Thirty (SP-30)

Referral Fees
Counselors must not accept referral fees. (See D.3.b.)

SECTION E: EVALUATION, ASSESSMENT, AND INTERPRETATION

Standard of Practice Thirty-one (SP-31)

Limits of Competence
Counselors must perform only testing and assessment services for which they are competent. Counselors must not allow the use of psychological assessment techniques by unqualified persons under their supervision. (See E.2.a.)

Standard of Practice Thirty-two (SP-32)

Appropriate Use of Assessment Instruments
Counselors must use assessment instruments in the manner for which they were intended. (See E.2.b.)

Standard of Practice Thirty-three (SP-33)

Assessment Explanations to Clients
Counselors must provide explanations to clients prior to assessment about the nature and purposes of assessment and the specific uses of results. (See E.3.a.)

Standard of Practice Thirty-four (SP-34)

Recipients of Test Results
Counselors must ensure that accurate and appropriate interpretations accom-

pany any release of testing and assessment information. (See E.3.b.)

Standard of Practice Thirty-five (SP-35)

Obsolete Tests and Outdated Test Results
Counselors must not base their assessment or intervention decisions or recommendations on data or test results that are obsolete or outdated for the current purpose. (See E.11.)

SECTION F: TEACHING, TRAINING, AND SUPERVISION

Standard of Practice Thirty-six (SP-36)

Sexual Relationships with Students or Supervisees
Counselors must not engage in sexual relationships with their students and supervisees. (See F.1.c.)

Standard of Practice Thirty-seven (SP-37)

Credit for Contributions to Research
Counselors must give credit to students or supervisees for their contributions to research and scholarly projects. (See F.1.d.)

Standard of Practice Thirty-eight (SP-38)

Supervision Preparation
Counselors who offer clinical supervision services must be trained and prepared in supervision methods and techniques. (See F.1.f.)

Standard of Practice Thirty-nine (SP-39)

Evaluation Information
Counselors must clearly state to students and supervisees in advance of

training, the levels of competency expected, appraisal methods, and timing of evaluations. Counselors must provide students and supervisees with periodic performance appraisal and evaluation feedback throughout the training program. (See F.2.c.)

Standard of Practice Forty (SP-40)

Peer Relationships in Training

Counselors must make every effort to ensure that the rights of peers are not violated when students and supervisees are assigned to lead counseling groups or provide clinical supervision. (See F.2.e.)

Standard of Practice Forty-one (SP-41)

Limitations of Students and Supervisees

Counselors must assist students and supervisees in securing remedial assistance, when needed, and must dismiss from the training program students and supervisees who are unable to provide competent service due to academic or personal limitations. (See F.3.a.)

Standard of Practice Forty-two (SP-42)

Self-growth Experiences

Counselors who conduct experiences for students or supervisees that include self-growth or self-disclosure must inform participants of counselors' ethical obligations to the profession and must not grade participants based on their nonacademic performance. (See F.3.b.)

Standard of Practice Forty-three (SP-43)

Standards for Students and Supervisees

Students and supervisees preparing to become counselors must adhere to the *Code of Ethics* and the *Standards of Practice* of counselors. (See F.e.3.)

SECTION G: RESEARCH AND PUBLICATION

Standard of Practice Forty-four (SP-44)

Precautions to Avoid Injury in Research

Counselors must avoid causing physical, social, or psychological harm or injury to subjects in research. (See G.1.c.)

Standard of Practice Forty-five (SP-45)

Confidentiality of Research Information

Counselors must keep confidential information obtained about research participants. (See G.2.d.)

Standard of Practice Forty-six (SP-46)

Information Affecting Research Outcome

Counselors must report all variables and conditions known to the investigator that may have affected research data or outcomes. (See G.3.a.)

Standard of Practice Forty-seven (SP-47)

Accurate Research Results

Counselors must not distort or misrepresent research data, nor fabricate or intentionally bias research results. (See G.3.b.)

Standard of Practice Forty-eight (SP-48)

Publication Contributors

Counselors must give appropriate credit to those who have contributed to research. (See G.4.a. and G.4.b.)

SECTION H: RESOLVING ETHICAL ISSUES

Standard of Practice Forty-nine (SP-49)

Ethical Behavior Expected
Counselors must take appropriate action when they possess reasonable cause that raises doubts as to whether counselors or other mental health professionals are acting in an ethical manner. (See H.2.a.)

Standard of Practice Fifty (SP-50)

Unwarranted Complaints
Counselors must not initiate, participate in, or encourage the filings of ethics complaints that are unwarranted or intended to harm a mental health professional rather than to protect clients or the public. (See H.2.f.)

Standard of Practice Fifty-one (SP-51)

Cooperation with Ethics Committees
Counselors must cooperate with investigations, proceedings, and requirements of the ACA Ethics Committee or ethics committees of other duly constituted associations or boards having jurisdiction over those charged with a violation. (See H.3.)

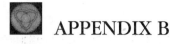

APPENDIX B

ETHICAL PRINCIPLES OF PSYCHOLOGISTS
AND CODE OF CONDUCT 2002

INTRODUCTION AND APPLICABILITY

The American Psychological Association's (APA's) Ethical Principles of Psychologists and Code of Conduct (hereinafter referred to as the Ethics Code) consists of an Introduction, a Preamble, five General Principles (A – E), and specific Ethical Standards. The Introduction discusses the intent, organization, procedural considerations, and scope of application of the Ethics Code. The Preamble and General Principles are aspirational goals to guide psychologists toward the highest ideals of psychology. Although the Preamble and General Principles are not themselves enforceable rules, they should be considered by psychologists in arriving at an ethical course of action. The Ethical Standards set forth enforceable rules for conduct as psychologists. Most of the Ethical Standards are written broadly, in order to apply to psychologists in varied roles, although the application of an Ethical Standard may vary depending on the context. The Ethical Standards are not exhaustive. The fact that a given conduct is not specifically addressed by an Ethical Standard does not mean that it is necessarily either ethical or unethical.

This Ethics Code applies only to psychologists' activities that are part of their scientific, educational, or professional roles as psychologists. Areas covered include but are not limited to the clinical, counseling, and school practice of psychology; research; teaching; supervision of trainees; public service; policy development; social intervention; development of assessment instruments; conducting assessments; educational counseling; organizational consulting; forensic activities; program design and evaluation; and administration. This Ethics Code applies to these activities across a variety of contexts, such as in person, postal, telephone, internet, and other electronic transmissions. These activities shall be distinguished from the purely private conduct of psychologists, which is not within the purview of the Ethics Code.

Membership in the APA commits members and student affiliates to comply with the standards of the APA Ethics Code and to the rules and procedures used to enforce them. Lack of awareness or misunderstanding of an Ethical Standard is not itself a defense to a charge of unethical conduct.

The procedures for filing, investigating, and resolving complaints of unethical conduct are described in the current Rules and Procedures of the APA Ethics Committee. APA may impose sanctions on its members for violations of the standards of the Ethics Code, including termination of APA membership, and may notify other bodies and individuals of its actions. Actions that violate the standards of the Ethics Code may also lead to the imposition of sanctions on psychologists or students whether or not they are APA members by bodies other than APA, including state psychological associations, other professional groups, psychology boards, other state or federal agencies, and payors for health services. In addition, APA may take action against a member after his or her conviction of a felony, expulsion or suspension from an affiliated state psychological association, or suspension or loss of licensure. When the sanction to be imposed by APA is less than expulsion, the 2001 Rules and Procedures do not guarantee an opportunity for an in-person hearing, but generally provide that complaints will be resolved only on the basis of a submitted record.

The Ethics Code is intended to provide guidance for psychologists and standards of professional conduct that can be applied by the APA and by other bodies that choose to adopt them. The Ethics Code is not intended to be a basis of civil liability. Whether a psychologist has violated the Ethics Code standards does not by itself determine whether the psychologist is legally liable in a court action, whether a contract is enforceable, or whether other legal consequences occur.

The modifiers used in some of the standards of this Ethics Code (e.g., *reasonably, appropriate, potentially*) are included in the standards when they would (1) allow professional judgment on the part of psychologists, (2) eliminate injustice or inequality that would occur without the modifier, (3) ensure applicability across the broad range of activities conducted by psychologists, or (4) guard against a set of rigid rules that might be quickly outdated. As used in this Ethics Code, the term *reasonable* means the prevailing professional judgment of psychologists engaged in similar activities in similar circumstances, given the knowledge the psychologist had or should have had at the time.

In the process of making decisions regarding their professional behavior, psychologists must consider this Ethics Code in addition to applicable laws and psychology board regulations. In applying the Ethics Code to their professional work, psychologists may consider other materials and guidelines that have been adopted or endorsed by scientific and professional psychological organizations and the dictates of their own conscience, as well as consult with others within the field. If this Ethics Code establishes a higher standard of conduct than is required by law, psychologists must meet the higher ethical standard. If psychologists' ethical responsibilities conflict with law, regulations, or other governing legal authority, psychologists make known their commitment to this Ethics Code and take steps to resolve the conflict in a responsible manner. If the conflict is unresolvable via such means, psychologists may adhere to the requirements of the law, regulations, or other governing authority in keeping with basic principles of human rights.

PREAMBLE

Psychologists are committed to increasing scientific and professional knowledge of behavior and people's understanding of themselves and others and to the use of such knowledge to improve the condition of individuals, organizations, and society. Psychologists respect and protect civil and human rights and the central importance of freedom of inquiry and expression in research, teaching, and publication. They strive to help the public in developing informed judgments and choices concerning human behavior. In doing so, they perform many roles, such as researcher, educator, diagnostician, therapist, supervisor, consultant, administrator, social interventionist, and expert witness. This Ethics Code provides a common set of principles and standards upon which psychologists build their professional and scientific work.

This Ethics Code is intended to provide specific standards to cover most situations encountered by psychologists. It has as its goals the welfare and protection of the individuals and groups with whom psychologists work and the education of members, students, and the public regarding ethical standards of the discipline.

The development of a dynamic set of ethical standards for psychologists' work-related conduct requires a personal commitment and lifelong effort to act ethically; to encourage ethical behavior by students, supervisees, employees, and colleagues; and to consult with others concerning ethical problems.

GENERAL PRINCIPLES

This section consists of General Principles. General Principles, as opposed to Ethical Standards, are aspirational in nature. Their intent is to guide and inspire psychologists toward the very highest ethical ideals of the profession. General Principles, in contrast to Ethical Standards, do not represent obligations and should not form the basis for imposing sanctions. Relying upon General Principles for either of these reasons distorts both their meaning and purpose.

Principle A: Beneficence and Nonmaleficence

Psychologists strive to benefit those with whom they work and take care to do no harm. In their professional actions, psychologists seek to safeguard the welfare and rights of those with whom they interact professionally and other affected persons, and the welfare of animal subjects of research. When conflicts occur among psychologists' obligations or concerns, they attempt to resolve these conflicts in a responsible fashion that avoids or minimizes harm. Because psychologists' scientific and professional judgments and actions may affect the lives of others, they are alert to and guard against personal, financial, social, organizational, or political factors that might lead to misuse of their influence. Psychologists strive to be aware of the possible effect of their own physical and mental health on their ability to help those with whom they work.

Principle B: Fidelity and Responsibility

Psychologists establish relationships of trust with those with whom they work. They are aware of their professional and scientific responsibilities to society and to the specific communities in which they work. Psychologists uphold professional standards of conduct, clarify their professional roles and obligations, accept appropriate responsibility for their behavior, and seek to manage conflicts of interest that could lead to exploitation or harm. Psychologists consult with, refer to, or cooperate with other professionals and institutions to the extent needed to serve the best interests of those with whom they work. They are concerned about the ethical compliance of their colleagues' scientific and professional conduct. Psychologists strive to contribute a portion of their professional time for little or no compensation or personal advantage.

Principle C: Integrity

Psychologists seek to promote accuracy, honesty, and truthfulness in the science, teaching, and practice of psychology. In these activities psychologists do not steal, cheat, or engage in fraud, subterfuge, or intentional misrepresentation of fact. Psychologists strive to keep their promises and to avoid unwise or unclear commitments. In situations in which deception may be ethically justifiable to maximize benefits and minimize harm, psychologists have a serious obligation to consider the need for, the possible consequences of, and their responsibility to correct any resulting mistrust or other harmful effects that arise from the use of such techniques.

Principle D: Justice

Psychologists recognize that fairness and justice entitle all persons to access to and benefit from the contributions of psychology and to equal quality in the processes, procedures, and services being conducted by psychologists. Psychologists exercise reasonable judgment and take precautions to ensure

that their potential biases, the boundaries of their competence, and the limitations of their expertise do not lead to or condone unjust practices.

Principle E: Respect for People's Rights and Dignity

Psychologists respect the dignity and worth of all people, and the rights of individuals to privacy, confidentiality, and self-determination. Psychologists are aware that special safeguards may be necessary to protect the rights and welfare of persons or communities whose vulnerabilities impair autonomous decision making. Psychologists are aware of and respect cultural, individual, and role differences, including those based on age, gender, gender identity, race, ethnicity, culture, national origin, religion, sexual orientation, disability, language, and socioeconomic status and consider these factors when working with members of such groups. Psychologists try to eliminate the effect on their work of biases based on those factors, and they do not knowingly participate in or condone activities of others based upon such prejudices.

ETHICAL STANDARDS

1. *Resolving Ethical Issues*

1.01 Misuse of Psychologists' Work

If psychologists learn of misuse or misrepresentation of their work, they take reasonable steps to correct or minimize the misuse or misrepresentation.

1.02 Conflicts Between Ethics and Law, Regulations, or Other Governing Legal Authority

If psychologists' ethical responsibilities conflict with law, regulations, or other governing legal authority, psychologists make known their commitment to the Ethics Code and take steps to resolve the conflict. If the conflict is unresolvable via such means, psychologists may adhere to the requirements of the law, regulations, or other governing legal authority.

1.03 Conflicts Between Ethics and Organizational Demands

If the demands of an organization with which psychologists are affiliated or for whom they are working conflict with this Ethics Code, psychologists clarify the nature of the conflict, make known their commitment to the Ethics Code, and to the extent feasible, resolve the conflict in a way that permits adherence to the Ethics Code.

1.04 Informal Resolution of Ethical Violations

When psychologists believe that there may have been an ethical violation by another psychologist, they attempt to resolve the issue by bringing it to the attention of that individual, if an informal resolution appears appropriate and the intervention does not violate any confidentiality rights that may be involved. (See also Standards 1.02, Conflicts Between Ethics and Law, Regulations, or Other Governing Legal Authority, and 1.03, Conflicts Between Ethics and Organizational Demands.)

1.05 Reporting Ethical Violations

If an apparent ethical violation has substantially harmed or is likely to substantially harm a person or organization and is not appropriate for informal resolution under Standard 1.04, Informal Resolution of Ethical Violations, or is not resolved properly in that fashion, psychologists take further action appro-

priate to the situation. Such action might include referral to state or national committees on professional ethics, to state licensing boards, or to the appropriate institutional authorities. This standard does not apply when an intervention would violate confidentiality rights or when psychologists have been retained to review the work of another psychologist whose professional conduct is in question. (See also Standard 1.02, Conflicts Between Ethics and Law, Regulations, or Other Governing Legal Authority.)

1.06 Cooperating With Ethics Committees

Psychologists cooperate in ethics investigations, proceedings, and resulting requirements of the APA or any affiliated state psychological association to which they belong. In doing so, they address any confidentiality issues. Failure to cooperate is itself an ethics violation. However, making a request for deferment of adjudication of an ethics complaint pending the outcome of litigation does not alone constitute noncooperation.

1.07 Improper Complaints

Psychologists do not file or encourage the filing of ethics complaints that are made with reckless disregard for or willful ignorance of facts that would disprove the allegation.

1.08 Unfair Discrimination Against Complainants and Respondents

Psychologists do not deny persons employment, advancement, admissions to academic or other programs, tenure, or promotion, based solely upon their having made or their being the subject of an ethics complaint. This does not preclude taking action based upon the outcome of such proceedings or considering other appropriate information.

2. *Competence*

2.01 Boundaries of Competence

(a) Psychologists provide services, teach, and conduct research with populations and in areas only within the boundaries of their competence, based on their education, training, supervised experience, consultation, study, or professional experience.

(b) Where scientific or professional knowledge in the discipline of psychology establishes that an understanding of factors associated with age, gender, gender identity, race, ethnicity, culture, national origin, religion, sexual orientation, disability, language, or socioeconomic status is essential for effective implementation of their services or research, psychologists have or obtain the training, experience, consultation, or supervision necessary to ensure the competence of their services, or they make appropriate referrals, except as provided in Standard 2.02, Providing Services in Emergencies.

(c) Psychologists planning to provide services, teach, or conduct research involving populations, areas, techniques, or technologies new to them undertake relevant education, training, supervised experience, consultation, or study.

(d) When psychologists are asked to provide services to individuals for whom appropriate mental health services are not available and for which psychologists have not obtained the competence necessary, psychologists with closely related prior training or experience may provide such services in order to ensure that services are not denied if they make a reasonable effort to obtain the competence required by

using relevant research, training, consultation, or study.

(e) In those emerging areas in which generally recognized standards for preparatory training do not yet exist, psychologists nevertheless take reasonable steps to ensure the competence of their work and to protect clients/patients, students, supervisees, research participants, organizational clients, and others from harm.

(f) When assuming forensic roles, psychologists are or become reasonably familiar with the judicial or administrative rules governing their roles.

2.02 Providing Services in Emergencies

In emergencies, when psychologists provide services to individuals for whom other mental health services are not available and for which psychologists have not obtained the necessary training, psychologists may provide such services in order to ensure that services are not denied. The services are discontinued as soon as the emergency has ended or appropriate services are available.

2.03 Maintaining Competence

Psychologists undertake ongoing efforts to develop and maintain their competence.

2.04 Bases for Scientific and Professional Judgments

Psychologists' work is based upon established scientific and professional knowledge of the discipline. (See also Standards 2.01e, Boundaries of Competence, and 10.01b, Informed Consent to Therapy.)

2.05 Delegation of Work to Others

Psychologists who delegate work to employees, supervisees, or research or teaching assistants or who use the services of others, such as interpreters, take reasonable steps to (1) avoid delegating such work to persons who have a multiple relationship with those being served that would likely lead to exploitation or loss of objectivity; (2) authorize only those responsibilities that such persons can be expected to perform competently on the basis of their education, training, or experience, either independently or with the level of supervision being provided; and (3) see that such persons perform these services competently. (See also Standards 2.02, Providing Services in Emergencies; 3.05, Multiple Relationships; 4.01, Maintaining Confidentiality; 9.01, Bases for Assessments; 9.02, Use of Assessments; 9.03, Informed Consent in Assessments; and 9.07, Assessment by Unqualified Persons.)

2.06 Personal Problems and Conflicts

(a) Psychologists refrain from initiating an activity when they know or should know that there is a substantial likelihood that their personal problems will prevent them from performing their work-related activities in a competent manner.

(b) When psychologists become aware of personal problems that may interfere with their performing work-related duties adequately, they take appropriate measures, such as obtaining professional consultation or assistance, and determine whether they should limit, suspend, or terminate their work-related duties. (See also Standard 10.10, Terminating Therapy.)

3. *Human Relations*

3.01 Unfair Discrimination

In their work-related activities, psychologists do not engage in unfair discrimination based on age, gender, gender identity, race, ethnicity, culture, national origin, religion, sexual orientation, disability, socioeconomic status, or any basis proscribed by law.

3.02 Sexual Harassment

Psychologists do not engage in sexual harassment. Sexual harassment is sexual solicitation, physical advances, or verbal or nonverbal conduct that is sexual in nature, that occurs in connection with the psychologist's activities or roles as a psychologist, and that either (1) is unwelcome, is offensive, or creates a hostile workplace or educational environment, and the psychologist knows or is told this or (2) is sufficiently severe or intense to be abusive to a reasonable person in the context. Sexual harassment can consist of a single intense or severe act or of multiple persistent or pervasive acts. (See also Standard 1.08, Unfair Discrimination Against Complainants and Respondents.)

3.03 Other Harassment

Psychologists do not knowingly engage in behavior that is harassing or demeaning to persons with whom they interact in their work based on factors such as those persons' age, gender, gender identity, race, ethnicity, culture, national origin, religion, sexual orientation, disability, language, or socioeconomic status.

3.04 Avoiding Harm

Psychologists take reasonable steps to avoid harming their clients/patients, students, supervisees, research participants, organizational clients, and others with whom they work, and to minimize harm where it is foreseeable and unavoidable.

3.05 Multiple Relationships

(a) A multiple relationship occurs when a psychologist is in a professional role with a person and (1) at the same time is in another role with the same person, (2) at the same time is in a relationship with a person closely associated with or related to the person with whom the psychologist has the professional relationship, or (3) promises to enter into another relationship in the future with the person or a person closely associated with or related to the person.

A psychologist refrains from entering into a multiple relationship if the multiple relationship could reasonably be expected to impair the psychologist's objectivity, competence, or effectiveness in performing his or her functions as a psychologist, or otherwise risks exploitation or harm to the person with whom the professional relationship exists.

Multiple relationships that would not reasonably be expected to cause impairment or risk exploitation or harm are not unethical.

(b) If a psychologist finds that, due to unforeseen factors, a potentially harmful multiple relationship has arisen, the psychologist takes reasonable steps to resolve it with due regard for the best interests of the affected person and maximal compliance with the Ethics Code.

(c) When psychologists are required by law, institutional policy, or extraordinary circumstances to serve in more than one role in judicial or administrative proceedings, at the outset they clarify role expectations and the extent of confidentiality and thereafter as changes occur. (See also Standards 3.04, Avoiding Harm, and 3.07, Third-Party Requests for Services.)

3.06 Conflict of Interest

Psychologists refrain from taking on a professional role when personal, scientific, professional, legal, financial, or other interests or relationships could reasonably be expected to (1) impair their objectivity, competence, or effectiveness in performing their functions as psychologists or (2) expose the person or organization with whom the professional relationship exists to harm or exploitation.

3.07 Third-Party Requests for Services

When psychologists agree to provide services to a person or entity at the request of a third party, psychologists attempt to clarify at the outset of the service the nature of the relationship with all individuals or organizations involved. This clarification includes the role of the psychologist (e.g., therapist, consultant, diagnostician, or expert witness), an identification of who is the client, the probable uses of the services provided or the information obtained, and the fact that there may be limits to confidentiality. (See also Standards 3.05, Multiple Relationships, and 4.02, Discussing the Limits of Confidentiality.)

3.08 Exploitative Relationships

Psychologists do not exploit persons over whom they have supervisory, evaluative, or other authority such as clients/patients, students, supervisees, research participants, and employees. (See also Standards 3.05, Multiple Relationships; 6.04, Fees and Financial Arrangements; 6.05, Barter With Clients/Patients; 7.07, Sexual Relationships With Students and Supervisees; 10.05, Sexual Intimacies With Current Therapy Clients/Patients; 10.06, Sexual Intimacies With Relatives or Significant Others of Current Therapy Clients/Patients; 10.07, Therapy With Former Sexual Partners; and 10.08, Sexual Intimacies With Former Therapy Clients/Patients.)

3.09 Cooperation With Other Professionals

When indicated and professionally appropriate, psychologists cooperate with other professionals in order to serve their clients/patients effectively and appropriately. (See also Standard 4.05, Disclosures.)

3.10 Informed Consent

(a) When psychologists conduct research or provide assessment, therapy, counseling, or consulting services in person or via electronic transmission or other forms of communication, they obtain the informed consent of the individual or individuals using language that is reasonably understandable to that person or persons except when conducting such activities without consent is mandated by law or governmental regulation or as otherwise provided in this Ethics Code. (See also Standards 8.02, Informed Consent to Research; 9.03, Informed Consent in Assessments; and 10.01, Informed Consent to Therapy.)

(b) For persons who are legally incapable of giving informed consent, psychologists nevertheless (1) provide an appropriate explanation, (2) seek the individual's assent, (3) consider such persons' preferences and best interests, and (4) obtain appropriate permission from a legally authorized person, if such substitute consent is permitted or required by law. When consent by a legally authorized person is not permitted or required by law, psychologists take reasonable steps to protect the individual's rights and welfare.

(c) When psychological services are court ordered or otherwise mandated, psychologists inform the individual of the nature of the anticipated services, including whether the services are court ordered or mandated and any limits of confidentiality, before proceeding.

(d) Psychologists appropriately document written or oral consent, permission, and assent. (See also Standards 8.02, Informed Consent to Research; 9.03, Informed Consent in Assessments; and 10.01, Informed Consent to Therapy.)

3.11 Psychological Services Delivered To or Through Organizations

(a) Psychologists delivering services to or through organizations provide information beforehand to clients and when appropriate those directly affected by the services about (1) the nature and objectives of the services, (2) the intended recipients, (3) which of the individuals are clients, (4) the relationship the psychologist will have with each person and the organization, (5) the probable uses of services provided and information obtained, (6) who will have access to the information, and (7) limits of confidentiality. As soon as feasible, they provide information about the results and conclusions of such services to appropriate persons.

(b) If psychologists will be precluded by law or by organizational roles from providing such information to particular individuals or groups, they so inform those individuals or groups at the outset of the service.

3.12 Interruption of Psychological Services

Unless otherwise covered by contract, psychologists make reasonable efforts to plan for facilitating services in the event that psychological services are interrupted by factors such as the psychologist's illness, death, unavailability, relocation, or retirement or by the client's/patient's relocation or financial limitations. (See also Standard 6.02c, Maintenance, Dissemination, and Disposal of Confidential Records of Professional and Scientific Work.)

4. *Privacy And Confidentiality*

4.01 Maintaining Confidentiality

Psychologists have a primary obligation and take reasonable precautions to protect confidential information obtained through or stored in any medium, recognizing that the extent and limits of confidentiality may be regulated by law or established by institutional rules or professional or scientific relationship. (See also Standard 2.05, Delegation of Work to Others.)

4.02 Discussing the Limits of Confidentiality

(a) Psychologists discuss with persons (including, to the extent feasible, persons who are legally incapable of giving informed consent and their legal representatives) and organizations with whom they establish a scientific or professional relationship (1) the relevant limits of confidentiality and (2) the foreseeable uses of the information generated through their psychological activities. (See also Standard 3.10, Informed Consent.)

(b) Unless it is not feasible or is contraindicated, the discussion of confidentiality occurs at the outset of the relationship and thereafter as new circumstances may warrant.

(c) Psychologists who offer services, products, or information via electronic transmission inform clients/patients of the risks to privacy and limits of confidentiality.

4.03 Recording

Before recording the voices or images of individuals to whom they provide services, psychologists obtain permission from all such persons or their legal representatives. (See also Standards 8.03, Informed Consent for Recording Voices and Images in Research; 8.05, Dispensing With Informed Consent for Research; and 8.07, Deception in Research.)

4.04 Minimizing Intrusions on Privacy

(a) Psychologists include in written and oral reports and consultations, only information germane to the purpose for which the communication is made.

(b) Psychologists discuss confidential information obtained in their work only for appropriate scientific or professional purposes and only with persons clearly concerned with such matters.

4.05 Disclosures

(a) Psychologists may disclose confidential information with the appropriate consent of the organizational client, the individual client/patient, or another legally authorized person on behalf of the client/patient unless prohibited by law.

(b) Psychologists disclose confidential information without the consent of the individual only as mandated by law, or where permitted by law for a valid purpose such as to (1) provide needed professional services; (2) obtain appropriate professional consultations; (3) protect the client/patient, psychologist, or others from harm; or (4) obtain payment for services from a client/patient, in which instance disclosure is limited to the minimum that is necessary to achieve the purpose. (See also Standard 6.04e, Fees and Financial Arrangements.)

4.06 Consultations

When consulting with colleagues, (1) psychologists do not disclose confidential information that reasonably could lead to the identification of a client/patient, research participant, or other person or organization with whom they have a confidential relationship unless they have obtained the prior consent of the person or organization or the disclosure cannot be avoided, and (2) they disclose information only to the extent necessary to achieve the purposes of the consultation. (See also Standard 4.01, Maintaining Confidentiality.)

4.07 Use of Confidential Information for Didactic or Other Purposes

Psychologists do not disclose in their writings, lectures, or other public media, confidential, personally identifiable information concerning their clients/patients, students, research participants, organizational clients, or other recipients of their services that they obtained during the course of their work, unless (1) they take reasonable steps to disguise the person or organization, (2) the person or organization has consented in writing, or (3) there is legal authorization for doing so.

5. *Advertising and Other Public Statements*

5.01 Avoidance of False or Deceptive Statements

(a) Public statements include but are not limited to paid or unpaid advertising, product endorsements, grant applications, licensing applications, other credentialing applications, brochures, printed matter, directory listings, personal resumes or curricula vitae, or comments for use in media such as print or electronic transmission, statements in legal proceedings, lectures and public oral pre-

sentations, and published materials. Psychologists do not knowingly make public statements that are false, deceptive, or fraudulent concerning their research, practice, or other work activities or those of persons or organizations with which they are affiliated.

(b) Psychologists do not make false, deceptive, or fraudulent statements concerning (1) their training, experience, or competence; (2) their academic degrees; (3) their credentials; (4) their institutional or association affiliations; (5) their services; (6) the scientific or clinical basis for, or results or degree of success of, their services; (7) their fees; or (8) their publications or research findings.

(c) Psychologists claim degrees as credentials for their health services only if those degrees (1) were earned from a regionally accredited educational institution or (2) were the basis for psychology licensure by the state in which they practice.

5.02 Statements by Others

(a) Psychologists who engage others to create or place public statements that promote their professional practice, products, or activities retain professional responsibility for such statements.

(b) Psychologists do not compensate employees of press, radio, television, or other communication media in return for publicity in a news item. (See also Standard 1.01, Misuse of Psychologists' Work.)

(c) A paid advertisement relating to psychologists' activities must be identified or clearly recognizable as such.

5.03 Descriptions of Workshops and Non-Degree-Granting Educational Programs

To the degree to which they exercise control, psychologists responsible for announcements, catalogs, brochures, or advertisements describing workshops, seminars, or other non-degree-granting educational programs ensure that they accurately describe the audience for which the program is intended, the educational objectives, the presenters, and the fees involved.

5.04 Media Presentations

When psychologists provide public advice or comment via print, internet, or other electronic transmission, they take precautions to ensure that statements (1) are based on their professional knowledge, training, or experience in accord with appropriate psychological literature and practice; (2) are otherwise consistent with this Ethics Code; and (3) do not indicate that a professional relationship has been established with the recipient. (See also Standard 2.04, Bases for Scientific and Professional Judgments.)

5.05 Testimonials

Psychologists do not solicit testimonials from current therapy clients/patients or other persons who because of their particular circumstances are vulnerable to undue influence.

5.06 In-Person Solicitation

Psychologists do not engage, directly or through agents, in uninvited in-person solicitation of business from actual or potential therapy clients/patients or other persons who because of their particular circumstances are vulnerable to undue influence. However, this prohibition does not preclude (1) attempting to implement appropriate collateral contacts for the purpose of benefiting an already engaged therapy client/patient or (2) providing disaster or community outreach services.

6. *Record Keeping and Fees*

6.01 Documentation of Professional and Scientific Work and Maintenance of Records

Psychologists create, and to the extent the records are under their control, maintain, disseminate, store, retain, and dispose of records and data relating to their professional and scientific work in order to (1) facilitate provision of services later by them or by other professionals, (2) allow for replication of research design and analyses, (3) meet institutional requirements, (4) ensure accuracy of billing and payments, and (5) ensure compliance with law. (See also Standard 4.01, Maintaining Confidentiality.)

6.02 Maintenance, Dissemination, and Disposal of Confidential Records of Professional and Scientific Work

(a) Psychologists maintain confidentiality in creating, storing, accessing, transferring, and disposing of records under their control, whether these are written, automated, or in any other medium. (See also Standards 4.01, Maintaining Confidentiality, and 6.01, Documentation of Professional and Scientific Work and Maintenance of Records.)

(b) If confidential information concerning recipients of psychological services is entered into databases or systems of records available to persons whose access has not been consented to by the recipient, psychologists use coding or other techniques to avoid the inclusion of personal identifiers.

(c) Psychologists make plans in advance to facilitate the appropriate transfer and to protect the confidentiality of records and data in the event of psychologists' withdrawal from positions or practice. (See also Standards 3.12, Interruption of Psychological Services, and 10.09, Interruption of Therapy.)

6.03 Withholding Records for Nonpayment

Psychologists may not withhold records under their control that are requested and needed for a client's/patient's emergency treatment solely because payment has not been received.

6.04 Fees and Financial Arrangements

(a) As early as is feasible in a professional or scientific relationship, psychologists and recipients of psychological services reach an agreement specifying compensation and billing arrangements.

(b) Psychologists' fee practices are consistent with law.

(c) Psychologists do not misrepresent their fees.

(d) If limitations to services can be anticipated because of limitations in financing, this is discussed with the recipient of services as early as is feasible. (See also Standards 10.09, Interruption of Therapy, and 10.10, Terminating Therapy.)

(e) If the recipient of services does not pay for services as agreed, and if psychologists intend to use collection agencies or legal measures to collect the fees, psychologists first inform the person that such measures will be taken and provide that person an opportunity to make prompt payment. (See also Standards 4.05, Disclosures; 6.03, Withholding Records for Nonpayment; and 10.01, Informed Consent to Therapy.)

6.05 Barter With Clients/Patients

Barter is the acceptance of goods, services, or other nonmonetary remuneration from clients/patients in return for psychological services. Psychologists may barter only if (1) it is not clinically contraindicated, and (2) the resulting arrangement is not exploitative. (See also Standards 3.05, Multiple Relationships, and 6.04, Fees and Financial Arrangements.)

6.06 Accuracy in Reports to Payors and Funding Sources

In their reports to payors for services or sources of research funding, psychologists take reasonable steps to ensure the accurate reporting of the nature of the service provided or research conducted, the fees, charges, or payments, and where applicable, the identity of the provider, the findings, and the diagnosis. (See also Standards 4.01, Maintaining Confidentiality; 4.04, Minimizing Intrusions on Privacy; and 4.05, Disclosures.)

6.07 Referrals and Fees

When psychologists pay, receive payment from, or divide fees with another professional, other than in an employer-employee relationship, the payment to each is based on the services provided (clinical, consultative, administrative, or other) and is not based on the referral itself. (See also Standard 3.09, Cooperation With Other Professionals.)

7. *Education and Training*

7.01 Design of Education and Training Programs

Psychologists responsible for education and training programs take reasonable steps to ensure that the programs are designed to provide the appropriate knowledge and proper experiences, and to meet the requirements for licensure, certification, or other goals for which claims are made by the program.

(See also Standard 5.03, Descriptions of Workshops and Non-Degree-Granting Educational Programs.)

7.02 Descriptions of Education and Training Programs

Psychologists responsible for education and training programs take reasonable steps to ensure that there is a current and accurate description of the program content (including participation in required course- or program-related counseling, psychotherapy, experiential groups, consulting projects, or community service), training goals and objectives, stipends and benefits, and requirements that must be met for satisfactory completion of the program. This information must be made readily available to all interested parties.

7.03 Accuracy in Teaching

(a) Psychologists take reasonable steps to ensure that course syllabi are accurate regarding the subject matter to be covered, bases for evaluating progress, and the nature of course experiences. This standard does not preclude an instructor from modifying course content or requirements when the instructor considers it pedagogically necessary or desirable, so long as students are made aware of these modifications in a manner that enables them to fulfill course requirements. (See also Standard 5.01, Avoidance of False or Deceptive Statements.)

(b) When engaged in teaching or training, psychologists present psychological information accurately. (See also Standard 2.03, Maintaining Competence.)

7.04 Student Disclosure of Personal Information

Psychologists do not require students or supervisees to disclose personal information in course- or program-related activities, either orally or in writing, regarding sexual history, history of abuse and neglect, psychological treatment, and relationships with parents, peers, and spouses or significant others except if (1) the program or training facility has clearly identified this requirement in its admissions and program materials or (2) the information is necessary to evaluate or obtain assistance for students whose personal problems could reasonably be judged to be preventing them from performing their training or professionally related activities in a competent manner or posing a threat to the students or others.

7.05 Mandatory Individual or Group Therapy

(a) When individual or group therapy is a program or course requirement, psychologists responsible for that program allow students in undergraduate and graduate programs the option of selecting such therapy from practitioners unaffiliated with the program. (See also Standard 7.02, Descriptions of Education and Training Programs.)

(b) Faculty who are or are likely to be responsible for evaluating students' academic performance do not themselves provide that therapy. (See also Standard 3.05, Multiple Relationships.)

7.06 Assessing Student and Supervisee Performance

(a) In academic and supervisory relationships, psychologists establish a timely and specific process for providing feedback to students and supervisees. Information regarding the process is provided to the student at the beginning of supervision.

(b) Psychologists evaluate students and supervisees on the basis of their actual performance on relevant and established program requirements.

7.07 Sexual Relationships With Students and Supervisees

Psychologists do not engage in sexual relationships with students or supervisees who are in their department, agency, or training center or over whom psychologists have or are likely to have evaluative authority. (See also Standard 3.05, Multiple Relationships.)

8. *Research and Publication*

8.01 Institutional Approval

When institutional approval is required, psychologists provide accurate information about their research proposals and obtain approval prior to conducting the research. They conduct the research in accordance with the approved research protocol.

8.02 Informed Consent to Research

(a) When obtaining informed consent as required in Standard 3.10, Informed Consent, psychologists inform participants about (1) the purpose of the research, expected duration, and procedures; (2) their right to decline to participate and to withdraw from the research once participation has begun; (3) the foreseeable consequences of declining or withdrawing; (4) reasonably foreseeable factors that may be expected to influence their willingness to participate such as potential risks, discomfort, or adverse effects; (5) any prospective research benefits; (6) limits of confidentiality; (7) incentives for participation; and (8) whom to contact for questions about the research and research participants' rights. They provide opportunity for the prospective participants to ask questions and receive answers. (See also Standards

8.03, Informed Consent for Recording Voices and Images in Research; 8.05, Dispensing With Informed Consent for Research; and 8.07, Deception in Research.)

(b) Psychologists conducting intervention research involving the use of experimental treatments clarify to participants at the outset of the research (1) the experimental nature of the treatment; (2) the services that will or will not be available to the control group(s) if appropriate; (3) the means by which assignment to treatment and control groups will be made; (4) available treatment alternatives if an individual does not wish to participate in the research or wishes to withdraw once a study has begun; and (5) compensation for or monetary costs of participating including, if appropriate, whether reimbursement from the participant or a third-party payor will be sought. (See also Standard 8.02a, Informed Consent to Research.)

8.03 Informed Consent for Recording Voices and Images in Research

Psychologists obtain informed consent from research participants prior to recording their voices or images for data collection unless (1) the research consists solely of naturalistic observations in public places, and it is not anticipated that the recording will be used in a manner that could cause personal identification or harm, or (2) the research design includes deception, and consent for the use of the recording is obtained during debriefing. (See also Standard 8.07, Deception in Research.)

8.04 Client/Patient, Student, and Subordinate Research Participants

(a) When psychologists conduct research with clients/patients, students, or subordinates as participants, psychologists take steps to protect the prospective participants from adverse consequences of declining or withdrawing from participation.

(b) When research participation is a course requirement or an opportunity for extra credit, the prospective participant is given the choice of equitable alternative activities.

8.05 Dispensing With Informed Consent for Research

Psychologists may dispense with informed consent only (1) where research would not reasonably be assumed to create distress or harm and involves (a) the study of normal educational practices, curricula, or classroom management methods conducted in educational settings; (b) only anonymous questionnaires, naturalistic observations, or archival research for which disclosure of responses would not place participants at risk of criminal or civil liability or damage their financial standing, employability, or reputation, and confidentiality is protected; or (c) the study of factors related to job or organization effectiveness conducted in organizational settings for which there is no risk to participants' employability, and confidentiality is protected or (2) where otherwise permitted by law or federal or institutional regulations.

8.06 Offering Inducements for Research Participation

(a) Psychologists make reasonable efforts to avoid offering excessive or inappropriate financial or other inducements for research participation when such inducements are likely to coerce participation.

(b) When offering professional services as an inducement for research participation, psychologists clarify the nature of the services, as well as the risks, obligations, and limitations. (See also Standard 6.05, Barter With Clients/Patients.)

8.07 Deception in Research

(a) Psychologists do not conduct a study involving deception unless they have determined that the use of deceptive techniques is justified by the study's significant prospective scientific, educational, or applied value and that effective nondeceptive alternative procedures are not feasible.

(b) Psychologists do not deceive prospective participants about research that is reasonably expected to cause physical pain or severe emotional distress.

(c) Psychologists explain any deception that is an integral feature of the design and conduct of an experiment to participants as early as is feasible, preferably at the conclusion of their participation, but no later than at the conclusion of the data collection, and permit participants to withdraw their data. (See also Standard 8.08, Debriefing.)

8.08 Debriefing

(a) Psychologists provide a prompt opportunity for participants to obtain appropriate information about the nature, results, and conclusions of the research, and they take reasonable steps to correct any misconceptions that participants may have of which the psychologists are aware.

(b) If scientific or humane values justify delaying or withholding this information, psychologists take reasonable measures to reduce the risk of harm.

(c) When psychologists become aware that research procedures have harmed a participant, they take reasonable steps to minimize the harm.

8.09 Humane Care and Use of Animals in Research

(a) Psychologists acquire, care for, use, and dispose of animals in compliance with current federal, state, and local laws and regulations, and with professional standards.

(b) Psychologists trained in research methods and experienced in the care of laboratory animals supervise all procedures involving animals and are responsible for ensuring appropriate consideration of their comfort, health, and humane treatment.

(c) Psychologists ensure that all individuals under their supervision who are using animals have received instruction in research methods and in the care, maintenance, and handling of the species being used, to the extent appropriate to their role. (See also Standard 2.05, Delegation of Work to Others.)

(d) Psychologists make reasonable efforts to minimize the discomfort, infection, illness, and pain of animal subjects.

(e) Psychologists use a procedure subjecting animals to pain, stress, or privation only when an alternative procedure is unavailable and the goal is justified by its prospective scientific, educational, or applied value.

(f) Psychologists perform surgical procedures under appropriate anesthesia and follow techniques to avoid infection and minimize pain during and after surgery.

(g) When it is appropriate that an animal's life be terminated, psychologists proceed rapidly, with an effort to minimize pain and in accordance with accepted procedures.

8.10 Reporting Research Results

(a) Psychologists do not fabricate data. (See also Standard 5.01a, Avoidance of False or Deceptive Statements.)

(b) If psychologists discover significant errors in their published data, they take reasonable steps to correct such errors in a correction, retraction, erratum, or other appropriate publication means.

8.11 Plagiarism

Psychologists do not present portions of another's work or data as their own, even if the other work or data source is cited occasionally.

8.12 Publication Credit

(a) Psychologists take responsibility and credit, including authorship credit, only for work they have actually performed or to which they have substantially contributed. (See also Standard 8.12b, Publication Credit.)

(b) Principal authorship and other publication credits accurately reflect the relative scientific or professional contributions of the individuals involved, regardless of their relative status. Mere possession of an institutional position, such as department chair, does not justify authorship credit. Minor contributions to the research or to the writing for publications are acknowledged appropriately, such as in footnotes or in an introductory statement.

(c) Except under exceptional circumstances, a student is listed as principal author on any multiple-authored article that is substantially based on the student's doctoral dissertation. Faculty advisors discuss publication credit with students as early as feasible and throughout the research and publication process as appropriate. (See also Standard 8.12b, Publication Credit.)

8.13 Duplicate Publication of Data

Psychologists do not publish, as original data, data that have been previously published. This does not preclude republishing data when they are accompanied by proper acknowledgment.

8.14 Sharing Research Data for Verification

(a) After research results are published, psychologists do not withhold the data on which their conclusions are based from other competent professionals who seek to verify the substantive claims through reanalysis and who intend to use such data only for that purpose, provided that the confidentiality of the participants can be protected and unless legal rights concerning proprietary data preclude their release. This does not preclude psychologists from requiring that such individuals or groups be responsible for costs associated with the provision of such information.

(b) Psychologists who request data from other psychologists to verify the substantive claims through reanalysis may use shared data only for the declared purpose. Requesting psychologists obtain prior written agreement for all other uses of the data.

8.15 Reviewers

Psychologists who review material submitted for presentation, publication, grant, or research proposal review respect the confidentiality of and the proprietary rights in such information of those who submitted it.

9. *Assessment*

9.01 Bases for Assessments

(a) Psychologists base the opinions contained in their recommendations, reports, and diagnostic or evaluative statements, including forensic testimony, on information and techniques sufficient to substantiate their findings.

(See also Standard 2.04, Bases for Scientific and Professional Judgments.)

(b) Except as noted in 9.01c, psychologists provide opinions of the psychological characteristics of individuals only after they have conducted an examination of the individuals adequate to support their statements or conclusions. When, despite reasonable efforts, such an examination is not practical, psychologists document the efforts they made and the result of those efforts, clarify the probable impact of their limited information on the reliability and validity of their opinions, and appropriately limit the nature and extent of their conclusions or recommendations. (See also Standards 2.01, Boundaries of Competence, and 9.06, Interpreting Assessment Results.)

(c) When psychologists conduct a record review or provide consultation or supervision and an individual examination is not warranted or necessary for the opinion, psychologists explain this and the sources of information on which they based their conclusions and recommendations.

9.02 Use of Assessments

(a) Psychologists administer, adapt, score, interpret, or use assessment techniques, interviews, tests, or instruments in a manner and for purposes that are appropriate in light of the research on or evidence of the usefulness and proper application of the techniques.

(b) Psychologists use assessment instruments whose validity and reliability have been established for use with members of the population tested. When such validity or reliability has not been established, psychologists describe the strengths and limitations of test results and interpretation.

(c) Psychologists use assessment methods that are appropriate to an individual's language preference and competence, unless the use of an alternative language is relevant to the assessment issues.

9.03 Informed Consent in Assessments

(a) Psychologists obtain informed consent for assessments, evaluations, or diagnostic services, as described in Standard 3.10, Informed Consent, except when (1) testing is mandated by law or governmental regulations; (2) informed consent is implied because testing is conducted as a routine educational, institutional, or organizational activity (e.g., when participants voluntarily agree to assessment when applying for a job); or (3) one purpose of the testing is to evaluate decisional capacity. Informed consent includes an explanation of the nature and purpose of the assessment, fees, involvement of third parties, and limits of confidentiality and sufficient opportunity for the client/patient to ask questions and receive answers.

(b) Psychologists inform persons with questionable capacity to consent or for whom testing is mandated by law or governmental regulations about the nature and purpose of the proposed assessment services, using language that is reasonably understandable to the person being assessed.

(c) Psychologists using the services of an interpreter obtain informed consent from the client/patient to use that interpreter, ensure that confidentiality of test results and test security are maintained, and include in their recommendations, reports, and diagnostic or evaluative statements, including forensic testimony, discussion of any limitations on the data obtained. (See also Standards 2.05, Delegation of Work to Others; 4.01, Maintaining Confidentiality; 9.01, Bases for Assessments; 9.06, Interpreting Assessment Results; and 9.07, Assessment by Unqualified Persons.)

9.04 Release of Test Data

(a) The term *test data* refers to raw and scaled scores, client/patient responses to test questions or stimuli, and psychologists' notes and recordings concerning client/patient statements and behavior during an examination. Those portions of test materials that include client/patient responses are included in the definition of *test data.* Pursuant to a client/patient release, psychologists provide test data to the client/patient or other persons identified in the release. Psychologists may refrain from releasing test data to protect a client/patient or others from substantial harm or misuse or misrepresentation of the data or the test, recognizing that in many instances release of confidential information under these circumstances is regulated by law. (See also Standard 9.11, Maintaining Test Security.)

(b) In the absence of a client/patient release, psychologists provide test data only as required by law or court order.

9.05 Test Construction

Psychologists who develop tests and other assessment techniques use appropriate psychometric procedures and current scientific or professional knowledge for test design, standardization, validation, reduction or elimination of bias, and recommendations for use.

9.06 Interpreting Assessment Results

When interpreting assessment results, including automated interpretations, psychologists take into account the purpose of the assessment as well as the various test factors, test-taking abilities, and other characteristics of the person being assessed, such as situational, personal, linguistic, and cultural differences, that might affect psychologists' judgments or reduce the accuracy of their interpretations. They indicate any significant limitations of their interpretations. (See also Standards 2.01b and c, Boundaries of Competence, and 3.01, Unfair Discrimination.)

9.07 Assessment by Unqualified Persons

Psychologists do not promote the use of psychological assessment techniques by unqualified persons, except when such use is conducted for training purposes with appropriate supervision. (See also Standard 2.05, Delegation of Work to Others.)

9.08 Obsolete Tests and Outdated Test Results

(a) Psychologists do not base their assessment or intervention decisions or recommendations on data or test results that are outdated for the current purpose.

(b) Psychologists do not base such decisions or recommendations on tests and measures that are obsolete and not useful for the current purpose.

9.09 Test Scoring and Interpretation Services

(a) Psychologists who offer assessment or scoring services to other professionals accurately describe the purpose, norms, validity, reliability, and applications of the procedures and any special qualifications applicable to their use.

(b) Psychologists select scoring and interpretation services (including automated services) on the basis of evidence of the validity of the program and procedures as well as on other appropriate considerations. (See also Standard 2.01b and c, Boundaries of Competence.)

(c) Psychologists retain responsibility for the appropriate application, interpretation, and use of assessment instruments, whether they score and interpret such tests themselves or use automated or other services.

9.10 Explaining Assessment Results

Regardless of whether the scoring and interpretation are done by psychologists, by employees or assistants, or by automated or other outside services, psychologists take reasonable steps to ensure that explanations of results are given to the individual or designated representative unless the nature of the relationship precludes provision of an explanation of results (such as in some organizational consulting, preemployment or security screenings, and forensic evaluations), and this fact has been clearly explained to the person being assessed in advance.

9.11. Maintaining Test Security

The term *test materials* refers to manuals, instruments, protocols, and test questions or stimuli and does not include *test data* as defined in Standard 9.04, Release of Test Data. Psychologists make reasonable efforts to maintain the integrity and security of test materials and other assessment techniques consistent with law and contractual obligations, and in a manner that permits adherence to this Ethics Code.

10. *Therapy*

10.01 Informed Consent to Therapy

(a) When obtaining informed consent to therapy as required in Standard 3.10, Informed Consent, psychologists inform clients/patients as early as is feasible in the therapeutic relationship about the nature and anticipated course of therapy, fees, involvement of third parties, and limits of confidentiality and provide sufficient opportunity for the client/patient to ask questions and receive answers. (See also Standards 4.02, Discussing the Limits of Confidentiality, and 6.04, Fees and Financial Arrangements.)

(b) When obtaining informed consent for treatment for which generally recognized techniques and procedures have not been established, psychologists inform their clients/patients of the developing nature of the treatment, the potential risks involved, alternative treatments that may be available, and the voluntary nature of their participation. (See also Standards 2.01e, Boundaries of Competence, and 3.10, Informed Consent.)

(c) When the therapist is a trainee and the legal responsibility for the treatment provided resides with the supervisor, the client/patient, as part of the informed consent procedure, is informed that the therapist is in training and is being supervised and is given the name of the supervisor.

10.02 Therapy Involving Couples or Families

(a) When psychologists agree to provide services to several persons who have a relationship (such as spouses, significant others, or parents and children), they take reasonable steps to clarify at the outset (1) which of the individuals are clients/patients and (2) the relationship the psychologist will have with each person. This clarification includes the psychologist's role and the probable uses of the services provided or the information obtained. (See also Standard 4.02, Discussing the Limits of Confidentiality.)

(b) If it becomes apparent that psychologists may be called on to perform potentially conflicting roles (such

as family therapist and then witness for one party in divorce proceedings), psychologists take reasonable steps to clarify and modify, or withdraw from, roles appropriately. (See also Standard 3.05c, Multiple Relationships.)

10.03 Group Therapy

When psychologists provide services to several persons in a group setting, they describe at the outset the roles and responsibilities of all parties and the limits of confidentiality.

10.04 Providing Therapy to Those Served by Others

In deciding whether to offer or provide services to those already receiving mental health services elsewhere, psychologists carefully consider the treatment issues and the potential client's/patient's welfare. Psychologists discuss these issues with the client/patient or another legally authorized person on behalf of the client/patient in order to minimize the risk of confusion and conflict, consult with the other service providers when appropriate, and proceed with caution and sensitivity to the therapeutic issues.

10.05 Sexual Intimacies With Current Therapy Clients/Patients

Psychologists do not engage in sexual intimacies with current therapy clients/patients.

10.06 Sexual Intimacies With Relatives or Significant Others of Current Therapy Clients/Patients

Psychologists do not engage in sexual intimacies with individuals they know to be close relatives, guardians, or significant others of current clients/patients. Psychologists do not terminate therapy to circumvent this standard.

10.07 Therapy With Former Sexual Partners

Psychologists do not accept as therapy clients/patients persons with whom they have engaged in sexual intimacies.

10.08 Sexual Intimacies With Former Therapy Clients/Patients

(a) Psychologists do not engage in sexual intimacies with former clients/patients for at least two years after cessation or termination of therapy.

(b) Psychologists do not engage in sexual intimacies with former clients/patients even after a two-year interval except in the most unusual circumstances. Psychologists who engage in such activity after the two years following cessation or termination of therapy and of having no sexual contact with the former client/patient bear the burden of demonstrating that there has been no exploitation, in light of all relevant factors, including (1) the amount of time that has passed since therapy terminated; (2) the nature, duration, and intensity of the therapy; (3) the circumstances of termination; (4) the client's/patient's personal history; (5) the client's/patient's current mental status; (6) the likelihood of adverse impact on the client/patient; and (7) any statements or actions made by the therapist during the course of therapy suggesting or inviting the possibility of a posttermination sexual or romantic relationship with the client/patient. (See also Standard 3.05, Multiple Relationships.)

10.09 Interruption of Therapy

When entering into employment or contractual relationships, psychologists make reasonable efforts to provide for orderly and appropriate resolution of responsibility for client/patient care in the event that the employment or contractual relationship ends, with paramount consideration given to the welfare of the client/patient. (See also Standard 3.12, Interruption of Psychological Services.)

10.10 Terminating Therapy

(a) Psychologists terminate therapy when it becomes reasonably clear that the client/patient no longer needs the service, is not likely to benefit, or is being harmed by continued service.

(b) Psychologists may terminate therapy when threatened or otherwise endangered by the client/patient or another person with whom the client/patient has a relationship.

(c) Except where precluded by the actions of clients/patients or third-party payors, prior to termination psychologists provide pretermination counseling and suggest alternative service providers as appropriate.

HISTORY AND EFFECTIVE DATE FOOTNOTE

This version of the APA Ethics Code was adopted by the American Psychological Association's Council of Representatives during its meeting, August 21, 2002, and is effective beginning June 1, 2003. Inquiries concerning the substance or interpretation of the APA Ethics Code should be addressed to the Director, Office of Ethics, American Psychological Association, 750 First Street, NE, Washington, DC 20002-4242. The Ethics Code and information regarding the Code can be found on the APA web site, *http://www.apa.org/ethics*. The standards in this Ethics Code will be used to adjudicate complaints brought concerning alleged conduct occurring on or after the effective date. Complaints regarding conduct occurring prior to the effective date will be adjudicated on the basis of the version of the Ethics Code that was in effect at the time the conduct occurred.

The APA has previously published its Ethics Code as follows:

American Psychological Association. (1953). Ethical standards of psychologists. Washington, DC: Author.

American Psychological Association. (1959). Ethical standards of psychologists. American Psychologist, 14, 279–282.

American Psychological Association. (1963). Ethical standards of psychologists. American Psychologist, 18, 56–60.

American Psychological Association. (1968). Ethical standards of psychologists. American Psychologist, 23, 357–361.

American Psychological Association. (1977, March). Ethical standards of psychologists. APA Monitor, 22–23.

American Psychological Association. (1979). Ethical standards of psychologists. Washington, DC: Author.

American Psychological Association. (1981). Ethical principles of psychologists. American Psychologist, 36, 633–638.

American Psychological Association. (1990). Ethical principles of psychologists (Amended June 2, 1989). American Psychologist, 45, 390–395.

American Psychological Association. (1992). Ethical principles of psychologists and code of conduct. American Psychologist, 47, 1597–1611.

Request copies of the APA's Ethical Principles of Psychologists and Code of Conduct from the APA Order Department, 750 First Street, NE, Washington, DC 20002-4242, or phone (202) 336-5510.

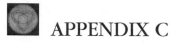 APPENDIX C

LISTING OF RELATED CODES OF ETHICS

American Association of Sex Educators, Counselors and Therapists (AASECT). (1993). *1993 Code of Ethics.* Chicago: Author. Retrieved March 2, 2001, from www.aasect .org/codeofethics.cfm.

American Counseling Association (ACA). (1997). *Policies and procedures for processing complaints of ethical violations.* Alexandria, VA: Author.

American Counseling Association (ACA). (1999). *Ethical Standards for Internet on-line counseling.* Alexandria, VA: Author. Retrieved March 10, 2004, from www.counseling.org.

American Mental Health Counselors Association. (2000). *Code of ethics for mental health counselors.* Alexandria, VA: Author. Retrieved February 28, 2001, from www .amhca.org/about2.html.

American Psychiatric Association. (1998). *Principles of medical ethics with annotations especially applicable to psychiatry.* Washington, DC: Author. Retrieved March 1, 2001, from www.psych.org/ apa_members/ethics.ctm.

American Psychological Association (APA). (1993). *Guidelines for providers of psychological services to ethnic, linguistic and culturally diverse populations.* Washington, DC: Author.

American Psychological Association (APA). (1993). *Record keeping guidelines.* Washington, DC: Author.

American Psychological Association (APA). (1994). Guidelines for child custody evaluations in divorce proceedings. *American Psychologist, 49,* 677–680.

American Psychological Association (APA). (1997). *Mental health patient's bill of rights.* Retrieved March 10, 2004, from www.apa .org/pubinfo/rights/rights.html.

American Psychological Association (APA). (1999). *Suggestions for psychologists working with the media.* Washington, DC: Author.

American Psychological Association Board of Professional Affairs.

(1999). Guidelines for psychological evaluations in child protection matters. *American Psychologist, 54,* 586–593.

American Psychological Association (APA), Committee on Legal Issues. (1996). Strategies for private practitioners coping with subpoenas or compelled testimony for client records or test data. *Professional Psychology: Research and Practice, 27,* 245 251.

American Psychological Association (APA), Committee on Professional Practice and Standards. (1995). Twenty-four questions (and answers) about professional practice in the area of child abuse. *Professional Psychology: Research and Practice, 26,* 377–383.

American Psychological Association, Committee on Professional Practice and Standards. (1994). Guidelines for child custody evaluations in divorce proceedings. *American Psychologist, 49,* 677–680.

American Psychological Association (APA), Committee on Women in Psychology. (1989). If sex enters into the psychotherapy relationship. *Professional Psychology: Research and Practice, 20,* 112–115.

American Psychological Association (APA), Division 44/Committee on Lesbian, Gay and Bisexual Concerns Joint Task Force. (2001). Guidelines for psychotherapy with lesbian, gay and bisexual clients. *American Psychologist, 55,* 1440–1451.

American Rehabilitation Counseling Association. (1987). *Code of professional ethics for rehabilitation counselors.* Arlington Heights, IL: Author.

American School Counselor Association (ASCA). (1998). *Ethical standards for school counselors.* Alexandria, VA: Author. Retrieved March 1,

2001, from www.schoolcounselor .org/ethics/standards/htm.

Association for Counselor Education and Supervision (ACES). (1993). Ethical guidelines for counseling supervisors. *Counselor Education and Supervision, 34,* 270–276.

Association for Specialists in Group Work (ASGW). (1998). *Best Practice Guidelines.* Available at www .asgw.educ.kent/diversity.htm.

Association for Specialists in Group Work. (1998). *Principles for Diversity-Competent Group Workers.* Retrieved February 25, 2004, from www.asgw.org-best .htm.

Association for Specialists in Group Work. (2000). *Professional Standards for the Training of Group Workers.* Retrieved February 25, 2004, from www.asgw.org/best .htm.

Association of State and Provincial Psychology Boards (ASPPB). (1991). *ASPPB code of conduct.* Montgomery, AL: Author.

Canadian Psychological Association. (2000). *Canadian code of ethics for psychologists. Revised.* Ottawa, ON: Author. Retrieved March 2, 2001, from www.cpa .ca/ethics2000.html.

Committee on Ethical Guidelines for Forensic Psychologists. (1991). Specialty guidelines for forensic psychologists. *Law and Human Behavior, 15,* 655–665.

International Association of Marriage and Family Counselors (IAMFC). (1993). *Ethical code for the International Association for Marriage and Family Counselors.* Alexandria, VA: Author. Retrieved March 2, 2001, from www.iamfc.org/ethicalcodes.htm.

National Association of School Psychologists (NASP). (2000). *Principles for professional ethics.* Silver Spring, MD: Author. Retrieved March 2, 2001, from www .naspweb.org/information/index .html.

National Association of Social Workers (NASW). (1999). *Code of ethics.* Silver Spring, MD: Author. Retrieved February 28, 2001, from www.naswdc.org/code.htm.

National Board for Certified Counselors. (1997). *National Board for Certified Counselors: Code of Ethics.* Alexandria, VA: Author. Retrieved February 28, 2001, www.nbcc.org/ethics/nbcc-code.htm.

National Career Development Association. (1991). *National Career Development Association Ethical Standards.* Alexandria, VA: Author. Retrieved March 1, 2001, from www.ncda.org/about/poles.html.

National Career Development Association. (1997). *NCDA guidelines for the use of the Internet for provision of career information and planning services* (Statement). Alexandria, VA: Author. Retrieved March 1, 2002, from www.ncda.org/about/polweb.html.

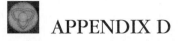

APPENDIX D

OUTLINE FOR WRITING
A COUNSELING SESSION CRITIQUE

Conducting counseling sessions with the support and feedback of a supervisor is an important part of a trainee's professional development. In most counselor education programs, sessions are recorded on either audio or videotape. Once a session is completed, the trainee plays back the recording, providing himself or herself with opportunity to review the quality of the counseling and the dynamics of the client. Information gained in the review can lead to ideas for future sessions and identify areas for improvement. Advanced counselors as well as trainees listen to or watch such tapes to develop a full picture of what happened in a session: important client emotions, beliefs, and personality characteristics not fully perceived during the session; significant moments or turning points; and notable things the counselor did or did not do. Receiving organized feedback from a supervisor and giving organized feedback to oneself are major vehicles both for improving one's work with a given client and for building one's professional skills.

Preparing a written critique of one's counseling sessions is an integral part of the supervisory process. We recommend that the trainee listen to each tape and prepare a written critique prior to supervision with either a field supervisor or university professor responsible for the internship experience. Each critique should show the counselor's thoughtful consideration of the progress of the counseling, with special attention to (1) the client's progress toward the resolution of counseling concerns and (2) the counselor's progress as the planner and facilitator of the counseling session.

A critique is similar to a case study in that it shows evidence of careful observation of a client and thought about the meanings of his or her behaviors. Rationales are needed when inferences are stated. A critique differs from a case study in that it is also a process report in which the counselor actively seeks formative feedback from the supervisor. It can also be regarded as a chapter in a work in progress, with prospects that subsequent events may alter current perceptions.

The following outline is offered as an aid for producing a written analysis of a counseling session, especially one that has been recorded. Used carefully, the outline can help a trainee organize thoughts about the client, the session, and the effectiveness of his or her work. A copy of the write-up will provide the supervisor with a quick yet intensive picture of the session and thus help him or her develop feedback that will be of greatest possible utility to both the counselor and the client. We assume that the supervisor will also listen to or view critical sections of the sessions when preparing written feedback and will at times watch parts of sessions with the trainee. The outline contains six major sections, along with indications of the kind of content that each section might contain. The content described for each category suggests what issues might be addressed, but each question need not be answered for each session and additional material ought to be included as appropriate. In continuing counseling, the critiques should be regarded as a series, and there is no need to repeat detail that has already been presented. Bridges from one critique to another that show new developments are helpful. The last section—headed "Help!"—reflects our experience as supervisors that a student's receptivity to feedback is directly related to his or her ability to clarify the kind of feedback that would be most helpful.

In presenting this template, we are offering one format that has worked well in our counselor education program. Of course, different supervisors might choose to organize differently, but we strongly urge that some form of written critique be included in the supervision process.

COUNSELING SESSION CRITIQUE

Background Information

Why did the client approach you (or why did you approach the client)? Was the client a walk-in or a referral? What were the important concerns and circumstances that brought the two of you together? If third parties were involved, what were the observations and concerns of the third party? What demographic information (such as age, grade in school, employment, family unit, and history) seems relevant to the presenting problem?

Overview of the Session

What did you talk about? What were the dominant issues and themes for this session? If the session was not the initial meeting, what were your process and outcome goals going into the session? Did you find it necessary to do something different because of the client's priorities? (This section should be fairly brief, leaving details of significant interactions for the following section).

Observations and Diagnostic Assessment

What observations and impressions do you have about your client and his or her life space? How intractable are the barriers to growth? How strong are the client's coping skills? What is the etiology of the client's present psychological capacity or incapacity? What is he or she trying to accomplish by various behaviors? What are the influences of significant others in the client's life? How effectively does the client handle relationships with significant others? What hypotheses do you have about the client that may form your counseling interventions? DSM diagnostic categories may be used if you believe they are appropriate. (Chapter 7 provides a structure for addressing many of these questions.) Also, what ethical or legal issues that have arisen or have the potential to arise? For example, if the client is severely depressed, the observations should include comment about the potential ethical responsibility to protect the client from any impulses to do harm to himself or herself.

Observations About the Self

What significant themes and patterns did you observe in your own behavior? In particular, what did you do that you considered especially effective and what areas were troublesome for you? What did you experience internally during the session, particularly at times or places where you felt confused, tense, disappointed, annoyed, disapproving, or controlling? Pay attention to any tendency to do for the client what the client needs to do for himself or herself. How did you implement the basic and advanced counseling skills that you have been working to improve?

Plans for the Next Session

How do you hope to follow up in subsequent sessions? What issues and concerns do you think will be worthwhile to explore? What process goals will you try to accomplish?

Help!

What kind of help you would like, either from your field supervisor, your university supervisor, or from fellow students in your supervision seminar? Focus both on the client's issues and on your helping efforts.

ILLUSTRATION OF A COUNSELING SESSION WRITE-UP

The following example is intended to show the nature of the content and the level of detail expected for a typical write-up submitted by a master's level intern working in a community mental health setting, with supervision on-site and at the university. It is a careful but imperfect presentation that would facilitate the supervision process. The critique analyzes the fourth counseling session with a client whose case has not previously been submitted for supervision.

COUNSELING SESSION CRITIQUE

Client's Name: Kenneth W
Agency Supervisor: Amy Loftus
Date of the Session: 7/23/03
Location of Counseling: Evergreen
  Mental Health
Fourth Session Counselor's Name:
  Chris Watkins
University Supervisor: Hudson Smith
Date Critiqued: 7/25/03

Background Information

Ken is a 20-year-old single male who lives at home with his divorced father after having dropped out of college. Ken's older brother and sister live out of town. His older brother also left college without finishing and is single; his older sister married upon graduation from high school. Ken's mother is remarried and lives in a nearby town. Ken reported that his relationships with both parents and his siblings are "okay" but that the family is not close. Ken is employed at the local library where he has been taught enough skills to work the desk, shelve books, catalog new acquisitions and enter them in the catalog. He likes the work, but the pay is low.

Ken came to counseling on his own because he felt that his life "was not going anywhere" and he thought he fit some of the symptoms of depression that he had seen in an anti-depressant ad on television. He had seen counselors both in high school and while at college and had found the time spent meaningful to him even though he never felt that he reached any conclusions or devised an action plan. In college he majored in European history, which he reports he liked. However, he found that the coursework and assignments "got in the way" of his freely pursuing study in his own way. He attended class less and less, finally leaving the university (a reputable urban state school) before he was thrown out. In the third session with this counselor, Ken talked about having few friends while living in a campus dormitory. He complained that he had found few people who were interested in serious pursuit of the study of history with whom to discuss his work. He also stated that he has never had a girlfriend, but that most of his friendships have been platonic relationships with females who were academically ambitious. Ken wondered whether his lack of sexual interest in women meant that he was gay. He said that he sometimes fantasized about guys who look good, but he has not had sex with men either and cannot imagine himself doing so.

In the initial counseling session, it was established that Ken does exhibit significant symptoms of depression, including a general feeling of sadness that becomes strong enough to lead to weeping at times, a tendency to sleep excessively, feelings of loneliness, a sense of being too tired all the time to do much, and some disturbance of eating patterns. He nevertheless is functional enough to meet his work schedule and actually looks forward to work, which provides his most meaningful human contact. A suicide assessment indicated that Ken had thought about "ending his misery," but that he has not developed a specific plan about when or how he would harm himself. He was referred to the psychiatrist at the clinic for assessment for antidepressant therapy and to consider the cause of his tiredness. The psychiatrist confirmed a diagnosis of dysthymic disorder, but recommended a period of counseling prior to making a decision about medication.

Overview of the Session

Having allowed mostly a free flow of information for the first three sessions and with results of the psychiatrist's consult in hand, I opened today's session by asking Ken what he would like to work on today. It seemed that the time was ripe for some priority setting so that Ken could begin to get a sense of movement with at least one of his set of interrelated concerns.

To my surprise, Ken was quick to say that he would like to talk about his living situation. When he decided to leave college, he had never considered any plan other than to return home. His dad, an accountant with a B.S. degree and a CPA license, had always been his source of support. Ken's dad was willing to have him come home, though he was deeply disappointed that for a second time a very bright son seemed to be throwing away the opportunity for an education. Ken's old room was there, and even though his mother had left while he was in college, the two men could "bach It."

In strictly practical terms, living at home had not worked out badly. Given Ken's low income, his dad had agreed not to charge rent, and Ken in turn had developed the habit of contributing by buying part of the groceries. The two men had no serious conflict, each occasionally cooking a meal and establishing a routine of cleaning up the house most Saturdays.

The problem that Ken had slowly come to understand was that he felt terribly inferior to his successful father and guilty for not becoming "a better man." Ken's dad has a busy professional life with some evening work, especially during income tax season. Even though it was his wife who ended the marriage, Ken's dad dates now that he is no longer married, leaving his "prime" son sitting at home alone. But even when the two men are home at the same time, Ken feels that his dad "keeps looking at me like I should be doing something." Ken's dad does not overtly criticize him and inquires about how things are going at work and so on, but Ken knows his dad is judging the way he is living. The remainder of the session was devoted to (1) exploring whether there is any way of improving the relationship/living situation between Ken and his dad and (2) discussing what other realistic choices Ken may be able to develop to live elsewhere.

Observations and Diagnostic Assessment

I considered it a positive sign that Ken was able to set a work agenda immediately when asked to do so. His ability to report on the dynamic situation with his dad showed insight into both his dad's attitudes and the sense that his own lack of progress with the transition to adulthood was too exposed and therefore painful when living in his dad's house. It had never occurred to Ken to try to talk with his dad about his feelings, and he wasn't sure it was a good idea. He didn't think his dad would openly ridicule him, but he was not sure his dad could understand how he feels. He agreed to think it over. Any shift to independent living at this

time will result in much diminished circumstances, but Ken wonders if he would feel better about himself if he were on his own. Ken reported feeling some excitement about tackling the problem of his living situation, whatever way it turns out.

Observations About the Self

I felt somewhat elated that Ken seemed to work so hard during the session. The previous sessions with him had left me feeling Ken's sense of malaise—almost sharing some of his hopelessness. In this session, it felt like we were really moving. I had some temptation to support the idea that Ken should get his own place, but I kept remembering, too, that there are advantages to his having the financial support of his dad to launch whatever plan Ken devises next. Overall, I was satisfied that we had a thorough discussion and that Ken had useful homework to do in considering both of his alternatives.

Plans for the Next Session

I'll try again to let Ken set the agenda by asking him where he would like to work today and I will follow his lead, while reserving at least half the session to return to his homework and his thoughts about his living situation. I expect that he will go there to begin with, but I'll give him control while remembering to work on the unfinished business. Still aware that the primary diagnosis is his mood disorder, I'll check on how he has been feeling.

Help!

Is it okay to work on the living situation as a first step? Future work needs to cover choices about Ken's life work and his sense of what will satisfy both what he likes to do and who he thinks he must be? In the final analysis, he needs employment that will meet his needs as he understands them. He probably needs help in establishing effective relationships with people his own age and achieving some kind of mature sexual gratification. I also wonder whether there is anything useful to salvage in his relationships with his family. If all this were done, his mood might take care of itself. With so much to be done, it feels almost trivial to spend time on whether he should be living at home. What do you think?

EXAMPLE OF A SUPERVISOR'S RESPONSE

The following response assumes that the session and critique were reviewed by the supervisor, and that, in this instance, feedback to the counselor was given in written form. Of course, an alternative procedure that occurs part of the time includes a face-to-face supervision conference that would address much of the same content.

SUPERVISOR'S RESPONSE

This was a good counseling session and a well-written critique. It seems that you have a good start with your client, and the precaution of seeking a consultation with the psychiatrist was appropriate. The decision to couch counseling as "work" in your opening lead proved to be a good choice, and it may help move your work beyond previous counseling where the client did not believe that much was accomplished in spite of his good feelings. It occurs to me that this client has so few successful relationships in his life that just spending time with a counselor who offers full attention may feel good, but is not likely in itself to be sufficient. One hypothesis might be that Ken has

never developed much facility at human relationships because of the family milieu where personal relationships were distant. The deficit seems to have extended to age mates as well. On the one hand, he might gain some insight about relationships by experiencing closeness and caring in his counseling sessions; on the other hand, his mood will likely improve if he gains more of a sense that he is in control of his future by making some decisions. As I viewed the session, I thought your leads were a good mixture of support and challenge.

My first impulse in responding to your "help" question is to ask you what else you would do if you did not work on the client's question about his living situation? Would you introduce another topic instead? Is there some way that you could tackle the complexity of his total situation all at once? I think not. Nevertheless, your feeling of wanting to be able to do more right away is understandable. But remember, with this client, you are trying to help him make up for lost time with the maturation process. Although you can facilitate his growth, it will take time for him to develop, and he will have to proceed a step at a time. It seems likely that specific action steps, if well planned, should give Ken a sense of increasing control over his life, with the result that his mood should begin to improve.

When you get back to talking about his living situation and the related issue of his relationship with his father, I think it would be useful for you to try a role-play of a conversation with his dad. I'd probably try it by taking the role of Ken's dad and letting Ken try to tell me how it feels living at home with him. But it would also be instructive to take the role of Ken and let him portray how he thinks his dad sees him. Either way, the process should help Ken clarify the relationship and how he wants to proceed.

Ken's need for help with career issues centers on the issue of how he can get paid enough (by his standards) to do things that he likes to do. This probably will require further schooling, given the kinds of interests he has, but it will be important to explore how he lost focus on his schooling. Ken's need for human contact, and ultimately relationships with age mates, remains on a future agenda as well.

It is important for you to ask Ken in each session how he has been feeling. With a dysthymic disorder diagnosis, the expectation would be that therapy would improve his mood as he gains control over his life. However, plateaus can be discouraging, and it is important to keep alert to his mood.

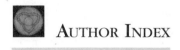

AUTHOR INDEX

Abrego, P. J., 48, 91, 112, 152, 169, 189
Achenbach, T. M., 159, 307
Addis, M. E., 188, 282, 283
Adelman, H. S., 141, 300
Adler, A., 216
Aguilera, D. C., 237, 238, 239, 240, 243, 244, 245, 247, 248
Ahern, J., 239
Alexander, F. M. 3, 216
Allen-Portsche, S. M., 110
American Association of University Women, 272, 279
American Counseling Association, 131, 132, 133
American Educational Research Association, 157
American Psychiatric Association, 156, 307
American Psychological Association, 131, 133, 138, 272, 275, 276
American Psychological Association Working Group on the Older Adult, 322, 323, 324, 328, 335, 336
Anastasi, A., 157
Anderson, J. R., 134
Arrendondo, P. M., 138, 257, 263, 264
Atkinson, D. R., 188, 256, 257, 264, 265, 266, 268, 270, 287, 288
Authier, J., 267

Bachelor, A., 3, 56
Baker, E. L., 216
Balogh, D. W., 141
Bandura, A., 311
Barker, P. 297, 299, 301
Barkham, M., 92
Barley, D. E., 1, 3, 9, 19, 35, 137, 152
Barret, B., 287, 288
Barret, R. L., 134
Beauchamp, T. L., 137
Beck, A. T., 4, 27, 53, 158, 221, 222
Bedi, D. E., 3, 7
Belenky, M. F., 271
Benefield, R. G., 88
Benjamin, A., 174
Bernard, J. M., 141
Bernard, M. E., 4, 221
Besner, H. F., 287

Beutler, L. E., 188, 197
Bleuer, J. C., 13
Bohart, A. C., 23, 52, 56, 150, 152
Bongar, B., 243
Bonsi, E. E., 110
Borgen, F., 158
Bouhoutsos, J. C., 142
Bradford, J., 289
Brady, C. A., 302
Bragdon, R. A., 120
Brammer, L. M., 28, 48, 91, 112, 152, 169, 189, 246
Brodsky, S. L., 197
Brooks, G. R., 281, 285
Broverman, D. M., 272
Broverman, I. K., 272
Brown, G. K., 158
Brown, S. P., 138, 263
Bucuvalas, M., 239
Budman, S. H., 121
Burke, J. E., 216, 218
Burnett, P. C., 159
Butcher, J. N., 157

Callanan, P., 36
Cangelosi, D., 302
Caplan, G., 244
Carkhuff, R. R., 3, 7, 33, 53
Carter, J. A., 35
Casper, L. M., 314
Cattell, A. K., 157
Cattell, H. E., 157
Cattell, R. B., 157
Celentana, M. A., 156
Chen, H., 322
Childress, J. F., 137
Christiani, T. S., 84
Clark, A. J., 87, 91, 92
Clarkson, R. E., 272
Claus, R. E., 141
Clinchy, B. M., 271
Cochran, S. V., 283
Cogar, M. M., 160
Committee on Women in Psychology, 142
Cooper, J. F., 232, 233
Corey, G. R., 36, 141, 169, 206, 217
Corey, M., 36, 141
Cormier, L. S., 4, 14, 33, 77, 101, 104, 122, 195
Costa, P. T., 157
Cottone, R. R., 141
Cowan, E. W., 189, 190

Cox, M. V., 307
Cramer, S. H., 174
Cristol, A. H., 232
Csikszentmihalyi, M., 3
Cumming, E., 334
Cummings, N. A., 121

Dahlstrom, W. C., 157
Danzinger, P., 338
Darrow, C., 321
deShazer, S., 233
Davenport, D. S., 189, 190, 195, 196
Deane, F. P., 120
Denman, D. W., 160
Deutsch, C. J., 15
DiClemente, C. C., 9, 186
Dinger, T. M., 120
Dinkmeyer, D. C., 84, 106, 307, 315, 317
Dinkmeyer, D. C., Jr., 84, 106, 315, 317
Doll, B., 299
Doyle, R. E., 185
Dryden, W., 221, 223
Duncan, B. D., 23, 39, 137
Dworkin, S. H., 287
Dyer, W. W., 186, 191

Egan, G., 3, 7, 33, 34, 37, 48, 53, 77, 78, 80, 83, 84, 110, 195
Eisenberg, S., 4, 53
Ellis, A., 4, 27, 221, 222, 223
Emery, G., 27, 221
Englar-Carlson, M., 283
Erikson, E., 216, 298, 325, 334
Estes, C. P., 271
Eysenck, H. J., 137

Fagan, J., 212
Faidley, A. J., 156
Fields, J., 314
Figley, C. R., 244
Fischer, A. R., 256
Fisher, C. B., 141
Fitts, W. H., 158
Fitzgerald, L. F., 138, 277
Forer, B., 142
Frank, J. B., 8, 92
Frank, J. D., 8, 92
Frauman, D., 76
Friedrich, W. N., 302
Freud, S., 3, 215
Fromm, E., 216

Galea, S., 239
Gallagher-Thompson, D., 321
Ganikos, M. L., 323, 330
Garbarino, J., 301
Garske, J. P., 92
Gatz, M., 322
Gelso, C. J., 35, 121, 122
George, R.L., 84
Gil-Rivas, V., 239
Gibson, W. T., 144, 288
Gilligan, C., 271, 298
Gilliland, B. E., 49, 196, 206, 238,
    239, 242, 243, 245, 247, 248
Gladding, S., 149
Gold, J., 239
Goldenberg, H., 317
Goldenberg, I., 317
Goldstein, A. P., 36
Good, G. E., 281, 283
Goodman, P., 212
Goodyear, R. K., 122, 123
Gough, H. G., 157
Goyette-Ewing, M., 312
Grady, K. A., 323, 330
Graham, J. R., 157
Grant, S. K., 268
Greenberg, L. S., 52, 56
Greenberg, M., 142
Guitierrez, F. J., 287
Gurman, A. S., 121
Gustafson, K. E., 141

Habben, C., 156
Hackney, H., 4, 33, 101, 104,
    122, 195
Hackett, G., 287, 288
Haley, W. E., 322
Hall, T. M., 302
Hammer, A., 158
Hancy, M., 320, 330
Hansen, J., 158
Harmon, L., 158
Harrison, R., 75
Haspel, K. C., 142
Havighurst, R. J., 326
Hawkins, E. J., 9
Hefferline, R., 212
Helms, J. E., 88, 92
Henry, W., 334
Herjanic, B., 307
Herlihy, B., 141
Hersh, J. B., 242, 244, 245, 248
Hill, C. E., 83, 88, 92, 111, 160,
    180, 181
Hillman, J., 238, 243, 245
Holland, J. L., 158
Holman, E. A., 239
Holroyd, J., 142
Horne, A. M., 280, 281, 282,
Horvath, A. O., 3, 7, 56
Hoyt, M. F., 232
Hubble, M. A., 23, 39, 137

Inhelder, B., 297
Ivey, A. E., 48, 53, 59, 62, 63, 73,
    75, 76, 84, 91, 168, 189, 258,
    259, 267

Ivey, M. B., 48, 53, 59, 62, 63, 73,
    75, 76, 84, 91, 168, 189, 259

Jackson, S. E., 15
James, R. K., 49, 196, 206, 238,
    239, 242, 243, 245, 247, 248
Johnson, B., 299
Joliff, D., 280, 281, 282
Jome, L. M., 256
Jones, J., 138, 263
Jordan, J. M., 263, 279
Jorgenson, L. M., 142
Jourard, S. M., 83
Jung, C. G., 216

Kaduson, H. G., 302
Kaemmer, B., 157
Kazantzis, N., 110
Kazdin, A. E., 26, 228, 299
Keith-Spiegel, P. S., 141
Kell, B. J., 123
Kelley, G. A., 26, 53
Kilpatrick, D., 239
Kitchener, K. S., 135, 140
Klein, E., 321
Kleinke, C., 119
Knight, B. G., 325
Kohlberg, L., 297
Koocher, G., 141
Korb, M., 212
Kottman, T., 304
Kovacs, A. L., 123
Krauskopf, C. J., 15
Krumboltz, L., 229
Kubler-Ross, E., 336
Kvale, H., 323

Lambert, M. J., 1, 3, 9, 19, 35,
    137, 152
Lampropoulos, G. K., 110
Landreth, G. L., 303
Lazarus, A. A., 156, 228, 307
Lebo, D., 303
Lee, C. C., 264
Leiter, M. P., 15
Leitner, L. M., 156
Lerman, H., 142
Levant, R. F., 281, 282, 284
Levinson, D. J., 321
Levinson, M., 321
Lichenstein, B., 197
Lindemann, E., 240
Locke, D., 138, 263
Logan, C., 287, 288
Lopez-Baez, S. I., 279
Lopez, S. J., 3
Lowenstein, S. F., 122
Lynn, S. J., 76

MacDonald, G., 28, 246
Mackey, E. F., 290
Mackey, R. A., 290
MacNeil, G., 244
Mahalik, J. R., 188, 282, 283
Martin, D. G., 77, 91, 121, 173
Martin, M. H., 186
Marx, J. A., 121, 122

Maslach, C., 15
McCrane, R. R., 157
McDavis, R. J., 257, 264
McDonald, P. A., 328, 330
McIntosh, D. N., 239
McKay, G. D., 315, 317
McKee, B., 321
McNamara, J. R., 141
Mecham, D., 159
Meehl, P., 157
Meichenbaum, D., 4, 27, 53, 221, 228
Melchert, T. P., 134
Meller, P. J., 268
Messer, S., 216
Michaels, S., 287
Miller, D. J., 139
Miller, M., 15
Miller, S. D., 23, 39, 137
Miller, W. R., 88
Millon, T., 157
Mintz, L. B., 188
Moleiro, C., 188, 197
Molnar, A., 233
Molteni, A. L., 92
Morten, G., 188, 256, 257, 264,
    265, 266, 270
Moyers, T. B., 195, 197
Mueller, W. J., 123
Muran, J. C., 16
Murray, H. A., 158
Myers, J. E., 322, 330, 335, 337
Muro, J. J., 307

Najavits, L. M., 14, 49
National Center for Health
    Statistics, 321
Nelson, R., 296, 298, 301
Niederehe, G., 321
Nielson, G. H., 323
Norman, S., 321
Norris, A., 334
Nurius, P. S., 4, 14, 77
Nutt, R., 138, 277
Nystul, M. S., 123, 307

O'Brien, B. A., 290
O'Brien, K. M., 83, 111, 180, 181
O'Grady, K. E., 88, 92
Okun, B. F., 55
O'Leary, E., 325
Olson, J. B., 323, 330
O'Neil, J. M., 188
Orton, G. L., 299, 300, 302, 307, 311

Parsons, F., 207, 225
Parsons, J. P., 142
Pate, R. H., 122
Patterson, C. H., 80, 81, 91, 169,
    206, 208, 218, 221, 222
Patterson, G. R., 316
Patterson, L. E., 4, 53, 299
Patterson, M. M., 134
Pedersen, P. B., 258, 261
Perkins, D. V., 141
Perls, F., 3, 85, 212
Perry, E. S., 88, 92
Piaget, J., 297

Pipes, R. B., 189, 190, 195, 196
Pleck, J. H., 281, 282
Pollack, W. S., 281
Polster, E., 3, 87, 212
Polster, M., 3, 87, 212
Ponterotto, J. G., 268
Pope, K. S., 131, 142, 143, 144, 288
Poulin, M., 239
Presbury, J. H., 189, 190
Prochaska, J. O., 9, 186, 206
Prout, H. T., 297, 298
Prouty, A. M., 156

Qualls, S. H., 321, 325
Quick, E. K., 233
Quintana, S. M., 123

Rabinowitz, F. E., 283
Rak, C. F., 299
Razzhavaikina, T. I., 110
Reich, W., 307
Remer, P., 278
Renk, K., 120
Resnick, J., 239
Rich, A., 288
Riordan, R. J., 186
Ritchie, M. H., 186
Robb, C., 322
Roberts, A. R., 244, 245, 248, 249
Robinson, F. P., 173, 174
Rogers, C. R., 3, 7, 23, 34, 52, 55,
    57, 60, 77, 150, 172, 206, 209
Roid, G. H., 158
Rollnick, S., 195, 197
Rooney, R. H., 186
Rorschach, H., 158
Rosencrantz, P. S., 272
Rosewater, L. B., 278
Rossberg, R., 174
Rudolph, L. B., 298, 299, 301, 312
Rush, A. J., 27, 221
Ryan, C., 289
Ryan, W., 268

Safran, J. D., 16
Samstag, L. W., 16
Sanchez, J., 138, 263
Sandoval, J., 244
Santoro, S., 338
Saunders-Robinson, M. A., 279
Schaefer, C. E., 302, 304
Schaie, W. K., 324
Scheel, M. J., 110
Schuerger, J., 105
Schweibert, V. L., 322, 330, 335, 337
Stott, F., 301
Scrutton, S., 335
Seay, T. A., 156
Segal, D. L., 321
Seligman, L., 120
Seligman, M. E. P., 3, 137
Sexton, T. L., 13

Shaffer, W. R., 149
Shamburg, B. S., 110
Shapiro, D., 92
Sharf, R. S., 206, 230, 232, 233
Shaw, B., 221
Shea, S. C., 243
Shepherd, I., 212
Sherman, E., 328, 330, 332, 333, 334
Shertzer, B., 173
Shostrum, E. L., 48, 91, 112, 152,
    169, 189
Shulman, L., 120
Sieber, J. E., 141
Silver, R. C., 239
Silverstein, L. B., 285
Simek-Morgan, L., 48, 189, 259
Simkin, J. S., 212
Sinacore-Guinn, A. L., 5
Skinner, B. F., 228
Skovolt, T. M., 16
Sloane, R. B., 232
Smart, D. W., 9, 35
Smyer, M., 322, 325
Snyder, C. R., 3
Sommers-Flanagan, J., 161, 162
Sommers-Flanagan, R., 161, 162
Sperry, L., 106
Spiegel, S. H., 88, 92
Spielberg, W., 281, 282
Sporakowski, M. J., 156
Spungin, C. I., 287
Stadler, H., 15, 138, 263
Staples, E. R., 232
Steer, R. A., 158
Stevan, L., 9, 35
Stevens, C., 16
Stewart, C., 244
Stewart, R., 312
Stiver, I., 149
Stone, S. C., 173
Stott, F., 301
Strupp, H. H., 14, 49
Sue, D., 258, 259, 260, 266, 267
Sue, D. W., 188, 256, 257, 258, 259,
    260, 264, 265, 266, 267, 270
Sue, S., 267
Sullivan, H. S., 216
Suzuki, L. A., 268
Swales, T., 307
Swensen, L., 142
Swenson, C. H., 156

Talebi, H., 188, 197
Tallman, K., 23, 52, 150, 152
Tannen, D., 271
*Tarasoff v. Regents of the University
    of California,* 141, 142
Tarule, J. M., 271
Taylor, L., 141, 300
Tellegen, A., 157
Thelen, M. H., 139
Thompson, B. J., 160

Thompson, C. E., 268
Thompson, C. L., 298, 299, 301, 312
Thoreson, R. W., 15
Thorman, G., 330, 334
Tichenor, V., 88, 92
Todd, D. M., 120
Toman, J. A., 287
Tonigan, J. S., 88
Toporek, R., 138, 263
Truax, C. B., 77

Urbina, S., 157
U. S. Bureau of the Census, 321

Van de Reit, V., 212
Vasquez, M. J. T., 131, 141
Vermeersch, D. A., 9, 35
Vetter, V. A., 143
Vlahov, D., 239
Vogel, S. R., 272
Vriend, J., 186, 191

Walker, L. E., 278
Wallace, W. A, 171
Walz, G. R., 13
Wampold, B. E., 1, 3, 19
Ward, D. W., 119, 121,123
Warnick, J., 232, 321, 322, 323, 324,
    325, 328, 330, 332, 336, 337
Warren C. S., 216
Watkins, C. E., 206, 208, 218, 221, 222
Watterson, D., 105
Weinberg, G., 122
Weiss, R. S., 122
Welfel, E. R., 10, 24, 30, 131, 139,
    141, 143, 170, 171, 272, 278,
    299, 300, 338
Wheeler, G., 212
Whipple, J. L., 9, 35
Whipple, K., 232
Whiston, S. C., 13
White, R. W., 123
Whitley, B. E., Jr., 141
Williamson, E. G., 4, 207, 225
Willis, S. L., 324
Wincze, J. P., 142
Wittig, A. F., 141
Wolinsky, M. A., 330, 336
Wolpe, J., 228, 230
Worrell, J., 278
Wrenn, C. G., 18, 262

Yalom, I. D., 30
Yontef, G. M., 212
Yorkston, N. J., 232
Young, K., 267

Zane, N., 267
Zarit, J., 325
Zarit, S. H., 325

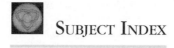

SUBJECT INDEX

ABC theory, 222
Ability-potential responses, 104,
    106, 108, 176
  and advice giving, 105
  definition, 104
  as encouragement, 106
  examples of, 104–105
  purpose of, 105
Acceptance, 175
Action plans, 109–119
  categories of, 112
  counselor skills in, 111–112
  definition, 110
  evaluating outcomes of,
    113–114
  homework for, 110
  obstacles to, 115–116
  organizational context of, 119
  revising, 114–115
  support for, 116–118
  and theoretical orientation, 109
  unsuccessful, 117
Additive responses, 54, 178
Advanced empathy, 31, 37, 48,
    68–72, 140, 143–144
Advice giving, 65–66
  And ability-potential
    responses, 106
Affirmation, 175
Ageism, 331–332
Alexithymia in men, 284
Anxiety, 24, 30
Assertiveness training, 110
Assessment (See also Diagnosis)
  BASIC ID, 156
  and behavioral observations,
    158–159
  of children, 305–311
  components of, 153–156
  in crisis intervention, 244–247
  definition, 149
  frame of reference for, 150–153
  and intake interviews, 161–162
  relation to theoretical
    orientation, 152–153
  and role playing, 159
  and standardized tests,
    157–158
  timing of, 160–162
  tools for, 156–159
Attending 33, 48–49

Beck Depression Inventory II, 158
Behavior
  cultural influences on, 258–259
  free and responsible, 29–30

importance of
    understanding, 3–4
  non-verbal, 47–50, 258–259
  self-defeating, 16–17
Behavior change, 24–25
Behavioral counseling, 228–234
Beliefs, change in 24–25
Beneficence, 137
Bisexual clients (*See* sexual
    minorities)
Blocks to communication,
    65–68
Body image, in women, 275
Brief therapy, 232–233
Burnout
  avoiding, 16
  definition, 15–16

California Personality
    Inventory, 157
Case studies
  advanced empathy, 79–80
  application of precepts, 11–12
  assessment, 163–164
  cognitive and behavioral
    change, 27–28
  confrontation, 89–90
  crisis intervention, 249–252
  culturally sensitive
    counseling, 267–268
  gender sensitive counseling
    with men, 286–287
    with women, 279–280
  interpretation, 93–94
  latchkey child, 308–311
  older Adult, 338–340
  oppositional client, 200–203
  undersocialized child,
    313–314
  role playing, 95–96
  specifying goals, 108
Catharsis, 46, 72–73, 302–303
Change
  as goal, 23–24
  secondary gains from
    avoiding, 115
Child abuse, 299, 308
Children
  assessing of, 305–311
  and blended families, 314,
    316–317
  cognitive development of,
    296–299
  communicating with, 299–305
  and confidentiality, 299–300
  and freedom, 298

and insight, 297, 303
latchkey, 311
misbehavior, reasons for, 317
moral development, 297–298
parental involvement, 314–317
psychosocial development
    of, 297–298
raised by grandparents,
    314–315
socialization of, 311–314
talking with, 300–302
use of play with, 302–304
Clients (*See also* children, older
    adults, reluctant clients,
    women)
  characteristics when beginning
    counseling, 46–47
Client change, 4–5
  readiness for, 186–187
Closed questions, 67–68, 181–182
Codes of ethics, 10, 130–135
Cognitive counseling, 221–225
Cognitive distortions, 222
Cognitive restructuring, 223
Communication
  blocks to, 65–69
  of caring and respect, 14
  of feedback, 74–76
  with children, 299–302
Compassion fatigue, 244
Concreteness, 34–35, 62–64,
    170, 173
Confidentiality, 130, 134, 143,
    170, 299–300, 338
  and duty to warn, 141–142
Confrontation, 37–38, 73, 77,
    83–89, 245–246,
  client defenses and, 87–88
  definition of, 83
  guidelines for, 88–89
  and mixed messages, 86
Congruence (*See also*
    genuineness), 7, 34, 60–62
Continuum of counseling
    theories, 207–209
Continuum of lead, 174–177
Control, locus of, 260–261
Coping skills, 10, 24, 25, 26, 28
  of clients in crisis, 244
Core conditions (*See* counseling
    core conditions)
Counseling
  and advice-giving, 7, 23, 64–65
  alternatives to, 36
  and conversation, 8
  core conditions of, 51–64

Counseling, (*continued*)
  definition, 23
  fundamental precepts of, 5–10
  goals of, 25–32
  model of, 2–4
  and negative feelings, 30–31
  and psychotherapy, 23–24
  purpose of, 1
  readiness for change, 9,
    186–187
  reasons for seeking, 46–47
  research on effectiveness, 1
  skills with culturally diverse
    clients, 266–269
  skills with gay, lesbian, and
    bisexual clients, 288–290
  skills with men, 283–285
  as work, 7–8, 34–35
Counseling process
  behavioral view of, 299–231
  brief therapy view of,
    232–233
  cognitive view of, 223–225
  effectiveness and efficiency, 1
  gender bias in, 278, 282–283
  gestalt view of, 213–215
  person-centered view of,
    210–211
  psychoanalytic view of,
    219–220
  with reluctant clients, 195–198
  stages of, 3–4
  trait-factor view of, 226–227
Counseling relationship,
    characteristics of, 7,
  concreteness, 62–64
  congruence, 60–62
  empathy, 52–57
  genuineness, 60–62
  positive regard, 57–60
  unconditionality, 57
Counseling theories
  behavioral, 228–232
  brief therapy, 232–233
  cognitive, 221–225
  continuum, 207–209
  gestalt, 212–215
  person-centered, 209–211
  psychoanalytic, 215–221
  trait-factor, 225–228
Counselor,
  characteristics of, 12–19
  emotions of, 15–16, 58–59
  expertise, 7
  licensing, 24
  nonverbal behavior of, 47–50
  predispositions of, 65
  stress, 15–16 (*See also*
    burnout and impairment)
  and value judgments, 16
Countertransference, 191–192
Crisis
  balancing factors in, 238–239
  definition of crisis, 238
  triggers of, 240–242
Crisis intervention
  action plans in, 247–249
  assessment of clients, 244–247
  assuring client safety in,
    243–244
  and core conditions, 242–243
  counseling process for, 242–249

and dangerous clients, 243–244
  goals of, 240
  supports for clients, 247
  termination of, 248–249
  vs. traditional counseling,
    237–238
Culture
  counselor understanding of,
    17–18
  emic perspective on, 258–259
  etic perspective on, 258
  importance in counseling,
    258–262
  and locus of control, 260–261
  and locus of responsibility, 188
  and older clients, 344
  and worldview, 260–262
Cultural diversity
  adapting generic model to,
    255–256
  and core conditions, 267
  counselor knowledge base
    for, 263–266
  counselor skills for, 266–269
  demographic trends, 256–257
  impact on counseling
    profession, 255
  and referral sources, 268
Cultural elitism, 262, 264–265
Cultural encapsulation, 18,
    262–263, 266
Cultural identity
  counselor, 262
  stage model of, 264–266
Cultural mistrust, 266
Cultural influences, 258–261
Cultural sensitivity
  and counselor self-
    awareness, 262–263
  and empathy, 55
  and racism, 260

Dangerous clients, 118–119,
    141–142, 243–244
Defenses and defense
    mechanisms, 71, 189, 213,
    216, 217, 218–219
  and confrontation, 84–85
  working with client's, 87–88
Desensitization, 230
Depression and the older
    client, 329
Diagnosis
  BASIC ID, 156
  and client defenses, 151–152
  criticisms of, 149
  dangers of, 4
  definition, 150
  and DSM-IV, 156, 157, 307
  formal systems for, 156
  medical versus counseling
    models of, 151–153
  mistakes in, 162–164
  proper timing of, 160–161
  tools for, 156–159
Direct intervention for
    dangerous clients, 118–119
Directiveness, counselor
  in goal setting, 106–109
Discrimination, 275, 276,
    278–279, 287
Dislike, for a client, 58–59

Dual relationships, 132–133, 278
Duty to warn, 141–142

Eating disorders, 275
Effective living, 2
Ego integrity, 325
Emic perspective, 258–259
Emotional distress, 24, 25, 28
Empathy, 7, 34, 37, 41, 42, 73,
    77–80, 190, 242, 267, 281,
    296, 318
  advanced, 77–80
  communication skills and, 53
  with culturally diverse
    clients, 267
  effects of, 55–56
  evocative, 77
  perceiving skills and, 53–55
  in person-centered
    counseling, 51, 210
  primary, 53–55, 77–79
  training with men, 284
Empowerment, 2, 278
Encouragement, 106 (*See also*
    ability-potential
    responses)
Environmental manipulation, 230
Erroneous thinking, 221–223
Ethical principles, 10, 135–140
  as basis of code, 135–136
  beneficence, 137
  fidelity, 139–140
  justice, 138
  nonmaleficence, 137–138
  respect for autonomy,
    136–137
Ethical theory, 140–141
Ethical violations
  motivation for, 144–145
  types, common, 142–144
Ethics
  and culturally diverse
    clients, 138
  importance to successful
    counseling 129–130
  relationship to the law, 141–142
  sexual misconduct, 142–143
  theories, 140–141
Ethics, Codes of, 8–9, 292–296
  and confidentiality, 133
  and dual relationships, 132,
    142–143
  duty to warn and protect,
    141–142
  and HIV status, 134–135
  and insurance payment, 133
  limitations of, 132–134
Etic perspective, 258
Examples
  ability potential responses,
    104–105
  concreteness, 63–64
  empathic responding, 56, 78
  ethical dilemmas, 130
  immediacy responses, 81–82
  interpretation, 93
  leading, 177–178
  primary vs. advanced
    empathy, 78
  questioning, 181–182
  selective reflection, 102
  structuring, 169

verbal encouragement to
disclose, 50–51
Exercises
age bias, 331
assessment of multiple
problems, 163–164
attending skills, 49–50
characteristics of effective
helpers, 12–13, 18
cultural awareness, 262–263
feedback, 73–74
genuineness, 62
recognizing gender bias,
273–274
use of selective reflections, 104
Exploration (*See* in-depth
exploration)

Family of older adults, working
with, 337–340
Fear of loss, 326–327
Feedback
principles of 74–76
use of, 73, 76–77
Fidelity, 139–140
Free association, 219
Freedom
with children and
adolescents, 29–30, 298
definition, 29
influence of culture on, 29
limitations, 229
role of counselors in client, 29

Gender bias (*See also* sexism)
and men, 282–283
and women, 274–277
Genuineness, 7, 34, 38, 47, 52,
60–62, 231, 242, 245, 267
Gestalt counseling, 212–215
Girls (*See* women)
Goal setting, 90–99
and ability-potential
responses, 104–106
brainstorming about, 97
client resistance to, 96
counselor directiveness in,
96–97
counselor responses to
guide, 91–96
division into subgoals, 97
as a part of in-depth
exploration, 64
influence of theory on, 97
and selective reflections,
102–103
suggesting goals, 96–97
techniques in, 92–96
timing of, 99–100
transition to, 91
Goals in counseling
choosing among, 36–37
discrepancy with behaviors, 77
outcome, 20–25
process, 25–27
Grief work with older adults,
253–254

Helping (*See also* counseling)
joys of, 19
HIV status, 135–136
Homework, 110, 111, 116

Homophobia, 287–288
Homosexual clients (*See* sexual
minorities)
Human nature
behavioral view of, 228–229
cognitive view of, 221–223
gestalt view of, 212–213
person-centered view of,
209–210
psychoanalytic view of, 216–219
trait-factor view of, 225–226

Immediacy, 7, 37–38, 73, 80–83,
175–176
Impairment, counselor, 15–16
(*See also* burnout)
In-depth exploration, 36–39
additive responses, 72, 77–80
advanced empathy and,
77–80
confrontation and, 83–90
counselor skills for, 73
feedback and, 74–77
goal setting in, 72
immediacy and, 80–83
insight and, 72–73
interpretation and, 90–94
role playing and, 94–96
Initial disclosure, 33–36, 47–70
attending skills and, 47–50
blocks to communication,
65–68
concreteness in, 62–64
core conditions for, 51–64
counselor's goal in, 57
empathy and, 52–57
genuineness and, 60–62
inviting communication in,
47–51
positive regard and, 57–60
purposes of, 45–46
relationship building in, 45
verbal encouragement of,
50–51
Insight, 72–73
sufficiency for change, 72
Intake interviews, 161–162
Interchangeable responses,
54–55, 177
Internalizing of feedback, 75–76
Interest inventories, 158
Interpretation, 40, 90–94, 178–179,
302–303, 333
Intervention,
crisis, 237–254
direct, 118–119
Introducing a new topic, 176

Journals, as assessment tools, 159
Joy of helping, 19
Judgment of ethical issues, 135
Justice, 138

Language
and cultural diversity, 266–267
Law and ethics, 141–142
Leading, 172–179
continuum of lead, 174–177
length of lead, 173
and stages of counseling,
177–179
Lecturing, 66

Lesbian clients (*See* sexual
minorities)
Licensing of counselors, 24
Life expectancy, 321–322
Life review, 334–335
Locus of control, 260–261
Locus of responsibility, 260–261
Loss, 20, 28, 237, 238,
241–242, 245

Managing anger
in men, 281, 284–285
in women, 273
Machismo, 289
Malpractice, 142
Medical conditions and diagnosis,
150–151, 162–163
Medication, 163
Men
alexithymia, 284
counseling skills with,
285–287
culturally stereotyped roles,
281–282
empathy training with, 283
gender role strain in, 282
managing anger in, 282–283
as reluctant clients, 188,
282–283
responsible sexuality in, 285
walling of emotions in, 281
younger men and boys,
284–285
Mental status examination, 161
*Millon Clinical Multiaxial
Inventory III*, 157
Minimal encouragers, 175
*Minnesota Multiphasic
Personality Inventory*, 157
Minnesota school of
counseling, 225
Mixed messages, 77
Modeling, 281–282, 284
Moral development, 216–217
Myers-Briggs Type Inventory, 125

Nondirective counseling, 209
Nonlinearity of counseling
process, 41–42
Nonmaleficence, 137–138
Nonverbal behavior, 47–50, 77, 168
and culture, 238, 239

Observation as assessment tool,
158–159
Observational checklists, 159
Older clients, 321–343
change potential, differences
in, 325
counseling agendas, 328–330
counseling procedures with,
300–337
normative life events, 325–328
physiological changes,
324, 326
reluctance to seek
counseling, 321–322
variability across life stage, 324
working with families of,
337–340
Open questions, 67–68, 181–182
Operant conditioning, 228

Oppositional clients, 185–205
  counselor emotions and, 191–193
  counselor responsibilities to, 193–196
  countertransference with, 191–193
  developing insight with, 187, 191
  and readiness for change, 186–187
  reluctance of, 185, 187–189
  resistance of, 185, 189–191
  self-fulfilling prophecy and, 189–190
  transference of, 189–190
  trust as an issue with, 185, 191, 196
Organizing lead, 175, 195–198
Outcome goals, 25–30

Paralinguistics, 48
Paraphrasing, 34
Parents, working with, 314–317
Personal constructs, 26–27, 53
Personality tests, 157–158
Person-centered counseling, 209–211
Pleasure principle, 216–217
Positive regard, 34, 57–60, 267, 332–333
Play media in counseling, 303–304
Precepts of effective helping, 5–12
Predispositions of counselor, 65
Primary empathy, 53–55, 77–79
Process goals, 25–27
Projective tests, 157–158
Psychoanalytic counseling, 215–224
Psychosexual development, 217
Psychosocial development, 217
Psychotherapy, 23–24

Questions,
  with children, 301
  closed, 67, 181–182
  in crisis intervention, 245
  excessive, 66–67
  and leading, 180–182
  open, 67–68, 181–182
  purposes of, 180

Racism, 264, 278
Rational emotive behavior therapy, 221–225
Reaching in and out, 13–16
Readiness for change, 109–111, 186–187
Reassurance, 176
Referral, 36, 126, 308
  working with referring third party, 198–203
Reframing, 91, 334
Relationship building, 45, 46–47
Reluctant clients, 46–47, 185–187, 189, 322–323
  men as, 188. 282–283
Resistance, 46, 185, 189–190
  to feedback, 46, 185, 189–190
  to goal setting, 106–407
  to referral, 36
  to termination 122–123,

Respect
  for autonomy, 136–137
  communication of, 7, 14
Responses,
  ability-potential, 104–106, 108, 176
  additive, 72, 77–80
  interchangeable, 54–55, 177
  leading, 172–177
  moment to moment decisions about, 168
  questioning, 180–182
  structuring, 169–172
Responsibility, locus of, 260–261
Responsible behavior, 29–30
Responsible sexuality in men, 285
Restatement, 175
Role-playing, 94–96, 159
Rorschach, 158

School records, as assessment tool, 306–307
Secondary post-traumatic stress, 244
Selective reflection, 102–104
Self-awareness
  by client, 2, 8–10
  by counselor, 14–16
  and cultural sensitivity, 262–263
Self-confrontation, 9
Self-defeating behavior, 16–17
Self-directed Search, 158
Self disclosure
  by client, 8–9, 45
  by counselor, 38, 61, 82
Self-help, 46
Self-perceptions
  and feedback, 74–75
Self-respect, 15
Self theory, 209–210
Sexism, (*See also* gender bias) 271, 272–275, 278, 279
Sexual harassment, 272, 276
Sexual minorities
  coming out issues, 289
  and committed relationships, 290
  counselor views of, 288–289
  family issues, 290
  heterosexist bias towards, 288–289
  societal attitudes towards, 287–288
"Should" statements, 58
Silence, 175
Stages of the counseling process
  commitment to action, 3, 39–41
  in-depth exploration, 3, 36–39
  initial disclosure, 2, 33–36
  non-linearity of, 41–42
Standardized tests, 157–158
  with culturally diverse clients, 268
Stereotyping, 262–263, 264, 269, 273, 281–282
Stress inoculation, 27
Storytelling, 68
Strong Interest Inventory, 158
Structuring techniques, 169–172
Substance abuse and the older adult, 330

Suicide
  and crisis intervention, 240, 241, 243–244
  and duty to warn, 141–142
  among sexual minorities, 287

Talking with children, 300–302
Tarasoff v. Regents of the University of California, 141
Target behaviors, 229
Tennessee Self-Concept Inventory, 157
Termination, 119–125
  client readiness for, 120–122
  client responses to, 122–123
  counselor goals for, 120
  counselor reluctance about, 123–124
  follow-up to, 125
  guidelines for positive, 124–125
  and interrupted counseling, 120
  and length of counseling, 119–120
  theoretical influences on, 123–124
Testing (*See* Standardized tests)
Thematic Apperception Test, 158
Therapeutic alliance, 3, 35
Theories (*See* counseling theories)
Third age clients, 331, 334, 335
Transference, 189, 220
Triggering events for crises, 240–242
Trust, 4, 6, 14, 34, 37, 47, 54, 60, 65, 71, 73, 75, 89
  and assessment, 151, 160
  conditions that promote, 33–34
  and diverse populations, 255, 256, 262, 279
  during goal setting, 106–107
  and intake interviews, 162
  violations of client, 142–144

Unconditional positive regard, 34, 57–60, 267, 332–333
Unconscious, 192, 217–218, 301

Value judgments, 16
Victimization, of women, 275–276

Walling off emotions and men, 284–285
Women
  body image in, 275
  counseling skills in, 277–278
  counselor attitudes towards, 274–275
  culturally diverse, 278–280
  and discrimination, 275–276
  and empowerment, 278
  and gender bias, 274, 276
  as unique population, 271
  and victimization, 142, 275–276
Work, counseling as, 7–8
Working alliance, 35
Worldview, 260–261
Wounded healer, 15

"Yes, but response," 106
Young men and boys, 284–285